PRECISION ATTACHMENTS IN DENTISTRY

CONTRIBUTORS

Peter Robert L'ESTRANGE, BDSc (Qld), MDSc (Qld), PhD (Lond),
Reader and Head of the Section of Prosthetic Dentistry,
Department of Dentistry, University of Queensland, Australia

Alan G. HANNAM, BDS, PhD, FDSRCS, FRACDS,
Professor, Department of Oral Biology, Faculty of Dentistry,
University of British Columbia, Canada

E. PULLEN-WARNER, FBIST, ARSH,
Chief Instructor, Department of Prosthetic Dentistry,
Institute of Dental Surgery, University of London

J. Saville ZAMET, MPhil, FDSRCS,
Consultant in Periodontology, University College Hospital, London

PRECISION ATTACHMENTS IN DENTISTRY

H. W. PREISKEL

MDS (Lond.), MSc (Ohio), FDSRCS (Eng.)
Consultant in Prosthetic Dentistry
Guy's Hospital, London

THIRD EDITION

THE C. V. MOSBY COMPANY

Saint Louis, Missouri

First edition 1968
Reprinted twice 1969

Second edition 1973
Reprinted with corrections 1974

Third edition 1979

1st Japanese edition published in 1970

2nd Japanese edition published in 1976

Spanish edition published in 1976

© 1979 H. W. Preiskel
Published by Henry Kimpton (Publishers) Ltd
7 Leighton Place, Leighton Road, London NW5 2QL

ISBN 0 85313 802 8

British Library Cataloguing in Publication Data
Preiskel, Harold Wilfred
    Precision attachments in dentistry – 3rd ed.
    1. Denture attachments
    I. Title
    617.6′92   RK656

Distributed in North America, including
Canada, South America and the Philippines by
The C. V. Mosby Company
Saint Louis, Missouri

Printed in Great Britain at the
University Press, Cambridge

Contents

Preface

The third edition contains three additional chapters. Both Alan Hannam's succinct explanation of the neuromuscular control of overdentures, and John Zamet's practical description of periodontal therapy before undertaking restorative dentistry must be of interest to any practising dental surgeon. The extra chapter on overdentures reflects the increasing importance of this type of therapy.

The advances that have taken place in the intervening years between editions are demonstrated by the numbers of new photographs, drawings, and updated references. However, the changes go far beyond illustrations alone and involve revision of the entire text. Some chapters have been completely rewritten, while others have been subjected to more subtle changes. I have refrained from exhibiting a plethora of shining, newly inserted restorations, gratifying though such spectacles are to the eye. Instead, I have gone out of the way to collect examples of failures from which valuable lessons can be learned.

Colleagues the world over have influenced the contents of this book. Wherever he works, today's practitioner requires both a broad-based education and the technical expertise with which to tackle the problems confronting him. An attempt has been made here to cater for both these needs, but there is no substitute for practical experience. Wherever possible, step-by-step guidance has been given and the clinical and technical information expanded. Readers are referred to standard works, when necessary, to avoid unnecessary enlargement of the text.

As in earlier editions, and in spite of radical alterations, this work is intended as a guide to the restoration of the partially dentate mouth and not as a catalogue of gadgets. However, the ever-widening use of attachments demonstrates their value and I hope that this book will aid the reader in evaluating the applications of these valuable devices in the planning and execution of prosthodontic treatment.

HAROLD PREISKEL

Acknowledgements

The production of this book has been a team effort to the extent that it is impossible to thank all concerned by name.

Colleagues from many countries have shared their knowledge with me, while the following have kindly lent me illustrations: Geoffrey Allan FDS (Figs. 560, 707); Neville Bass Dip.Orth., FDS (Figs. 26–35 and 38–46); Harry Gelfant DDS (Figs. 197–200); John McLean O.B.E., D.Sc., MDS (Figs. 627 and 628); and Martin Seymour, BDS (Figs. 630, 631), and William R. Scott, DDS (Figs. 282, 284 and 287–289).

My particular thanks are also due to those who have shared their most precious secrets – information about their failures.

Both Mr J. O. Forrest and Dr D. Preiskel have spent many hours correcting the manuscript, and Drs A. Koper, F. Kratochvil, M. Mensor and W. Scott have all read parts of the text. Most of the attachment manufacturers have checked the proofs concerning their own products.

Cendres et Métaux S.A. have made me welcome on several occasions and provided a wealth of technical information. I have also received valuable help, courtesy and co-operation from Ceka p.v.b.a., and Métaux Precieux S.A. Messrs A. P. M. Sterngold and Messrs Jelenko have demonstrated their continued interest.

The Editors of the *British Dental Journal, Dental Practitioner,* and *Journal of Prosthetic Dentistry* have kindly allowed me to reproduce illustrations from papers I have published in these journals.

Many of the new restorations have been constructed by Messrs Paul Portanier, Brian Reardon and Brian Dance, and the dental technicians of Guy's Hospital and Dental School have never failed to help me.

Mrs Gillian Lee has drawn most of the new illustrations and I am grateful for the time and care she has taken over the task. I would also like to express my thanks to Miss P. Archer and all the members of the Medical Illustration Department at Guy's who have so willingly come to my assistance on numerous occasions. Miss J. Hodgkin and the staff of the Dental Photographic Department have cheerfully carried a very heavy burden while Mr G. Rytina and his staff of the Medical Photographic Department have gone well beyond their normal bounds of duty to help with awkward problems.

Mrs Elsie Crook has done far more than type the manuscripts and organise the illustrations. She cajoled me into re-writing the book, encouraged me when the task seemed never-ending, and worked extremely hard when unwell.

My thanks are also due to Professor D. J. Neill for his co-operation.

David Beardsley BDS, Mrs H. Calaidzis and all who work with me in practice have given invaluable help in collecting information and material for this book.

My wife and family have suffered from my preoccupation with work on this project and I am grateful for their forebearance.

Finally, my thanks to the publishers, Messrs Henry Kimpton, for their patience and co-operation.

H. W. PREISKEL
25 Upper Wimpole Street,
London W1

CHAPTER 1

Treatment Planning

The establishment of rapport with a patient is essential to the success of any prosthodontic treatment. This vital factor may develop during the early stages of treatment, an important ingredient being the ability to reconcile what is feasible with the patient's expectations. Complete dentures are likely to tax the operator in this respect.

In some instances, rapport cannot be achieved, possibly due to the patient's temperament or other reasons. Continuing therapy under these conditions can only be described, in the words of Dr Samuel Johnson, as a triumph of hope over experience.

In arriving at a decision to undertake preliminary therapy and to make a prosthesis, six important questions must be answered, though other factors play a part:

1. Is the patient healthy?
2. Is a prosthesis necessary?
3. Is the patient suitable for a prosthesis?
4. How large a space is to be restored?
5. By what structures is the prosthesis to be supported?
6. How is the prosthesis to be made?

Answers to these questions cannot be found by a few polite enquiries and a cursory glance inside the mouth. Nor can any type of examination or planning be carried out in this manner. The examination of the patient is one of the most important aspects of treatment by prosthetic restorations, and it is noticeable that the most experienced operators are those who spend the greatest amount of time on this step.

IS THE PATIENT HEALTHY?

The dental practitioner must be concerned with the general well-being of his patient.

Prosthodontic replacement of missing teeth can hardly have anything but a beneficial effect and many of the procedures can be carried out even upon moderately sick patients, should the need arise.

Should any surgical procedure be required, it will have to be considered, together with the attendant type of anaesthesia, in relation to the patient's health and any medical treatment he is receiving. Account must also be taken of the emotional strain involved in the treatment.

Patients with heart disease are probably the most frequently at risk. They may require antibiotic protection against bacterial endocarditis, while others may be on anticoagulant or anti-hypertensive therapy. It is, therefore, wise to work in co-operation with the patient's physician. Routine blood pressure evaluation is now being advocated for the age group to which many of these patients belong.

Apart from potential hazards to the patient during the treatment, the dentist must be aware of possible dangers to himself, and other patients. Hepatitis B, also known as serum hepatitis, is diagnosed by detection in the blood of Australia antigen, now called hepatitis B antigen. The incubation period is long, between six weeks and six months, and the antigen may be present in the blood for six weeks or more before the onset of symptoms. The antigen is present in saliva in serum positive patients. The problem is that the virus can be transmitted between a patient and the dental surgeon. It is also possible for a dental surgeon who is positive to infect his patient. There is evidence that the incidence of hepatitis is higher in dentists than in a comparable population of lawyers. Furthermore, at least one report has suggested that transmission by the dentist was responsible for an outbreak of viral hepatitis in a community in the United States.

In order to reduce risk to himself the dentist should be wary of patients with a history of jaundice, multiple blood transfusions, and renal dialysis. Patients who may be drug addicts or male homosexuals also appear to have higher carrier rates.

Infection is spread by the virus in the blood of the patient, bloodstained saliva, and possibly normal saliva. The common route is by inoculation or accidental abrasion of the skin or mucosa. Since the dentist cannot hope to identify incubating cases it is prudent to take precautions such as careful examination of the hands and covering them, wearing eye protectors and a mask.

IS A PROSTHESIS NECESSARY?

This is a most important, yet one of the more difficult decisions to be made. Both the patient and his oral conditions require consideration.

A detailed history should be taken, paying particular attention to the reasons for the loss of teeth and, if extractions took place in phases over several years, a record should be made of the sequence in which these were carried out. Should the patient be wearing a partial denture a great deal can be learnt from an assessment of the prosthesis and the patient's reaction to it. If this denture must be replaced, it may still have value, in modified form, as a transitional prosthesis.

The examination should start with a general investigation of the mouth, noting the number and distribution of the remaining teeth together with any apparent discrepancy between centric jaw relation and the centric occlusion of the teeth (see chapter 3 on occlusal surfaces). The individual teeth should naturally be checked for caries. Since all partial prostheses derive support from the periodontal structures, it is important that these tissues should be sound and healthy before the prosthesis is made. It is also essential that the prosthesis be designed carefully to cause only the minimal interference with the periodontal structures. An assessment of the periodontal condition should, therefore, be made ensuring that the gingivae are pink, firm, and stippled with the gingival margins knife-edged. The crevice should not exceed one or two millimetres, and probing should not cause bleeding. If there is evidence of periodontal disease, as is commonly the case, this must be treated before any restorative work is carried out. This treatment always includes bringing the patient's plaque control up to a satisfactory standard. The appearance of the soft tissues including the floor of the mouth, cheeks, and tongue should be noted. Even at this early stage, lack of denture space or other problems may become apparent.

The patient's co-operation during this course of treatment may be a useful pointer to the way ahead.

If necessary, a halt may be called before patient and operator are involved in unnecessary expenditure.

Two important diagnostic aids are necessary to complete the examination – full-mouth radiographs and mounted diagnostic casts. Full-mouth radiographs should show the level of the alveolar bone around the teeth, the width of the periodontal ligament space, and periapical structures, and any retained roots or other pathological structures.

Diagnostic casts should include details of the entire denture-bearing area as well as of the natural teeth, for the shape of these areas plays an important part in the design of the restoration.

A centric relation record will be required. Of the common methods used, the horseshoe-shaped piece of wax is least likely to give acceptable results. A method recommended by Dawson (1974) has now been found simple to employ and to give excellent results. There are many alternative methods, the result not the technique being the important factor. Diagnostic casts of each jaw are made and an occlusal rim made on the upper. Where sufficient teeth are standing the wax is built across the occlusal surfaces of the premolar and molar teeth, out of contact with areas representing soft tissues and clear of the upper anterior teeth (Fig. 1). One

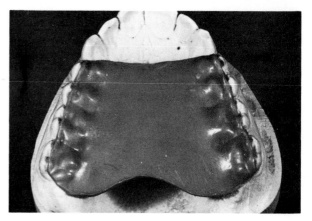

Fig. 1   Where sufficient teeth are standing the wax rim is built across the occlusal surfaces of the premolar and molar teeth, out of contact with areas representing soft tissues.

important feature is to cut the wax back so that it is flush with the buccal cusps. (An extremely hard base wax must be employed such as Moyco Extra Hard Beauty Wax*.) Three thicknesses of wax is the maximum that should be employed. When it has been adapted it will probably be somewhat thinner.

* J. Bird Moyer Co., Philadelphia, PA 19132, U.S.A.

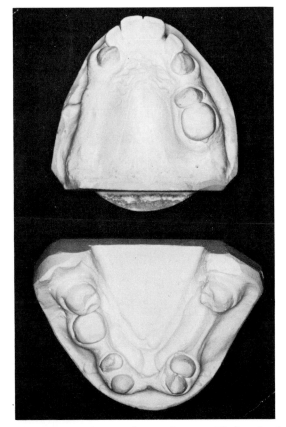

Fig. 2 Upper and lower diagnostic casts. Their value for treatment planning is greatly increased if they are mounted on an adjustable articulator.

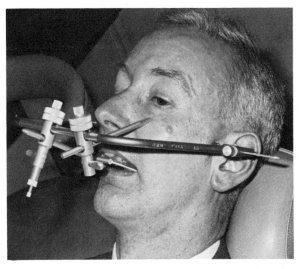

Fig. 3 The facebow record with the infra-orbital marker in position.

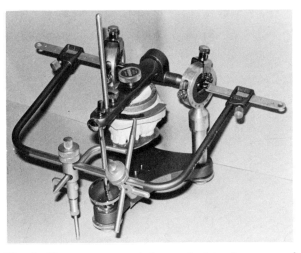

Fig. 4 Upper cast mounted on articulator by means of facebow record.

Before placing the rim in the mouth only the outer sections are softened. The upper teeth are dried, so that the record will tend to adhere to them while the wet lower teeth will separate from the record without dislodging it. The operator is then free to manipulate the jaw with both hands. This technique is described in the next chapter.

Once the record has been made it is cooled with air, removed, and chilled in ice water. Care should be taken that no penetration of the wax has occurred. Any excess wax that has flowed over the buccal cusps is cut back with a disposable scalpel blade. The record is now tested again in the mouth, and after subsequent chilling can be used for mounting the diagnostic casts. The record must fit these casts as it fits the mouth, otherwise it will need to be remade and a new jaw relation made. Since this type of centric relation record must be made at an increased vertical relation of occlusion, a facebow record is essential. The centric relation record should be made at a vertical relation just sufficient to prevent contact of the teeth. Dawson (1974) has also described a modification of this technique, useful where mobility patterns are demonstrated in posterior teeth or where patients find it difficult to hold their mandibles still. An anterior stop is made with compound or acrylic resin at the desired vertical relation. This anterior stop will help stabilize the mandible while the record material of choice is setting or hardening.

Where a quadrant of teeth is missing or insufficient remain to allow an entirely tooth supported rim to be made, a conventional rim will be required, supported by the mucosa in the edentulous regions.

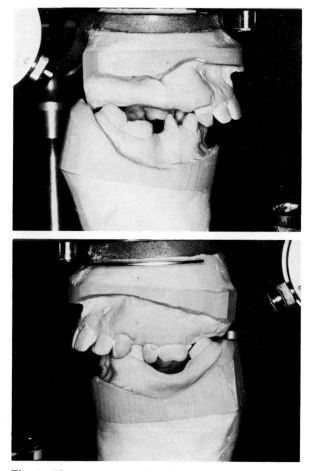

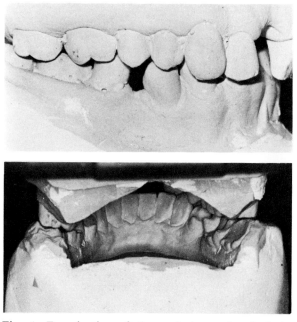

Fig. 6 Examination of the occlusion and articulation from the buccal aspect alone can be deceptive.

Fig. 5 The casts mounted on the articulator. A thorough examination of the occlusion can now be made, and the difficulties of restorative procedures assessed.

The centric relation record is again made with the natural teeth just separated and a facebow record is again essential.

It is a pity that adjustable articulators are surrounded with an aura of mystery by some practitioners. Others appear to worship the instrument and regard it as the raison d'être for the treatment, rather than as a tool. Sensibly employed, adjustable articulators simplify treatment. Trying to occlude two hand-held casts is a difficult procedure and the result may be hopelessly inaccurate. If casts are to be mounted on an articulator (Figs. 2–4), it takes no longer to mount them on an adjustable one than on a plane-line type. An adjustable articulator allows examination of the casts mounted in positions corresponding with centric relation or centric occlusion (Fig. 5), and in addition it enables an assessment to be made of lateral and protrusive excursions that would otherwise have to be carried out by guesswork. Examination of the casts on the articulator allows an assessment to be made of the relationship of palatal and lingual cusps. Looking at the buccal aspect alone can be deceptive (Fig. 6). Planning the appearance is also simplified, as the infra-orbital marker of the facebow ensures that the occlusal plane of the casts mounted on the articulator is the same as that in the mouth, when the head is level. There is certainly a place for more complex methods of occlusal analysis employing 'hinge-axis' locating facebows and gnathological articulators that allow more comprehensive adjustments, but not for routine use.

The method outlined for mounting diagnostic casts is a compromise. It is simple and quick to use and provides an accuracy that will match the jaw relation records that most operators can obtain. No articulator can be more accurate than the records used in it. However, of the various jaw relations made, by far the most important is that of centric relation.

WHY MAKE A PROSTHESIS?

A prosthesis may be required to restore appearance and speech, to improve chewing, or to spread occlusal load over a wider area. It may also be used to correct the occlusion of natural teeth. Constructing a restoration may prevent migration of teeth adjacent to a space, or overeruption of the opposing teeth. A restoration may also help prevent the development of abnormal speech habits or jaw postures.

On the other hand, construction of a prosthesis is time-consuming, it may require tooth preparation and will probably involve coverage of some of the gingival margins and mucosa. Wearing a prosthesis makes good plaque control imperative, while the prosthesis itself will require periodic inspection. The only firm rule to guide the operator in his decision is to ensure that he is in possession of all the facts.

HOW LARGE A SPACE IS TO BE RESTORED?

The span of the restoration is the key to the treatment plan. It determines the work the prosthesis will do as well as the loads to which the prosthesis and the structures supporting it will be subjected. Articulated diagnostic casts are necessary when making this decision, and their value is enhanced if lateral and protrusive records have been made. It is important to realise that with most articulators these records are only accurate at the particular positions in which the records have been made. Intermediate positions are an approximation. Wear facets on the remaining teeth are a useful guide to the magnitude and direction of forces that may be applied to the prosthesis. At this stage, it is convenient to examine the opposing occlusal surfaces and to make a note of any reshaping that may

be required (Fig. 7). Overeruption of opposing teeth can usually be corrected by grinding, which should be planned at this stage. It may be necessary to alter the cusps and fossae of the remaining teeth to conform with centric jaw relation, in which case the occlusal surfaces of the teeth of the prosthesis should also be made to correspond with this position. The time to make this decision is at the beginning of the treatment.

Typical spaces to be restored are anterior or posterior gaps bounded by natural teeth, or spaces with no distal abutment. Various types of prostheses for restoring these spaces are described in the chapters on prefabricated attachments. If the prosthesis chosen requires prefabricated attachment, these should be selected and measured against the teeth on the diagnostic casts before any tooth preparation is carried out. It is easy to misjudge the space (especially vertical space) required for an attachment, and it is important to discover any error as early as possible so that either the treatment plan can be changed, or another attachment substituted.

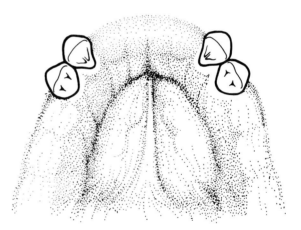

Fig. 8 A typical situation favouring a combined lower anterior fixed prosthesis and a removable bilateral distal extension denture.

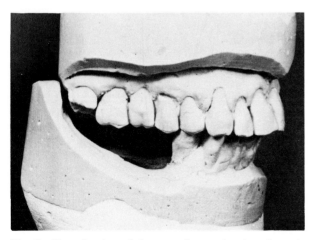

Fig. 7 Examination of the opposing occlusal surfaces is essential to enable reshaping to be planned.

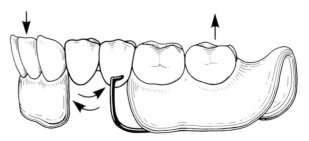

Fig. 9 A partial denture restoring all these gaps has a tendency to rotate about the abutment teeth.

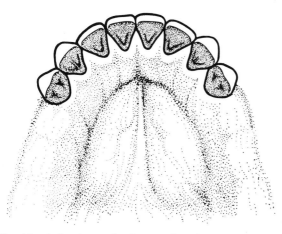

Fig. 10   A fixed prosthesis restoring the anterior space splints both groups of abutments.

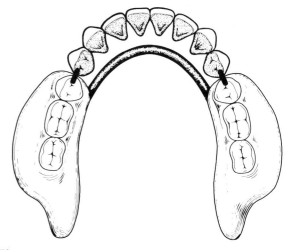

Fig. 12   An attachment-retained denture made in conjunction with the anterior restoration.

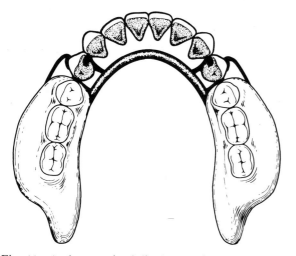

Fig. 11   A clasp-retained distal extension denture made in conjunction with an anterior fixed prosthesis.

Frequently, several gaps are found in one jaw. They may be restored with one prosthesis such as a partial denture, one or more fixed prostheses, or a combination of fixed and removable restorations. Such a combination may be used where there is an anterior gap and bilateral posterior distal spaces (Fig. 8).

A partial denture restoring all these gaps would have a tendency to rotate about the abutment teeth (Fig. 9). A better approach is to construct a fixed prosthesis for the anterior teeth (Fig. 10). The posterior spaces can then be restored with a bilateral distal extension partial denture, that can be clasp-retained (Fig. 11) or attachment-retained (Fig. 12).

Combined restorations of this nature frequently result in problems with the articulation, particularly when opposed to a complete denture. The development of a balanced articulation is important if the stability of the complete denture is to be ensured. It is tempting to complete the construction of the fixed restoration first before considering the dentures. However, it may then be quite impossible to produce the arrangement of the teeth and compensating cures required for a balanced articulation. The fixed restoration determines the vertical relation of occlusion, the occlusal plane, and the position of the anterior teeth. A trial insertion is necessary to determine the position of all the teeth before the denture framework is made.

The fixed prosthesis is normally the restoration of choice for missing anterior teeth (Fig. 13). However, aesthetic requirements may dictate the use of artificial mucosa to replace lost tissues (Fig. 14) while the edentulous span may be sufficiently long to require mucosal support (Figs. 15, 16). Spaced teeth may be necessary for other patients. These are just a few examples of the indications for removable prostheses. Where splinting across the edentulous space is required, bar attachments may be employed to connect the abutments either side, and it is also possible to make removable labial flanges for certain fixed prostheses. Decisions relating to the design, however, can only be made with the aid of mounted diagnostic casts. Where just a few teeth, or roots, remain the assessment of vertical space is especially important. The planning of the restoration depends upon the room available (Fig. 17).

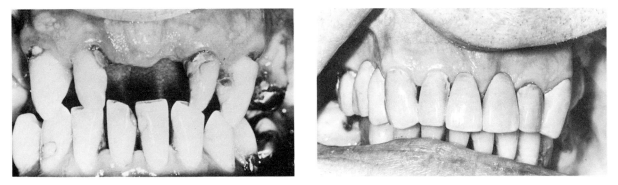

Fig. 13   A fixed prosthesis is normally the restoration of choice for anterior teeth.

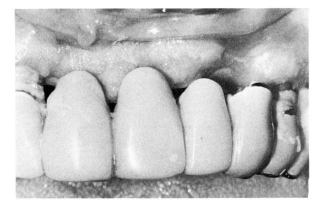

Fig. 14a   Note bone loss in canine region following root removal from this fixed prosthesis. This loss will dictate a removable replacement prosthesis if the canine eminence is to be restored.

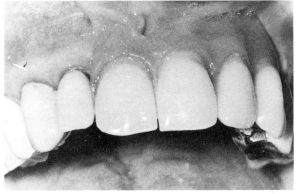

Fig. 14b   Edentulous span restored with a removable prosthesis.

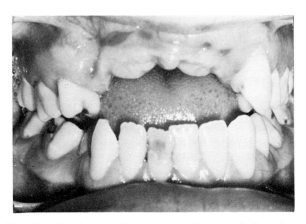

Fig. 15a   The degree of bone loss and length of edentulous span will require a removable restoration for appearance and to gain some mucosal support.

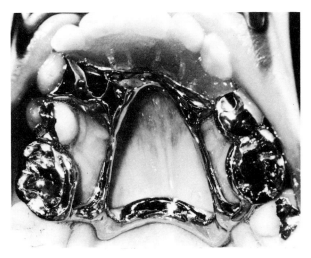

Fig. 15b   Restoration in place following mucogingival surgery.

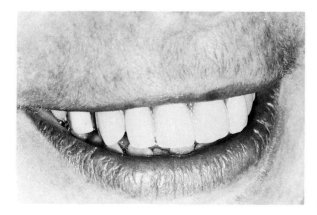

Fig. 16   Note labial support, particularly to margin of lip. Artificial mucosa is essential in this instance to allow correct positioning of anterior teeth.

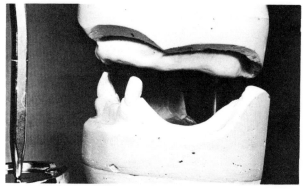

Fig. 17   Vertical space available is the key to planning overdentures or similar prostheses.

BY WHAT STRUCTURES IS THE PROSTHESIS TO BE SUPPORTED?

Once a decision has been made on restoring a space, the manner in which the prosthesis will be supported against vertical and horizontal forces must be considered. A partial prosthesis may be tooth-borne, tooth- and mucosal-borne, or mucosal-borne. The principles involved are simple. Loads falling on the prosthesis must be reduced to a minimum; any loads that do fall on it should be spread as widely as possible. Reduction of occlusal load is achieved by keeping the artificial occlusal surfaces small, by reshaping the opposing occlusal surfaces if necessary, and by ensuring there is even contact with the opposing dentition. The occlusal requirements of various types of prostheses are discussed in the chapter on occlusal surfaces.

Loads falling on the prosthesis should be spread over as many natural teeth as possible, and maximum support from the mucosa obtained by wide mucosal coverage, where necessary. However carefully the restoration is made, some additional load is likely to be placed on the abutment teeth and their prognosis must be evaluated with care.

Distal extension and complete overlay dentures raise the problem of load distribution between teeth and mucosa. Once it is understood that a correctly designed and constructed prosthesis has only the slightest tendency to move around the abutment teeth in function, the way is clear to understand the controversy over 'stress-breaking'. Prefabricated attachments allowing movement between the two components have many uses; however, it is gener-

ally their shape and size rather than the 'stress-breaking' properties claimed for them that allow their use where a more rigid unit would be contra-indicated. A 'stress-breaker' may be used as a safety valve, but never as a means of anchoring an unstable denture to a rigid abutment. Perceptible movements of a prosthesis in function are potentially harmful to the abutment teeth, to the underlying mucosa, and to the edentulous ridge. The aim must always be to design and construct an inherently stable denture and to pay attention first to the prosthetic principles involved before considering technical details of the various attachments.

HOW IS THE PROSTHESIS TO BE MADE?

1. The path of insertion

With the aid of a surveying instrument, the casts could be inspected to determine the most favourable path of insertion for the prosthesis. When prefabricated attachments are used, the path of insertion is critical, so that it is important to ensure there are no mucosal undercuts relative to this path. It is usually necessary to give a lower distal extension denture a path of insertion that approaches from the distal aspect in order to extend the lingual flanges into the retromylohyoid fossae (Fig. 18): removable anterior restoration commonly requires a path of insertion inclined to approach from the labial aspect.

2. Retention and stability

Once in place, a prosthesis has to resist displacing forces along its path of insertion. Anterior, posterior, and lateral displacing forces acting

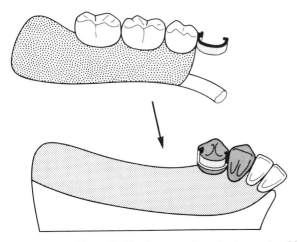

Fig. 18 A bilateral distal extension denture should normally be given a path of insertion that approaches from the distal aspects of the abutments.

individually or in combinations tend to rock and rotate the prosthesis out of position.

Direct retention can be considered to be the force resisting removal of the prosthesis along its path of insertion. The resistance of a clasp arm to deformation, friction between the denture components and the natural teeth, or friction between the sections of an attachment may all provide direct retention. Mucosal coverage by the denture base provides direction retention as well. The forces of adhesion, cohesion, and surface tension acting between the denture base, saliva, and mucosa, cause a pressure reduction under the denture base when the base is slightly displaced. Further denture movement is thereby resisted.

Resistance to lateral displacing forces is provided by rigid bracing components of the prosthesis, and by mucosal support. If a bilateral prosthesis is constructed, lateral displacing forces can be shared between the teeth and the mucosa of both sides, while a force tending to dislodge one side is resisted by the retainer on the opposite side. These retainers act with a mechanical advantage corresponding to the width of the dental arch (Fig. 19). A bilateral prosthesis is, therefore, inherently more stable than a unilateral restoration.

Anterior and posterior displacing forces are normally resisted by the natural teeth. However, the anterior removable prosthesis frequently needs additional support from the mucosa. When clasp retainers are employed for distal extension prostheses, posterior displacing forces must be resisted by rigid components of the metal framework. It is

insufficient to rely on mucosal coverage and the clasp arm, for the flexible retaining arm is likely to flex under distal displacing forces (Fig. 20). An attachment in this position must be designed to resist these displacing forces (Fig. 21).

It is more difficult to provide resistance to forces tending to rock and rotate the prosthesis out of place, yet this is commonly the manner in which a patient tends to dislodge a prosthesis.

Resistance to these displacing forces is provided by the forces of retention, and the mechanical efficiency with which these retaining forces act is determined by the stability of the prosthesis. The more precise the path of insertion of a prosthesis the better it will resist displacing forces tending to rock it out of place, while it will be understood from previous discussion that a denture with several widely spaced retainers is likely to prove more stable than one in which the retainers are close together.

A distal extension prosthesis has a tendency for the posterior section of the denture base to lift away from the mucosa when sticky foods are chewed. Some types of clasp-retained dentures do not prevent this movement, as the denture pivots around the tip of the clasp arm (Fig. 22). This tendency to rotate around the clasp can be prevented by incorporating a structure known as an indirect retainer. An indirect retainer is a rigid component of the denture and becomes the point around which the denture tends to rotate. As a result, the tip of the clasp arm is now in an undercut relative to this movement which it can therefore prevent (Fig. 23). The greater the distance between the indirect retainer and the clasps, the more efficient is its action. Although an improved clasp design engaging the distal undercuts of the abutment teeth may minimise rotational movements of the denture base, where there are only six anterior teeth remaining in a somewhat square arch it may be impossible to provide enough indirect retention to make the denture stable (Fig. 24).

Prostheses with prefabricated attachments have precise paths of insertion and so the need for indirect retention is reduced. Many extracoronal units specifically incorporate a device to prevent tipping of the base. It is, however, essential to select sturdy attachments, and splinted abutments are usually necessary.

If attachments are to be employed, the amount of vertical and buccolingual space available needs to be examined with care. This is best carried out with the aid of mounted diagnostic casts (Fig. 25). A minimum of 4 mm vertical space is usually required for prefabricated attachments. Where less space is

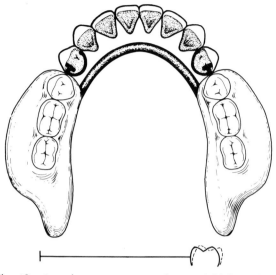

Fig. 19   A major connector, such as a rigid lingual bar, allows lateral displacing forces to be shared by the teeth and mucosa of both sides of the jaw. A rotational load applied to the artificial teeth of one side will be resisted by the retainers of the opposite side acting with a considerable mechanical advantage.

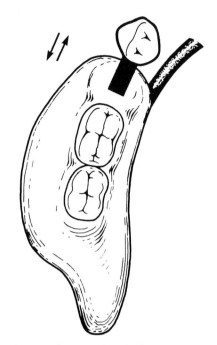

Fig. 21   An attachment placed distally in position must be able to withstand displacing forces.

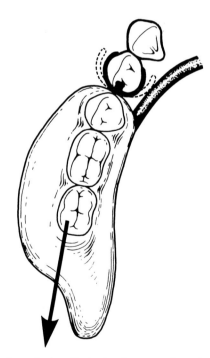

Fig. 20   A posterior displacing force tends to 'open up' this type of clasp arm. A mesial occlusal rest is usually to be preferred.

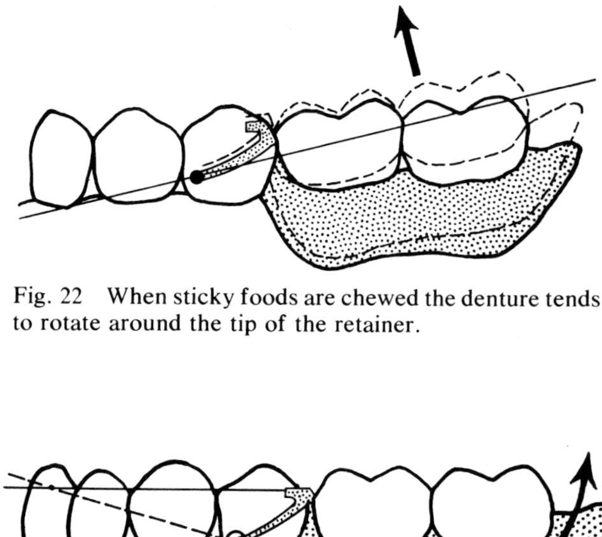

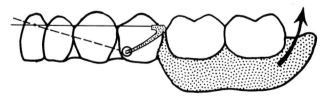

Fig. 22   When sticky foods are chewed the denture tends to rotate around the tip of the retainer.

Fig. 23   An indirect retainer becomes the point around which the denture tends to rotate. The tip of the clasp is now in an undercut relative to this movement which it can therefore prevent.

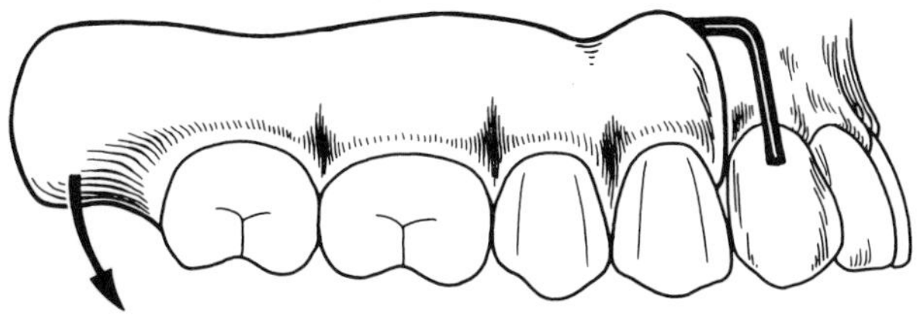

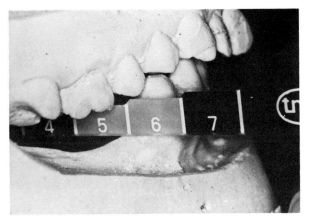

Fig. 24 With only six anterior teeth remaining in a square-shaped arch, it may be impossible to provide enough indirect retention to make the denture stable.

Fig. 25 Vertical space available for attachments can be measured on the diagnostic casts by means of a gauge (EM Gauge, Bell International, Inc. 1320 Marston Road, Burlingame, CA90401). Buccolingual room should be assessed as well.

available, laboratory-produced units can be constructed; simpler semi-precision rests, in conjunction with retention arms in ball and socket joints, should also be considered.

When prefabricated attachments are used, the retention between the abutment crowns and the tooth preparations should be planned as well; it is pointless having a retentive denture if the abutment crowns are dislodged when it is removed. Abutment preparations should, therefore, be restricted to full coverage, unless a three-quarter coverage restoration is indicated and can be made with adequate retention and strength.

3. The major connector

The major connector is the chassis of a bilateral prosthesis to which all other components are joined. Since it connects the bases on each side, the major connector acts as a load distributor and makes a large contribution to the stability of the prosthesis. Significant flexibility within the framework will detract from its ability to carry out these tasks. Equally apparent is the fact that the connector should cover the least possible area of gingivae, and that its overall bulk be as small as possible. The high modulus of elasticity of chrome cobalt alloys compared with yellow golds has advantage in this respect, but the design of the connector must be considered with care. Some major connectors, such as palatal plates, may themselves transmit occlusal loads to the mucosa, in which case the weight of the structure may become important.

The principles of major connector design vary little between clasp-retained and attachment-retained dentures. For a detailed consideration the reader is referred to a standard text on partial denture construction. Suggested reading is provided at the end of this chapter and those succeeding it. Attachments introduce additional complications that can only be overcome with proper understanding of the clasp retainer.

(a) Compatibility of denture base components

Many intracoronal attachments require to be soldered to the major connector. Soldering a precious metal attachment to a chrome cobalt framework is possible, but technically exacting. Where space considerations permit, a precious metal major connector is easier to employ. It also simplifies construction of the lingual bracing arm.

Where attachments may be buried in the acrylic resin of the denture base, as with most extracoronal attachments, chrome cobalt alloys produce few problems. On the contrary, their reduced weight and bulk confer considerable advantages assuming the laboratory is equipped with suitable facilities for investing, casting, and polishing the alloy.

(b) Adaptation of the framework to the abutments

Recent improvements with investment material, matched with new alloys of chrome cobalt have gone a long way to improve the accuracy of castings. Nevertheless, gold alloys are far easier to employ when anything other than a simple lingual arm is contemplated. The difference in hardness between a gold crown and a chrome cobalt denture is a factor that is normally overrated. Problems, when they occur, usually result from inaccuracy of adaptation.

(c) Indirect retention

Since many attachments incorporate effective tilt preventing components, the major connector design can be simplified accordingly. Since all the components of a removable prosthesis are joined to the major connector, its importance cannot be over emphasised. Apart from function, patient tolerance and appearance need to be considered as well. Mounted diagnostic casts are invaluable in making this decision.

PRELIMINARY TREATMENT

The health of the periodontal structures is one of the most important influences on the success or failure of the entire treatment. Thorough scaling and plaque control are essential for nearly every patient. There is much to be said for accepting patients on a probationary basis until their plaque control practice is adequate and their mouths are healthy. No tooth preparation should be started until the periodontal structures are sound. Muco-gingival surgery may be necessary to eliminate pocketing and to restore an adequate zone of attached gingiva. Short clinical crowns may require to be lengthened and small irregularities of the denture-bearing mucosa removed. Any necessary root canal therapy should be carried out as part of the preliminary therapy rather than as emergency endodontics when preparing the abutment crowns.

Preparation of the tissues covering the edentulous areas is overlooked all too frequently. An impression made over inflamed tissues can only produce a restoration that maintains the structures in this state. Mildly abused tissues may recover if the denture causing the problem is left out for about three days. More extensive problems will require the use of tissue conditioners. Where problems of this nature are associated with problems of jaw postures, the existing partial denture may be connected into a transitional denture by means of base extension and correction of the occlusal surfaces.

Nowadays, there is seldom need to accept malaligned or malpositioned teeth as a basis for prosthodontic therapy. While crowns can be used to mask small rotations of the teeth, or to make minor corrections to their alignment, tooth preparation can never be an effective substitute for tooth position. Ross (1974) has described minor tooth movements without appliances.

Preliminary orthodontic therapy can drastically change the problems of prosthodontics (Figs. 26, 27). The diastema between central incisors is difficult to obliterate by oversized crowns if the restoration is to remain good looking. Simple appliances can be employed in some instances. Retraction of incisors, quite apart from placing them in a more stable position, will remove unwanted spaces, improve angulation, periodontal health and facilitate subsequent restorative dentistry (Figs. 28–32).

Apart from the problems of the orthodontic therapy, considerable care in planning is essential to prevent awkward spaces that cannot be restored in a pleasing manner (Figs. 33, 34). Another point to consider is the root relationships of adjoining teeth. If these roots are close together it will be impossible to provide adequate proximal space between the crowns when the teeth are subsequently restored (Fig. 35).

Where loss of posterior occlusal support has been combined with spreading of the incisors, a simple plan is to restore the posterior occlusion with transitional acrylic resin prostheses made with gold collars around the teeth. Small hooks can be inserted in these prostheses and elastic used for retraction. This retraction is really a tipping movement rather than a bodily movement of the teeth. As a safety measure, a small orthodontic wire ligature covered with acrylic resin can be placed around the neck of one of the teeth to be retracted,

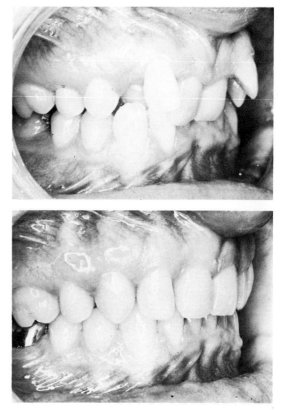

Fig. 26 Preliminary orthodontic therapy can change the problems of prosthodontics.

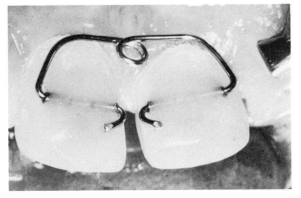

Fig. 27   Simple orthodontic treatment may be used to appose some spaced incisors.

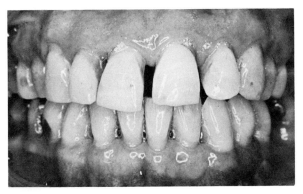

Fig. 28   Adult with spaced incisors before orthodontic treatment.

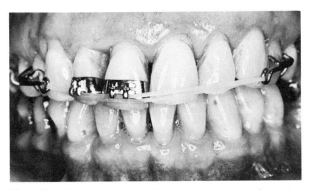

Fig. 29   The patient during the course of active treatment.

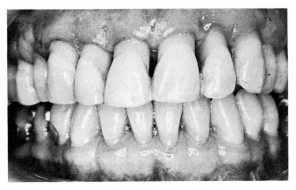

Fig. 30   The same patient after six weeks of treatment and with a provisional splint.

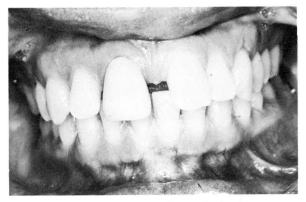

Fig. 31   Another example before orthodontic therapy.

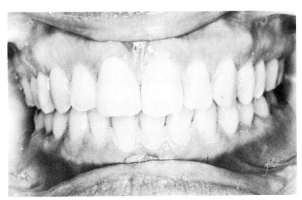

Fig. 32   After orthodontic therapy.

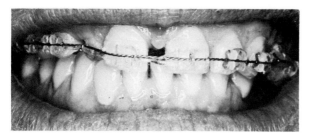

Fig. 33   Retraction and realignment of anterior teeth.

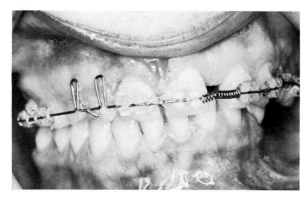

Fig. 34   Subsequent distal movement of the upper left lateral incisor to provide space for a pontic.

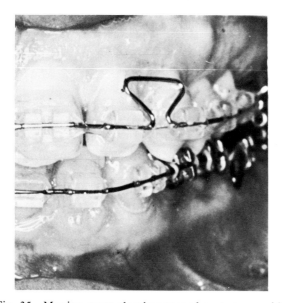

Fig. 35   Moving apart closely opposed roots to provide proximal space between the crowns.

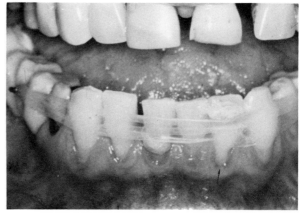

Fig. 36   When loss of posterior occlusal support has caused the incisors to spread out, the occlusal table can be built up with acrylic resin temporary bridges. These restorations form a base for retraction of the incisors.

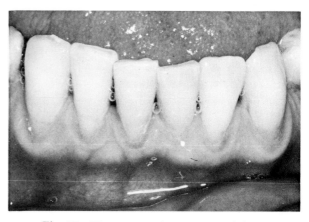

Fig. 37   The same patient one month later.

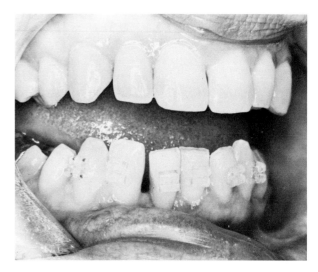

Fig. 38   Bands applied to labial surfaces.

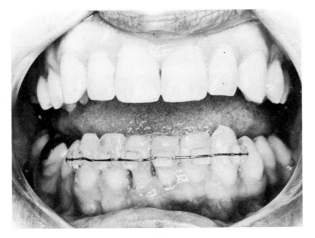

Fig. 39   Active treatment.

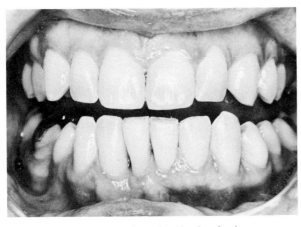

Fig. 40   Completion of orthodontic therapy.

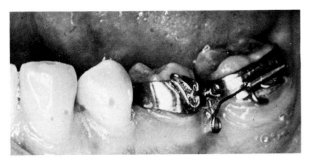

Fig. 41   The realignment of a tilted distal abutment.

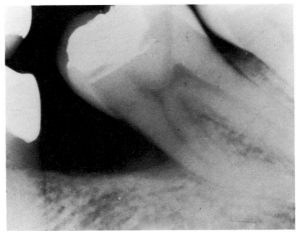

Fig. 42   Another example showing mesial infra-osseous pocket before therapy.

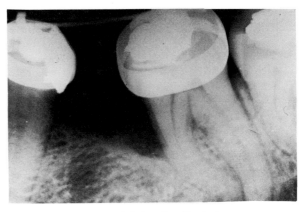

Fig. 43   Uprighting the distal abutment.

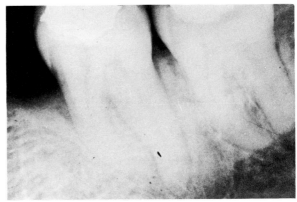

Fig. 44   Note the improvement in the infra-osseous pocket. The tooth is now in a far better position, and at a better angle, to act as a retainer.

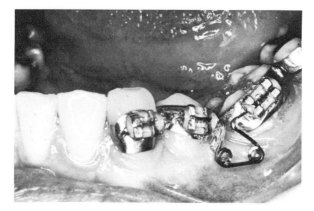

Fig. 45   The apices of a tilted molar being rotated mesially.

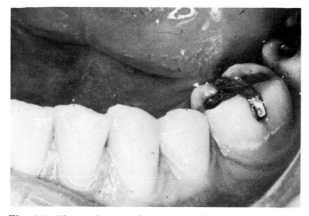

Fig. 46   The molar now in contact with the premolar. A new restoration will be required for the tooth.

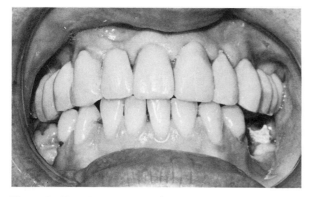

Fig. 47   For large restorations, a temporary acrylic resin prosthesis allows a patient to become accustomed to a restored occlusion, and therefore simplifies recording centric jaw relation subsequently. Adjustments to occlusal surfaces are easy to make and the appearance can be decided upon before the permanent restoration is completed.

and a similar ligature placed near the incisal edge of another tooth (Fig. 36). These ligatures will prevent the tubing from sliding onto the gingivae or jumping off the teeth (Fig. 37).

Simplified techniques now available with orthodontic bands have made possible a range of therapy that might otherwise have been dismissed as too complex. The modern bands are far better looking and can be applied with adhesive to the labial surfaces of the teeth. As a result, combinations of rotations and malangulations can be corrected (Figs. 38–40).

Tilted distal abutments are another common complication to prosthodontic therapy. While mechanical answers are available to ease the problems of malalignment, they do not solve the associated periodontal problems. It is far better to restore the tilted abutment to an upright position (Fig. 41). If this is carried out, the preparation of the tooth is simplified, and additional retention for the crown may be obtained. Furthermore, loads will be applied at a more favourable angle, while the changes in angulation of the tooth may well contribute to removal of a mesial infra-osseous pocket (Figs. 42–44).

A modified approach can be employed where there is little space between tilted molars and the more mesial teeth. The apices of the molar tooth are brought forward so that while the tooth is made upright there is no space between it and the adjacent premolar (Figs. 45, 46).

The examples illustrated are only a few of the possibilities available with adult orthodontics today. Specialist help is recommended and it should be understood that the periodontal condition should be reassessed after orthodontic therapy.

Once a patient has become accustomed to his restored posterior occlusion he frequently reverts to centric jaw relation, or a position nearby. If the occlusion of the restoration had been adapted to an acquired protruded mandibular posture, most of the posterior teeth of a removable prosthesis may need to be replaced. A fixed prosthesis, however, may need to be completely reconstructed as the crown preparations may have to be modified. For this reason, transitional prostheses are desirable. Where fixed prostheses are concerned, a transitional acrylic resin restoration allows occlusal adjustments to be made at an early stage, and acts as an occlusal template. The appearance can also be decided upon before the final prosthesis is made (Fig. 47).

Ideally, transitional acrylic restorations should be adapted onto a metal framework. This type of construction allows accurate adaptation of the gingival margins and wide proximal spaces.

REFERENCES AND FURTHER READING

ADAMS, D. and ZWINK, R. (1976) Treating Australia Antigen Positive Patients. Practical Experience. *Brit. dent. J.*, *141*, 341

DAWSON, P. E. (1974) *Evaluation, Diagnosis, and Treatment of Occlusal Problems*. C. V. Mosby, St Louis, Mo.

HENDERSON, D. and STEFFEL, V. L. (1977) *McCracken's Removable Partial Prosthodontics*. 5th ed. C. V. Mosby, St Louis, Mo.

NAGINGTON, J. and VARLEY, E. W. B. (1976) Hepatitis B and the dental surgeon. *Brit. dent. J.*, *141*, 337

NEILL, D. J. and WALTER, J. D. (1977) *Partial Denture Prosthetics*. Blackwell Scientific Publications, London.

ROSS, I. F. (1974) Tooth Movement and Repositioning of the Mandible without Appliances. *J. prosthet. dent.*, *31*, 290

ZARB, G. A., BERGMAN, B., CLAYTON, J. A. and JACKAY, H. F. (1978) *Prosthodontic Treatment for Partially Edentulous Patients*. C. V. Mosby Company, St Louis, Mo.

CHAPTER 2

Periodontal Therapy before Restorative Dentistry

J. Saville Zamet

Periodontal disease is responsible for the majority of tooth loss, yet it is seldom treated. This fact must present modern dentistry with one of its greatest challenges. There is conclusive evidence to show that bacteria within dental plaque are responsible for the disease (Sockransky 1970), but as yet there is no chemotherapy available that can be used on a permanent basis. The disease has to be controlled by mechanical means such as toothbrushing, woodsticks and floss.

Restorative dentistry may influence the pattern of health and disease in three ways. Firstly, inadequate restorations and attachments placed in a healthy mouth may distort the anatomy of the tissues to the extent that good plaque control can no longer be maintained and periodontal breakdown will start to occur. Secondly, the underlying periodontal problems may have escaped recognition during the examination, diagnosis and treatment planning phase. Indeed it may have been the major reason for tooth loss, for which the patient is now seeking replacement. Thirdly, all well-made restorations should exert a protective function to the surrounding healthy periodontal tissues and should allow easy access for plaque control.

THE CONTROL OF DISEASE

Nearly all epidemiological studies have shown a close correlation between dental plaque and periodontal disease. Experimental gingivitis has been induced in healthy subjects by withdrawing oral hygiene over a number of weeks. The disease has then been eliminated by the re-institution of good plaque control, without the need for any further treatment (Löe et al. 1965). An analogy can be drawn between periodontal disease and diabetes. Neither disease can be cured, but both diseases are amenable to control – diabetes by means of diet and insulin, periodontal disease by the total elimination of plaque

from the teeth every day. In the same way that diabetes can be monitored by the assessment of blood sugar levels, a method has to be found to monitor the plaque control abilities of the patient. One advantage of this method is the development of a base-line of oral hygiene ability before the onset of treatment. This will allow an accurate representation of failure or improvement, rather than using the vague description of 'poor' or 'good', which are too general to have meaning for either the patient, hygienist or dentist.

MEASUREMENT OF PLAQUE AND GINGIVAL INDEX SCORES

Representative diagrams of the maxillary and mandibular dental arches are required (Figs. 48a and 48b). Each tooth surface is sub-divided into four parts, the dotted outlines of the teeth are left unchanged where they are missing and blocked in where the teeth are present.

The plaque index is based on the presence or absence of plaque on four surfaces of each tooth after staining with erythrosin. The surfaces involved are shaded. The gingival index is established by the presence or absence of oedema, bleeding, or redness adjacent to the four surfaces on each tooth. The tooth surfaces involved are again shaded as required. The percentage of tooth surfaces with plaque or adjacent gingival inflammation out of the total number of surfaces present can be measured on a chart (Fig. 49). The number of teeth in the mouth are plotted against the number of tooth surfaces involved and by following the oblique lines downwards the percentage of tooth surfaces with either plaque or adjacent gingival inflammation can be obtained.

The advantage of this type of charting is its simplicity compared with the more complex indices that have been used in the past. The patient will also

Plaque Index   **76** %

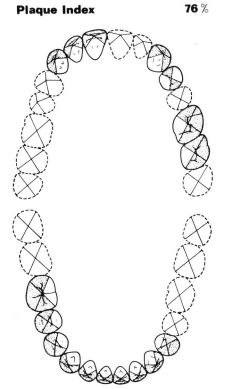

Gingival Index   **89** %

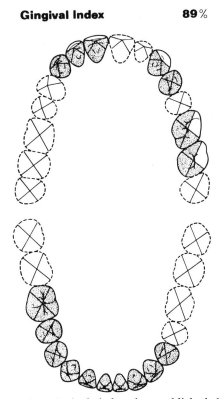

Fig. 48a The plaque index is based on the presence or absence of plaque on four surfaces of each tooth after staining with erythrosin. The surfaces involved are shaded.

Fig. 48b The gingival index is established by the presence or absence of oedema, bleeding or redness adjacent to the four surfaces of each tooth. The tooth surfaces involved are shaded.

CHART FOR CALCULATING PERCENTAGE SURFACES INVOLVED

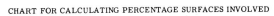

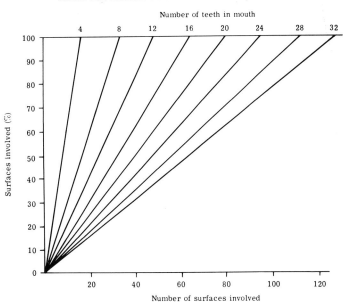

Fig. 49 The number of teeth in the mouth are plotted against the number of tooth surfaces involved and by following the oblique line downwards the percentage of tooth surfaces with either plaque or adjacent gingival inflammation can be obtained.

readily appreciate the meaning of a percentage system based on the presence or absence of plaque or inflammation and this can be used as an instructional tool during the course of oral hygiene teaching. In addition, the diagrams demonstrate the distribution of plaque or inflammation and again can be compared from visit to visit, highlighting the areas where the patient's plaque control is inadequate or where alternative methods may need to be tried.

A considerable divergence of opinion exists as to whether the plaque control programme should be undertaken as a separate entity or as part of the overall initial preparation of the mouth which will include scaling, and root planing. Some clinicians also recommend that the plaque control programme be undertaken on five consecutive days; others advocate longer intervals. It should be emphasised that there is no scientific data to prove that any particular regime is superior to the other. The long term goal is a permanent change of behaviour. However, in many cases this cannot be expected even from a successful plaque control programme. The problem is that many factors which are beyond control of the practising dentist are decisive in the attitude that the patient has to preventive health and behaviour. Nevertheless, nearly all the studies on oral hygiene show that repeated motivation is likely to give positive results. The dentist will, therefore, have to arrange for an on-going plaque control programme over the long term.

ANATOMICAL RELATIONSHIPS OF TEETH AND RESTORATIVE DENTISTRY

The normal interdental papilla between teeth which are in contact is never truly peg-shaped nor even pyramidal. Its shape is determined by the interdental embrasure, which in the healthy mouth should be completely filled by gingival tissue. The crest of this gingiva is knife-edged and directed towards the contact points or areas between approximating teeth. Diagrams of normal interdental gingiva between incisor and molar teeth are shown in Figs. 50, 51. Cohen (1959) has described the shape as a 'col'.

The shape of the interdental col is like a 'U' between the gingival peaks when teeth are grossly overcrowded (Fig. 52). With the crowns instanding or outstanding from the arch, the contacts between teeth are nearer to the cervical regions of the crown and occasionally part of the roots may also be in contact. The space for inaccessible bacterial plaque between the teeth is much larger than between teeth

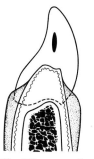

Fig. 50   Diagram of a vertical labiolingual section through the contact points of lower incisors, with clinically normal gingiva. The gingival col is short and dips only slightly between the peaks.

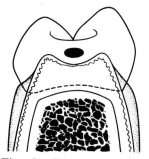

Fig. 51   Diagram of the normal col between premolar or molar teeth. This col is long and dips below the contact zones.

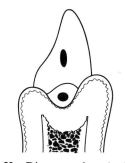

Fig. 52   Diagram of a gingival col between overcrowded lower incisors. This dips deeply between the gingival peaks, providing considerable space between the teeth for undisturbed growth of bacterial plaque.

in regular alignment. This 'U' may well be further enlarged if swelling of the buccal and lingual gingival peaks has resulted from bacterial inflammation. Although the problems of overcrowding and malalignment of teeth can be found in any part of the mouth; the classic areas are between the maxillary central and lateral incisor, the disto-buccal root of the maxillary first molar and the mesio-buccal root of the maxillary second molar, the mandibular lateral and canine teeth and the mandibular incisor teeth. A difference of opinion exists as to whether tooth irregularity is a major predisposing factor in the development of periodontal disease. There is no disagreement that it poses a severe problem to the construction of effective restorations. Further encroachment on remaining embrasure space inevitably occurs, together with the inflammatory swelling of the buccal and lingual gingival peaks, resulting from the presence of inaccessible plaque between the teeth. This is particularly true of full coverage porcelain to gold restorations, where the tendency is to under-prepare the gingival third of the tooth and to overcontour this area of the restoration, in order to retain a sufficient width of porcelain and the correct shade (Parkinson 1976).

The early extraction of posterior teeth, especially in the mandible, may eventually result in tilting of one or more of the remaining molar teeth (Figs. 53, 54). This presents a problem in treatment planning because on many occasions the mesial surface of the tilted tooth shows an area that is inaccessible to plaque control and inevitably a progressive periodontal lesion, usually infra-bony in type, will occur. The construction of a restoration on this tooth will locate the mesial margin in a periodontal pocket, there would also be inadequate vertical space for the use of a precision attachment. The periodontal lesion in such cases is a direct extension of the tissue morphology that has resulted from the tilted position of the tooth. Pocket elimination procedures will therefore fail, as the periodontal structures will return to their original form. The best solution where tilted molar teeth are to be used as abutments, is to upright them by means of minor tooth movement (Brown 1973). This has the following advantages:

1. An easier path of insertion.

2. Increased retention, since all the crown is now available for preparation.

3. The margins of the restoration can be made supra-gingival.

4. The bone and soft tissue morphology change as the tooth is uprighted. This will often lead to the elimination of the mesial bony defect and an increased zone of attached gingiva, as the epithelium of the pocket wall becomes evaginated and keratinized.

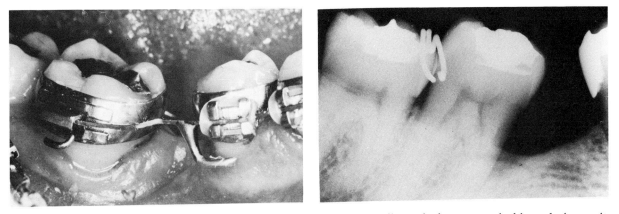

Fig. 53 The second molar tooth is tilted mesially and the intra-oral radiograph shows a vertical bony lesion on its mesial surface.

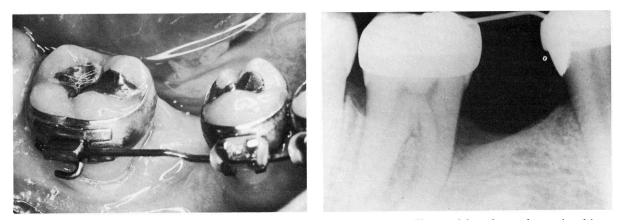

Fig. 54 The second molar tooth is uprighted by an orthodontic appliance. The mesial pocket and associated bony defect is eliminated as the bony morphology changes and the area is debrided with intermittent curettage.

THE EFFECT OF RESTORATIONS ON THE PERIODONTIUM

G. V. Black's concept that proximal restorations should always be placed beneath the free gingivae is no longer acceptable. Both animal and human studies have shown that the extension of restorations into the gingival crevice is a contributing factor in causing periodontal breakdown (Marcum 1967, Silness 1970, Valderhaug 1972, Newcomb 1974, Leon 1975). Scanning electron microscopic studies have shown that the irregularities in the margins of restorations, microporosities and cement margins, all attract plaque sufficient to cause gingival inflammation.

It is often stated in the dental literature that a convexity in the gingival third of the crown is essential for protection of the gingival sulcus area from the impaction of food (Wheeler 1962). Evidence against this theory has been advanced by Yuodelis et al. (1973), who contend that perfectly healthy gingival tissues can be maintained without the protection of crown contours, providing that plaque control is adequate. The commonest mistake is to make bulging rounded crowns (Eissmann et al. 1971). Such an over-contour interferes with the sealing of the gingival cuff around the neck of the tooth and enhances both supra- and sub-gingival plaque accumulation.

The proximal contour of fillings, crowns and pontics should maintain sufficient space for a normal interdental papilla. The tendency is for these restorations to be overcontoured during construction. A long area of contact corono-apically will result in a distortion of the col area, which becomes deeply U-shaped as swelling of the displaced buccal and lingual papillae progresses (Fig. 55). At right angles, a wide contact area bucco-lingually will distort the col area into a wide shallow U-shape, as the buccal and lingual peaks are displaced. This situation will again be exaggerated by inflammation as plaque control becomes increasingly difficult (Fig. 56).

THE EFFECT ON THE PERIODONTIUM OF PARTIAL DENTURES

The concept that a partial denture is a device for losing one's teeth slowly, painfully and expensively, has received support from a number of studies (Koivumaa 1956, Tomlin et al. 1961, Carlsson et al. 1965, Derry et al. 1970). The correlation between caries and periodontal injury to the residual dentition on one hand and the patient's oral hygiene on

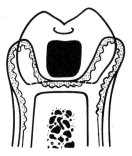
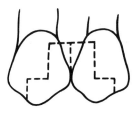

Fig. 55 A long contact point between restorations corono-apically resulting in a distortion of the col area, which becomes deeply 'U' shaped.

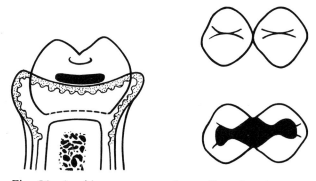

Fig. 56 A wide contact area bucco-lingually distorting the col area into a wide but shallow 'U' shape.

the other, has been well demonstrated by Koivumaa et al. (1960). If oral hygiene was unsatisfactory, denture construction contributed to carious lesions in the abutment teeth and gingivitis around them within one year, even if metal based teeth and mucosal borne partial dentures were designed according to accepted principles.

Fortunately, a more hopeful picture begins to emerge when a concerted effort is made to improve and maintain oral hygiene. Bergman et al. (1977) found no deterioration to the denture-supporting structures in a six year study. Patients had undergone periodontal treatment that included concentrated instruction and motivation in oral hygiene. Subjects were reviewed at yearly intervals when remotivation, scaling and prosthetic adjustments were carried out.

MANAGEMENT OF SOFT TISSUE AND HARD TISSUE DEFORMITIES AROUND ABUTMENT TEETH

Patients must be able to remove plaque from around and between the necks of the teeth if periodontal disease is to be controlled. Pocket formation or deformities in the underlying bone will frustrate adequate plaque control and progressive periodontal breakdown will begin. The surgical procedures available to treat these problems vary according to the depth of pockets present, the need for osseous correction, and the amount of attached gingiva.

Gingivectomy

The resection of the pocket wall, using a 45° incision to the long axis of the teeth, provides a useful method for eliminating pocket depth (Fig. 57). This technique should only be used when there is an adequate width of attached gingiva, so that a functional zone of attached tissue will remain post-operatively and also when there are no under-lying bony deformities. The gingivectomy incision can be embellished by gingivoplasty, accentuating the knife edge of the gingival margin and interdental grooving. Gingivectomy is particularly useful in correcting hyperplastic marginal and interdental areas prior to the construction of new restorations; in addition, gingivectomy will expose additional tooth structure where altered passive eruption is resulting in a shortened clinical crown, and it will also expose carious lesions at the amelo-cemental junction. It should be remembered that as the gingivectomy wound heals, the reforming gingival tissue will tend to cuff out coronally, and allowance will have to be made for the change in level of the gingival tissues if the margins of restorations are to remain supra-gingival.

Flap curettage (The Modified Widman flap) (Fig. 58)

This method of treating pocket depths lies mid-way between that of curettage and the full resective methods of flap surgery. The original technique was described by Widman in 1918, but has been modified and used extensively by the Ann Arbor group in Michigan (Ramfjord and Nissle 1974). The internally

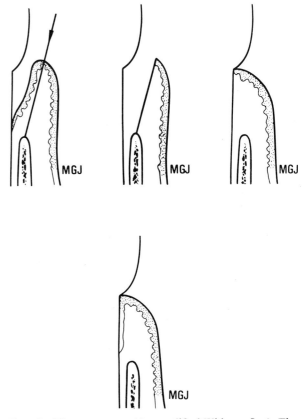

Fig. 58 Flap curettage (the modified Widman flap). The internally bevelled incision is made from the gingival margin labially (an exaggerated scallop is made on the palatal side to allow for good tissue approximation interdentally). Flap reflection is conservative and sufficient to allow the resection of the marginal wedge of tissue and debridement of the area. The flap is replaced to its original position and secured with interrupted sutures. Osseous surgery may sometimes be necessary to ramp interdental areas to allow for better approximation of labial and palatal flaps.

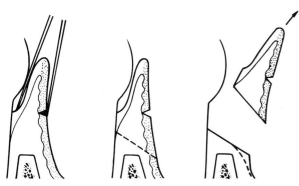

Fig. 57 The gingivectomy incision showing the Krane Caplan pocket marking forceps in situ. The incision starts apically to the puncture marks in order to achieve a 45° angle to the long axis of the tooth. The pocket wall is resected and a physiologic contour achieved.

bevelled incision follows the scalloped outline of the gingival crest and the entire outer wall of the pocket is retained (Fig. 58). On the palatal side the internally bevelled incision has an exaggerated scallop and should also allow for some thinning of the palatal mucosa by undermining dissection.

The interdental collar of tissue is carefully incised and curetted away and the root surfaces and adjacent bone debrided. No osseous reshaping is carried out unless the interdental bone is thickened and will not permit accurate flap adaption interdentally.

Maintaining the full height of gingival tissue labially or buccally and with the exaggerated scallop and thinned tissue palatally, good approximation of tissue can usually be obtained interdentally without the formation of a soft tissue interdental crater. The flaps are stabilised with interrupted sutures.

The flap curettage technique is valuable in maxillary anterior parts of the mouth, where aesthetic factors are important. In deep lesions where resective techniques are not feasible, flap curettage again provides an alternative method of treatment. The inductive potential with the filling-in of vertical bony defects following this technique has recently been demonstrated in a comparative clinical trial of various methods of pocket elimination by Rosling et al. (1976).

The replaced flap

Where the pocket depths are well within the zone of attached gingiva, but underlying bony deformities are present and require treatment, the gingivectomy approach would result in bone exposure, slow healing and soreness, especially on the palate. The internally bevelled incision provides the ideal alternative, allowing the corrected bony form to be covered by mature gingival tissue. The bone is then protected against further resorption and healing is rapid. The internally bevelled incision is made at about 20° to the long axis of the tooth, and is used both to remove the ulcerated sulcular lining of the pocket (leaving a fresh connective tissue edge) and also to thin the gingival tissue at the same time. The starting point of the internally bevelled incision is judged by taking soundings of the crest of the bone, using a periodontal probe, once the local anaesthetic has been administered. The incision is made 2 mm coronal to the crest of the bone and the flap is not dissected beyond the muco-gingival junction, so that no apical displacement occurs. Under these circumstances the flap margin will go back in an optimal position for healing in relation to the crest of the

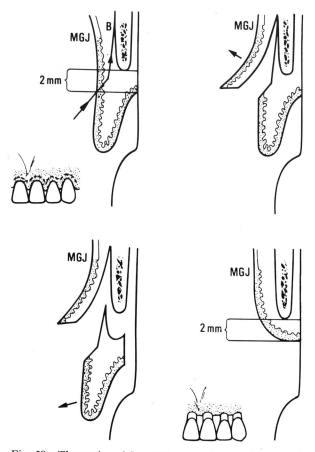

Fig. 59   The replaced flap. Where pocket depths are well within the zones of attached gingiva (usually in the maxilla) the position of the internally bevelled incision on the labial or buccal is made 2 mm coronal to the crest of the bone that can be sounded by pushing a probe through the base of the pocket.

bone (Fig. 59). Pocket depth, of course, will be eliminated by the removal of the coronal cuff of gingiva. The same procedure is carried out on the palate (Fig. 60).

The apically positioned flap

Pocket depths may extend close to or beyond the muco-gingival junction; either an externally bevelled gingivectomy, or an internally bevelled incision related to the crest of the bone would result in incisions being placed in alveolar mucosa and with little or no gingiva remaining post-operatively. Under these circumstances, the entire gingival wall of the pocket is retained on the labial or buccal side. The internally bevelled incision is carried out around the necks of the involved teeth, keeping the incision

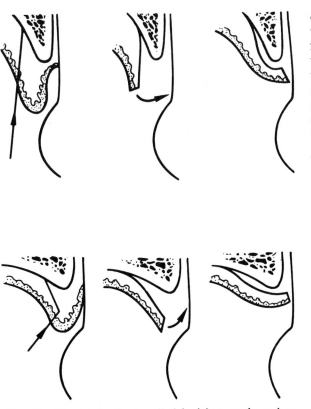

extent of bone exposure usually depends on the visibility that is required for osseous correction. If further detachment of the flap is required beyond this point to obtain adequate apical positioning, then the dissection can be split thickness, leaving periosteum to protect the underlying bone. The apically positioned flap, therefore, is really a three part flap: split thickness to thin the flap coronally, full thickness to expose the underlying bony deformities, and split thickness again to obtain depth for the flap to be positioned apically (Fig. 61). On the palatal side the reverse bevel incision is carried out 2 mm coronal to the crest of the bone and a similar procedure can often be used lingually in the mandibular molar areas, where the gingival width is greater. Circumferential or continuous sutures are used to suspend the flap around the necks of the teeth. Periosteal sutures improve the reliability of the procedure by preventing a coronal displacement of the flap.

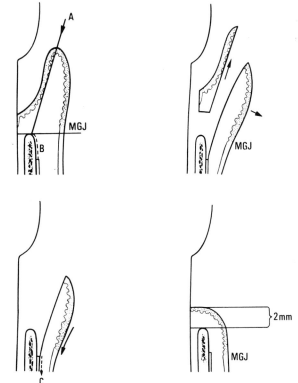

Fig. 60 The internally bevelled incision on the palate. When the gingival tissue is thin and the palatal vault deep, the internally bevelled incision to eliminate pocket depth is made 2 mm coronal to the crest of the bone and angulated to thin the flap at the same time. When the internal wedge of tissue is resected away, the margin of the flap is displaced along the same horizontal plane to fit tightly around the neck of the tooth and to cover the underlying bone. When the palate is shallow and the gingiva thick and detached, the crown of the tooth will restrict the positioning of the scalpel blade. Accordingly an initial incision some 2 or 3 mm deep is made using a B.P. No. 15 scalpel blade. This incision is then re-entered using a Goldman Fox No. 7 knife, which will allow the secondary incision to be angulated, so thinning the flap. Following the removal of the cervical wedge of tissue, the flap margin is adapted to cover the crest of the bone. It should be noted however, that the flap margin is displaced through the arc of a circle, in contrast to the steep palate and therefore an increased length of flap will be required for adequate coverage of the crestal bone and close contact with the necks of the teeth.

close to the gingival margin. It is *not* related to the underlying bone. The split thickness incision will thin the gingival tissue and ends at the crest of the bone. The flap is then detached from the underlying bone with a periosteal elevator in an apical direction. The muco-gingival junction will be freed and the

Fig. 61 The apically positioned flap. When pocket depths extend close to or beyond the mucogingival junction, the internally bevelled incision is kept close to the gingival margin. The thinned outer wall of the pocket is reflected beyond the mucogingival junction and apically positioned 2 mm coronal to the crest of the bone.

The importance of a functional zone of attached gingiva

The attached gingiva, under normal conditions, appears as a ribbon of keratinized tissue, firmly bound down to the underlying bone and cementum around the necks of the teeth, and with a marginal cuff of about 2 mm that is detached and forms the gingival sulcus. The function of attached gingiva is to accept the shearing stresses of mastication and to dissipate muscle pull on the marginal tissues. It has been suggested that the dense, closely packed collagen fibre groups found in zones of attached gingiva are better deterrents to the infiltration of inflammation than the loosely arranged fibre apparatus of alveolar mucosa. Support for this contention was given by Lang and Löe (1972) in their study of attached gingiva. They found that areas with a band of attached gingiva of less than 2 mm had more persistent gingival inflammation. The restorative implications can readily be drawn: that an inadequate gingival band may not withstand the trauma resulting from tooth preparation, impression taking and the close proximity of restoration margins. A minimal zone of attached gingiva may be increased by one of two methods: the split thickness apically displaced flap, or soft tissue grafts.

The split thickness apically displaced flap

This procedure can be used to increase the zone of attached gingiva and eliminate pocket depths that are close to or beyond the mucogingival junction, provided that there is an adequate depth to the vestibular fornix. In order to conserve all the existing gingiva, an internally bevelled incision is made close to the gingival margin. A vertical releasing incision will often be helpful in providing a plane of dissection for the scalpel blade in an apical coronal direction. The marginal cuff is curetted away and the muco-periosteal flap apically positioned to the desired level and securely stabilized with sutures. During healing, granulation tissue covers the exposed periosteum and matures to form keratinized attached gingiva; depending on the level to which the flap was positioned, an overall gain in gingival width will result (Fig. 62). The split thickness apically displaced flap is used most commonly in the mandibular labial and buccal areas, where gingival width is inherently small. The mandibular lingual area presents a more difficult problem because of the difficulties of split thickness dissection. A full thickness flap is therefore employed, apically positioned, to expose a small area of marginal bone.

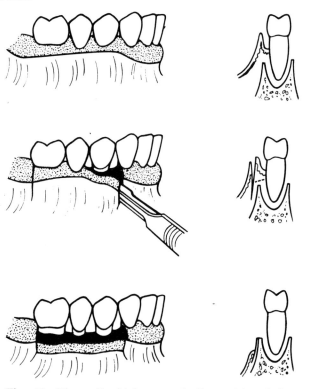

Fig. 62 The split thickness apically positioned flap. Where gingival width needs to be increased and sufficient vestibular depth exists, a split thickness flap is displaced apically to the crest of the bone. New attached gingiva is formed over the exposed periosteum and blends in with the existing gingival tissue to give an increased width of attached gingiva.

Pedicle grafts

Grupe and Warren (1956), were the first to introduce pedicle graft procedures in periodontics and later modifications have been suggested by Corn (1964) and Cohen and Ross (1968). The laterally repositioned flap can be used where there is a lack of attached gingiva on one particular tooth (Figs. 63, 64). It is essential that adequate vestibular depth is present and that donor tissue is of adequate width and quality. Prominent root surfaces on palpation and thin gingival tissue may point to an underlying dehiscence in the donor area and in such instances the lateral graft is contraindicated.

A gingivectomy incision is made along the margins of the defect and, where necessary, is extended apically to include frena and muscle attachments that are encroaching on the area. The bevel of the gingivectomy incision on the stable side of the recipient area should be long to provide for a good

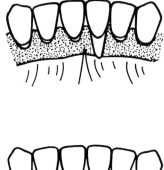

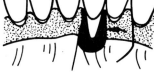

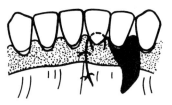

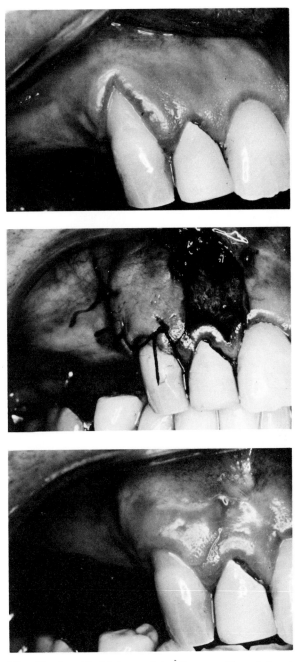

Fig. 63   The laterally positioned flap. This form of repair can be used to treat isolated areas of recession, providing vestibular depth is adequate, sufficient gingival tissue is present laterally and underlying bony dehiscences or fenestrations are not suspected. Opinions vary in the literature as to whether this flap should be full thickness, split thickness, or a combination of the two, leaving periosteum over the donor area, but also providing periosteum to cover the exposed root surface, which will be of benefit during healing.

overlap with the donor flap. The root surface is planed to remove the surface layer of cementum, with its entrapped endotoxin and plaque. Where the root surface is prominent, reduction may be required with a fine diamond stone in an air turbine to bring the root prominence within the boundaries of the alveolus. The donor flap is then dissected using an internally bevelled incision marginally and a vertical incision 1½ tooth widths lateral to the recipient site. The donor tissue is dissected on a partial thickness basis to ensure adequate periosteal and connective tissue protection of the exposed area. A cut back incision in the direction to which the flap is to be repositioned will ensure adequate mobility and lessen tension on the flap in its new position. The flap is then sutured into place with a circumferential

Fig. 64   A split thickness laterally repositioned flap to repair recession on the maxillary right canine. A marginal cuff of tissue is left around the neck of the tooth in the donor area to avoid unnecessary recession. In this instance the thin delicate tissue that was present in the saddle area did not represent good donor tissue and the more anterior area was preferred. The post-operative result shows good root coverage prior to restorative dentistry, but a small amount of gingivoplasty would be an advantage to thin the tissues at this stage.

suture around the neck of the recipient tooth and interruptal sutures at the area of overlap.

The double papilla flap provides a useful alternative form of treatment for repairing isolated areas of recession (Fig. 65). In this technique the donor tissue is mobilized solely from the adjacent papillae. The ideal situation for its use would be found in treating a narrow cleft with insufficient donor tissue to construct a lateral flap, or where the possibility of dehiscence may exist over the root surface in the potential donor area. The distal papilla is bevelled to expose connective tissue, which will be covered by the overlap of the mesial portion of the flap, thereby avoiding a butt joint. The papillae are then sutured together, a delicate operation, and then stabilized with periosteal sutures at their lateral margins. A sling suture is also employed around the neck of the tooth.

The edentulous area pedicle graft was described by Corn (1964). The modification of the laterally repositioned flap makes use of keratinized tissue from an edentulous saddle area. With careful dissection and use of a cut back incision to improve

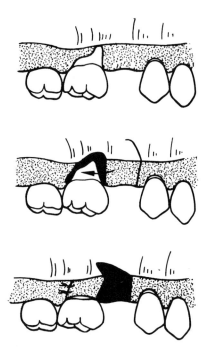

Fig. 66   The edentulous area pedicle graft utilizes tissue from an adjacent saddle area, which can be apically and laterally positioned to cover an area of isolated recession.

mobility, the muco-periosteal flap can be positioned both apically and laterally to cover the prepared root surface (Figs. 66, 67).

Free gingival grafts

Free autogenous grafts have been used with great success in plastic surgery for many years. Their application in periodontal therapy is more recent and can be attributed to King and Pennel (1964) and the well documented studies of Sullivan and Atkins (1968). The particular indications for the use of free gingival grafts are where there are inadequate bands of attached gingiva, often with high muscle attachments, in the presence of a shallow vestibule. In contrast to the flap procedures mentioned above, the free gingival graft can be effectively used to deepen the vestibule as well as increasing the zone of attached gingiva. The problems associated with muscle attachments will be eliminated when these fibres are dissected away from the area covered with mature gingival tissue. The free gingival graft is unpredictable when attempts are made to cover exposed root surfaces. The graft will usually necrose over the avascular root surface unless the defect is narrow and the periodontal membrane on each side close together to provide a good blood supply. The

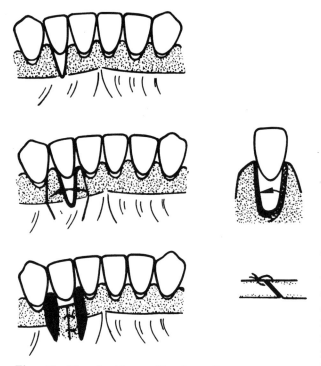

Fig. 65   The double papilla flap allows the use of papillary tissue mesially and distally to the defect and avoids the exposure of marginal bone. The delicate flaps should be full thickness and overlapped to avoid a butt joint.

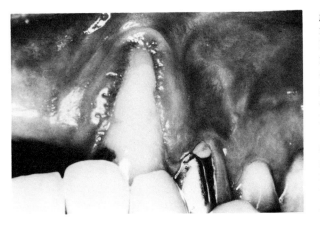

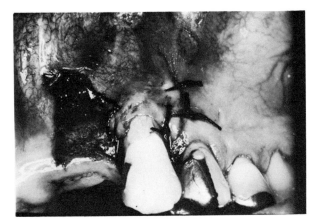

gingival graft should also be avoided in areas requiring osseous surgery. The danger here is that lack of adjacent periosteum may compromise the revascularization of the graft. In these cases the establishment of a functional zone of attached gingiva is usually carried out as a two-stage procedure, the graft being carried out either before or after pocket elimination.

Gingival grafts may be considered marginal or submarginal (Figs. 68–70). Where the marginal gingiva is narrow and perpetually inflamed, despite initial treatment, the graft should completely replace the marginal tissue. If, on the other hand, the gingival sulcus is clinically healthy and there is a narrow pre-existing zone of gingiva, this tissue is left in situ, but extended apically by means of a submarginal graft. The recipient site is prepared by means of a split thickness dissection, together with careful removal of all muscle and connective tissue down to the firm base of periosteum. The donor area for the graft is the masticatory mucosa of the hard palate and, if necessary, a foil template may be used to ensure the accurate size and shape of the graft. Soehren et al. (1973) have suggested that the optimal thickness of gingival grafts should be 1 to 1.5 mm, based upon functional, healing, mechanical and aesthetic factors. The graft should be completely immobilized during healing. Immobilization is achieved by holding the graft under pressure for several minutes, to ensure a uniformly thin fibrin

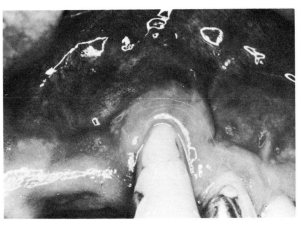

Fig. 67 Isolated recession on a maxillary canine caused by a partial denture. The edentulous area pedicle graft is used to cover the root surface that has not been restored and a good overlap is made on the stable side. The final result shows an adequate zone of attached gingiva, prior to the completion of restorative procedures.

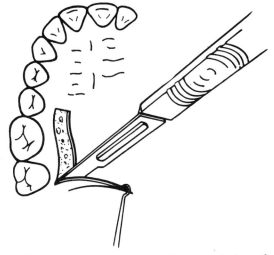

Fig. 68 A split thickness dissection of graft tissue from the palate. This should be 1 to 1.5 mm in thickness. The shape of the graft can be outlined with a B.P. No. 15 scalpel blade and either dissected off using the same instrument, or a Goldman Fox No. 7 knife, which has an excellent angulation for this palatal procedure.

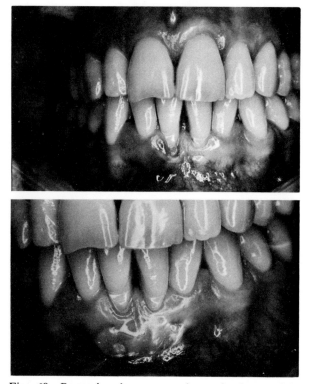

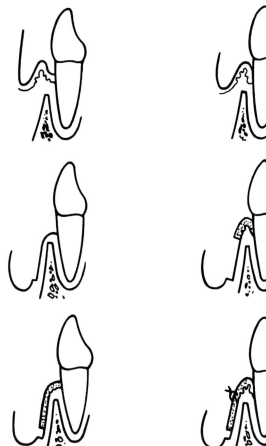

Fig. 69 Recession has occurred on the lower right mandibular incisor, leaving little or no attached gingiva. There is also a muscle pull. Some marginal tissue is still available on the lower left incisor tooth. A free gingival graft has been utilized replacing the gingival margin on the right incisor, but being submarginal on the left incisor tooth.

Fig. 70   Where the marginal tissues are formed of mucosa or where the gingival width is very narrow and perpetually inflamed, a marginal graft would be used to completely replace these tissues (left).

Where the marginal gingiva is healthy but gingival width needs to be increased and vestibular depth is shallow, the marginal tissues can be left intact and the submarginal graft used (right).

clot, then a minimal number of sutures can be inserted, or the coronal and lateral margins of the graft covered with cyanoacrylate. To reduce the area of the wound, the mucosa apical to the graft can be sutured to the underlying periosteum. On no account should it be sutured to the graft itself, because of the movement that will ensue. Both the recipient and donor sites are covered with surgical dressing.

The treatment of edentulous ridge areas

A simple gingivectomy/gingivoplasty technique can be used to correct distorted ridge areas, provided that adjacent pocket depth is shallow and there is an adequate zone of attached gingiva. The gingivectomy incision is carried right along the crest of the ridge, from one abutment tooth to the other. Following this the ridge can be embellished by gingivoplasty, either by means of scraping with the

gingivectomy knife (Fig. 71) or by using a pair of surgical nippers. The removal of fibrous tissue from the crest of the ridge will produce more vertical space, so making for better and stronger pontic design.

If pocket depths are more severe and underlying bony deformities exist, a flap approach should be used. Providing that there is an adequate zone of attached gingiva, two parallel and converging incisions are made along the crest of the ridge. The distance apart of these incisions will vary according to the pocket depths on the abutment teeth. The central wedge is removed and lateral wedges of tissue dissected free by undermining incisions. The

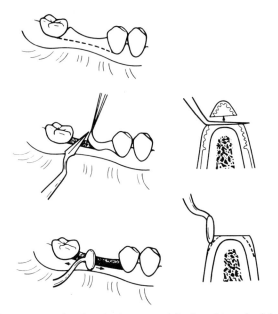

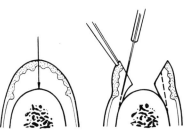

Fig. 73 Where gingival widths are barely adequate in relation to ridge areas, pocket depths should be eliminated by apically positioning the tissue, so that none of the gingival width is sacrificed. Ridge-plasty procedures should be blended in with surgery in adjacent areas.

Fig. 71 A simple gingivectomy/gingivoplasty incision can be used to correct distorted ridge areas, providing pocket depth is shallow and there is an adequate zone of attached gingiva. Either a Bard Parker No. 15 scalpel blade, or Goldman Fox No. 11 knife, can be used for the marginal resection and a Goldman Fox No. 7 knife used to scrape the tissue to provide the marginal bevelling.

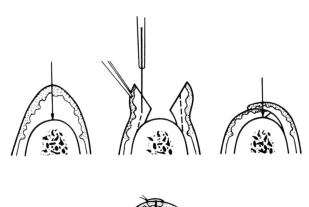

Fig. 72 If pocket depths are more severe and underlying bony deformities are present, a flap procedure should be used to eliminate pocket depths in relation to ridge areas. Where a more than adequate zone of attached gingiva is present, a linear incision is made along the crest of the ridge, the flaps partially reflected and thinned on their inner surface. The flaps are then overlapped and the excess tissue removed. The two flaps are then approximated with interrupted sutures.

flaps are then elevated as far as necessary to expose the underlying bony deformities, which can then be reshaped, the flaps are then approximated and sutured (Fig. 72). Where the edentulous ridge has only a narrow zone of attached gingiva, it is wise to conserve this as far as possible. A linear incision is therefore made, passing along the crest of the ridge, the two flaps are elevated into a vertical plane and thinning incisions made allowing the wedges of thickened tissue to be removed. In order to facilitate the apical repositioning of the gingiva in the saddle area, the flaps are reflected beyond the mucogingival junction. Vertical relieving incisions may be necessary on the distal and mesial aspects of abutment teeth. This will depend on the periodontal procedures being carried out in adjacent areas. Following osseous surgery, the flaps are approximated and sutured. The gingival tissue in the saddle area, now occupying a more apical position, allows for an increase in clinical crown height and an optimal ridge contour for good pontic adaption (Fig. 73).

Tuberosity and retromolar areas

The presence of excessive amounts of thick fibrous tissue is common in both these areas. Pocket depths are due more to the exaggerated soft tissue morphology than to a down-growth of the epithelial attachment onto cementum. The shortened clinical crowns that result from these deformities in tuberosity and retromolar areas complicates tooth

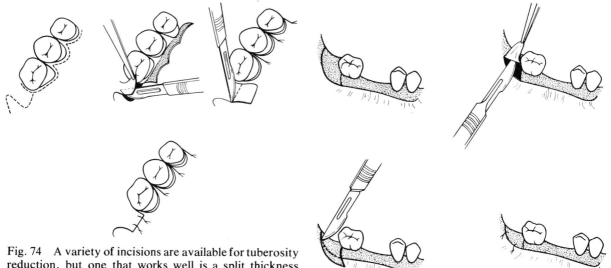

Fig. 74   A variety of incisions are available for tuberosity reduction, but one that works well is a split thickness lateral flap, reflected as part of the buccal gingival wall. The underlying area is debrided and osseous lesions treated as required and then the flap replaced over the area. The excess overlap can then be removed. Tuberosity procedures are again blended in with surgery that is being carried out around adjacent teeth.

Fig. 75   Pocket reduction in retromolar areas can be achieved by a split thickness flap distal to the last molar tooth. This allows the underlying connective tissue to be removed and osseous deformities exposed and treated. The flap is then collapsed back over the area and the excess tissue removed. This form of surgery is again blended in with surgical procedures in adjacent areas.

preparation, impression taking, and establishing a margin to the restoration that is supra-gingival. In addition, the shortened clinical crown provides inadequate retention. Surgical reduction of thickened tuberosity and retromolar areas follows the same principles as those outlined for ridge areas (Figs. 74, 75). A word of caution should be given about the excessive reduction of tuberosity tissue, because of the inherent problems that will occur if a partial denture is required at some time in the future. In these circumstances, a partial reduction of the tuberosity area may be carried out and the remaining pocket maintained by means of curettage. Where the first molar tooth is available, it may be more prudent to sacrifice the second molar when pocket depths related to tuberosity areas are excessively deep and involve the furcation.

The management of periodontal abnormalities by root removal

The pattern of alveolar and supporting bone loss in periodontal disease may be unequal, even in relation to the different roots of a molar tooth. Removal of the offending root or roots will allow the tooth to be retained and, if necessary, to function as an abutment (Fig. 76). In some instances the roots of posterior teeth are in close proximity, making for

difficulties in oral hygiene and treatment. This type of situation is often found where the disto-buccal root of the first maxillary molar flares towards the mesio-buccal root of the second maxillary molar (Fig. 77). In addition to the problems of plaque control, no space remains for an adequate embrasure if these teeth are to be restored. The removal of one or both of these roots will allow for a manageable embrasure form.

Following periodontal disease, the furcation areas of molar teeth may become exposed. Such areas are not amenable to plaque control and are often the site of periodontal abscess formation. Such teeth are therefore not satisfactory as abutments. Removal of one root in relation to mandibular molar teeth, or one or two roots in relation to maxillary molars (Fig. 78), will allow access to these areas and carefully designed restorations will allow for adequate plaque control.

THE MAINTENANCE PROBLEM

The inherent susceptibility of the periodontal tissues to recurrent disease must always be borne in mind. However, many studies have now demonstrated that

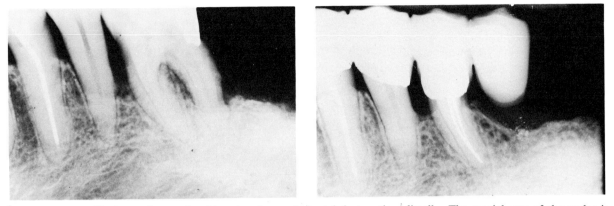

Fig. 76 A mandibular molar tooth with extensive periodontal destruction distally. The mesial root of the molar is retained and treated endodontically, the distal root removed by hemisection. Following periodontal therapy, the mesial root provides excellent support for fixed bridgework.

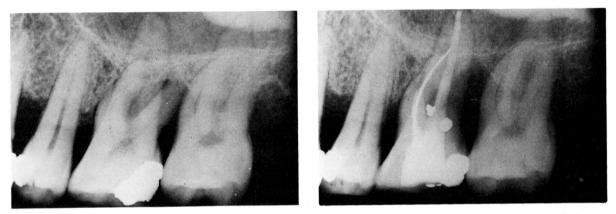

Fig. 77 Vertical alveolar bone loss is associated with the close proximity of the disto-buccal root of the first molar and the mesio-buccal root of the second molar. Root amputation of the disto-buccal root of the first molar together with endodontic therapy, will often allow for definitive pocket elimination. In some instances the mesio-buccal root of the second molar may also need removal.

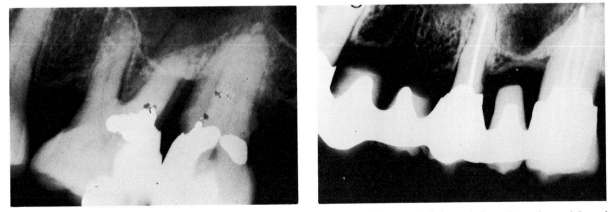

Fig. 78 Furcation involving maxillary first molar. The furcation could be probed through from buccal, mesial, and distal aspects. The mesio-buccal root with good bony support is retained as an abutment for a fixed bridge. The remaining two roots are sectioned and removed, during periodontal surgery in this quadrant of the mouth.

it is possible, by comprehensive plaque control programmes, to prevent the progression of periodontitis. In young adults a frequency of one or two prophylactic visits per year may be sufficient to prevent periodontitis (Lightner et al. 1971, Suomi et al. 1971, Bergman et al. 1977). A divergence of opinion would seem to exist as to how frequently patients should be recalled for professional tooth cleaning and reinforcement of oral hygiene. The results above contradict those reported by Nyman et al. (1975), where it was found that a six month recall programme for scalings failed to achieve an adequate oral hygiene and thereby to avoid a relapse of periodontal treatment. A possible explanation for this divergence of opinion would be the depth of motivation given both prior to and in conjunction with oral hygiene instruction. The finding that improved oral home care, rather than the mechanical cleaning of teeth once a month, could maintain a high standard of gingival health has been shown by Lang et al. (1973) and Glavind (1977).

When planning partial dentures and restorations, it is essential that the design facilitates plaque control procedures. Crown margins should be kept supragingival, proximal areas should allow proper cleansing and the denture materials should be placed as far away from the marginal gingivae as possible. The problems of oral hygiene may be further compounded by restorations with precision attachments that distort the anatomy of abutment teeth. Despite the greatest care in the planning and execution of treatment, the results of periodontal therapy may result in anatomical deformities that are difficult to maintain. Available information has shown that gingivitis can be prevented buccally and lingually by the correct use of a tooth brush (Lindhe and Koch 1967), but the effect of the tooth brush alone has only a limited effect in interdental areas. A series of studies (Gjermo and Flotra 1970, Wolffe 1976, Nyak and Wade 1977) has shown that ancillary methods of interdental cleaning are absolutely essential if periodontal health is to be maintained. The choice of which agent to use seems to depend on the individual needs and capabilities of the subject in question. Thus wood sticks, floss, Proxa-brushes and interspace brushes were all of value, though none demonstrated a clear superiority. However, in wide open interproximal areas following periodontal destruction, the interdental brush proved to be the most efficient.

The well-worn phrase 'that familiarity breeds contempt' could not be more apt than when applied to the problems of maintenance. Dentists by nature are attracted to new patients with new and taxing problems and are often negligent about picking up the subtle tissue changes that may occur in patients who have been under their care over a long period. In the true sense of the word, periodontal disease is never cured but is only controlled, and there will be instances when further treatment will be required, possibly of a surgical nature. It is perhaps better to discuss these possibilities with the patient at the end of the treatment phase, rather than explain them at one of the recall appointments. The frequency of maintenance treatment should be based on tissue response. A frequent recall (every two to four months) is needed by patients whose plaque formation is heavy and where oral hygiene procedures, despite constant motivation, remain only moderate. On the other hand, patients who have excellent plaque control and form minimal deposits on their teeth, can be seen at yearly intervals.

Periodontal probing in areas that are presenting problems should be carried out at each recall visit. A full periodontal probing should only be required every year. Particular attention should be paid to furcation involvements and areas of gingival recession should be re-assessed; tooth mobilities and occlusal relationships should also be recorded. A full mouth, long cone, radiographic survey need only be repeated once every three years. However, in areas of particular concern, a more frequent assessment may be required.

REFERENCES AND FURTHER READING

BERGMAN, B. HUGOSON, A. and OLSSON, C. O. (1977) Caries and periodontal status in patients fitted with removable partial dentures. *J. Clin. Periodont.*, 4, 134

BROWN, I. S. (1973) The effect of orthodontic therapy on certain types of periodontal defects. I: Clinical findings. *J. Periodont.*, 44, 727

CARLSSON, S. E., HEDEGÅRD, B. and KOIVUMAA, K. K. (1965) Studies in partial dental prosthesis. IV. Final results of a 4-year longitudinal investigation of dentogingivally supported partial dentures. *Acta odont. scand.*, 23, 443

COHEN, B. (1959) Morphological factors in the pathogenesis of periodontal disease. *Brit. dent. J.*, 107, 31

COHEN, D. W. and ROSS, S. E. (1968) The double papillae repositioned flap in periodontal surgery. *J. Periodont.*, 39, 65

CORN, H. (1964) Edentulous area pedicle graft in mucogingival surgery. *Periodontics*, 2, 229

DERRY, A. and BERTRAM, V. (1970). A clinical survey of removable partial dentures, after two years usage. *J. prosth. dent.*, 16, 721

EISSMANN, H. F., RADKE, R. A. and NOBLE, W. A. (1971) Physiologic design criteria for fixed dental restorations. *Dent. Clin. N. Amer.*, *15*, 543

GJERMO, P. and FLOTRA, L. (1970) The effect of different methods of interdental cleaning. *J. Periodont. Res.*, *5*, 230

GLAVIND, L. (1977) The effect of monthly professional mechanical toothcleaning on periodontal health in adults. *J. Clin. Periodont.*, *4*, 100

GRUPE, H. and WARREN, R. (1956) Repair of gingival defects by sliding lateral flap. *J. Periodont.*, *27*, 92

KING, K. and PENNEL, B. (1964) Free autogenous gingival grafts. Paper presented at the Annual Meeting of the *Philadelphia Society of Periodontology.*

KOIVUMAA, K. (1956) Changes in periodontal tissues and supporting structures connected with partial dentures. *Suom. hammaslääk. toim.*, *52*, Suppl. 1

KOIVUMAA, K., HEDEGARD, B. and CARLSSON, G. (1960) Studies in partial denture prosthesis. I. An investigation of dentogingivally supported partial dentures. *Suom. hammaslääk. toim.*, *56*, 248

LANG, N. P., CUMMING, B. R. and LÖE, H. (1973) Tooth brushing frequency as it relates to plaque development and gingival health. *J. Periodont.* 44, 396

LANG, N. P. and LÖE, H. (1972) The relationship between the width of keratinized gingiva and gingival health. *J. Periodont.*, *43*, 623

LEON, A. (1975) A clinical study of the effect of Cl. II amalgam fillings on the periodontium. *M.D.S. Thesis.* University of London

LIGHTNER, L. M., O'LEARY, T. J., DRAKE, R. D., CRAMP, P. P. and ALLEN, M. F. (1971) Preventive periodontic procedures: results over 46 months. *J. Periodont.*, *42*, 555

LINDHE, J. and KOCH, G. (1967) The effect of supervised oral hygiene on the gingivae of children: Lack of prolonged effect of supervision. *J. Periodont. Res.*, 2, 215

LINDHE, J. and NYMAN, S. (1975) The effect of plaque control and surgical pocket elimination on the establishment and maintenance of periodontal health. A longitudinal study of periodontal therapy in cases of advanced disease. *J. Clin. Periodont.*, *2*, 67

LÖE, H. THEILADE, E. and JENSEN, S. B. (1965) Experimental gingivitis in man. *J. Periodont.*, *36*, 177

LÖVDAL, A., ARNO, A., SCHEI, O. and WAERHAUG, J. (1961) Combined effect of supragingival scaling and controlled oral hygiene on the incidence of gingivitis. *Acta odontol. scand.*, *19*, 537

MARCUM, J. S. (1967) The effect of crown marginal depth upon gingival tissues. *J. prosth. Dent.*, *17*, 479

NEWCOMB, J. M. (1974) The relationship between the location of subgingival crown margins and gingival inflammation. *J. Periodont.*, *45*. 151

NYAK, R. P. and WADE, A. B. (1977) The relative effectiveness of plaque removal by the Proxa brush and rubber cone stimulator. *J. Clin. Periodont.*, *4*, 128

NYMAN, S., ROSLING, B. and LINDHE, J. (1975) The effect of professional tooth cleaning on healing after periodontal surgery. *J. Clin. Periodont.*, *2*, 80

PARKINSON, C. D. (1976) Excessive crown contours facilitate endemic plaque niches. *J. prosth. Dent.*, *35*, 424

RAMFJORD, S. P. (1959) Indices for prevalence and incidence of periodontal disease. *J. Periodont.*, *30*, 51

RAMFJORD, S. P., KNOWLES, J. W., NISSLE, R. R., SCHICK, R. A. and BURGITT, F. G. (1973) A longitudinal study of periodontal therapy. *J. Periodont.*, *44*, 66

RAMFJORD, S. P. and NISSLE, R. R. (1974) The modified Widman flap. *J. Periodont.*, *45*, 601

ROSLING, B., NYMAN, S., LINDHE, J. and JERN, B. (1976) The healing potential of the periodontal tissues following different techniques of periodontal surgery in plaque free dentitions. A two year clinical study. *J. Clin. Periodont.* 3, 233

SILNESS, J. (1970) The periodontal condition in patients treated with dental bridges. III. The relationship between the location of crown margins and periodontal conditions. *J. Periodont. Res.*, *5*, 225

SOCKRANSKY, S. S. (1970) The relationship of bacteria to the etiology of periodontal disease. *J. Dent. Res.*, *Supplement No. 2*

SOEHREN, S. E., ALLEN, A. L., CUTRIGHT, D. E. and SEIBERT, J. S. (1973) Clinical and histologic studies of donor tissues utilized for free grafts of masticatory mucosa. *J. Periodont.*, *44*, 727

SULLIVAN, H. and ATKINS, J. (1968) Free autogenous gingival grafts. II. Principles of successful grafting. *Periodontics*, *6*, 121

SUOMI, J. D., GREENE, J. C., VERMILLION, J. R., DOYLE, J., CHANG, J. J. and LEATHERWOOD, E. C. (1971) The effect of controlled oral hygiene procedures on the progression of periodontal diseases in adults. Results after the third and final year. *J. Periodont.*, *42*, 152

TOMLIN, H. R. and OSBORNE, J. (1961) Cobalt chromium partial dentures. A clinical survey. *Brit. dent. J.*, *110*, 307

VALDERHAUG, J. (1972) Prepaver ingsgrensens beliggenhet krone/bro synspunkter. *Norske Tandlaegeforen. Tidende*, *82*, 386

WHEELER, R. C. (1962) Complete crown form and the periodontium. *J. prosth. Dent.*, *11*, 722

WIDMAN, L. (1920). The operative treatment of pyorrhea alveolaris, a new surgical method. Stockholm, 1918. *Reviewed in the Brit. dent. J.*, *S1*, 293

WOLFFE, G. N. (1976) An evaluation of proximal surface cleansing agents. *J. Clin. Periodont.*, *3*, 148

YUODELIS, R. A., WEAVER, J. D. and SAPHOS, G. (1973) Facial and lingual contours of artificial complete crown restorations and their effect on the periodontium. *J. prosth. Dent.*, *29*, 61

CHAPTER 3

The Occlusal Surfaces

The occlusal surfaces of a restoration are its working surfaces. Masticatory and occlusal forces are transmitted through these areas, which need to be planned with care and constructed with accuracy.

Dentures are normally constructed to place artificial teeth in the mouth. It is surprising, therefore, that in practice one so often finds these artificial teeth added apparently as an afterthought. Components of partial dentures may interfere with the articulation of the opposing teeth. By their irregularities these opposing teeth may play havoc with the denture when eccentric jaw movements are attempted. Had these problems been diagnosed, correction at an early stage of treatment would have been relatively straightforward. Instead, we all too frequently see desperate and mutilating 'correction' in which an attempt is made to adapt a prosthesis to a hopeless situation. At best, the prognosis, function, and appearance of the restoration is jeopardised.

Important as it may be, careful analysis of individual diagnostic casts alone is inadequate. These casts must be correctly related to one another requiring an intermaxillary record. Since the intermaxillary record may involve a change in vertical dimension, a facebow should be employed. Even if centric relation were recorded at the vertical relation of occlusion, the facebow would still be necessary as an aid in the assessment of lateral jaw movements. Furthermore, the infra-orbital marker will relate the occlusal plane to the Frankfort plane, a factor that may help in planning the appearance of the restoration. Precise hinge axis location is not always necessary so that relatively simple facebows like the Dentatus, Hanau, or Whipmix will suffice. Matsumoto (1976) has classified deficient occlusions into three groups:

Group 1 The vertical dimension of occlusion is determined by occlusal stops.

Group 2 No occlusal stops but teeth present in both jaws.

Group 3 Teeth are present in one jaw only. Depending on the patient's dentition the vertical dimension of occlusion may be assessed by:
1. Direct measurement.
2. Indirect measurement.

The vertical relation of occlusion

If this essential relationship is determined by the natural teeth a major difficulty is overcome. One can proceed as follows:

1. Direct apposition of casts

This simple and accurate method may be employed where there are adequate teeth remaining in contact to make the existing jaw relationship obvious. One provision is essential: a previous occlusal analysis in centric relation and the correction of any interferences.

2. Overlay occlusal rims

This procedure may be used where there are widely spaced occlusal stops but insufficient teeth present to allow direct cast opposition. The Dawson type occlusal rim is constructed on the upper cast covering the premolar and molar teeth. It should not touch the areas representing the mucosa. This wax is chilled and cut away from the buccal cusps so that the seating of the cast in the record is easily checked. An extra-hard base wax is required.

3. Mucosal-borne occlusal rims

Closely spaced occlusal rims are to be placed in the edentulous areas. This is often necessary for distal extension spaces. Hard wax bases will suffice if handled with care. A soft recording index such as fast setting stone or zinc oxide is desirable.

The distal extension base is particularly prone to

errors in jaw relation recording owing to the forces that may be exerted by the opposing natural teeth. The entire design may be influenced where vertical space is short so that time spent at an early stage is well rewarded. Far better to spend a few extra moments early in the therapy, than to be faced with hours of frustration later on.

Unlike a complete denture in which the condylar pathway is virtually the only factor outside the operator's control, the partial denture will have to conform to an established occlusal plane. Careful jaw relation recordings will show the modifications necessary to the opposing teeth.

Without occlusal stops the problem is more complex. Efforts at measuring the vertical relation of occlusion by maximum biting force or other means have not yet proved reliable in clinical practice. It is therefore necessary to make indirect assessments by first measuring the vertical relation of rest.

The vertical relation of rest

The original Brodie and Thompson concept of a stable vertical dimension of rest throughout life was convenient for prosthodontics as removal of the teeth was not considered to affect the rest position of the mandible. Unfortunately the theory has not stood the test of time. Nairn (1976) has pointed out that removal of teeth or occlusal stops is often followed by the adoption of a new rest position, usually with the jaws closer together. Tallgren (1967) showed that dentures can be constructed to a variety of occlusal vertical dimensions all demonstrating an inter-occlusal (freeway) space. Demonstrations of inter-occlusal space were not by themselves reliable guides to the occlusal vertical dimension of the dentures.

Factors influencing the vertical dimension of rest may include higher centres, mechanoreceptor activity in the periodontal ligament, oral mucosa, and temporomandibular joint, together with possible monosynaptic stretch reflexes. Möller (1976) has put forward evidence suggesting that the rest position is subject to a servo-control mechanism. Yemm (1976), however, postulated that the position is determined by the tendency of structures to come to physical rest because of their visco-elastic properties.

Whatever the outcome of these controversies, the best the clinician can achieve is to seat his patient comfortably and upright. An assessment should be made with the minimum of fuss and with no more than one occlusal rim in the mouth. The occlusal rims are mucosal borne and usually constructed of extra-hard base wax.

With the vertical dimension of rest established an inter-occlusal space needs to be provided. As a general rule this space will measure about 4 mm in the first premolar region – slightly larger for patients with Angles Class II Division II malocclusions and slightly smaller for those with Class III malocclusions. Swallowing and phonetic guides are often useful.

Patients who have only roots present in one jaw are treated as edentulous. The occlusal rims cover the roots.

Where teeth are present, jaw relation problems may be considered in two situations:
1. Teeth present in both jaws.
2. Teeth present in one jaw alone.

In both situations over-erupted or tilted teeth may complicate the determination of the occlusal plane. To overcome these problems, steps will need to be cut in the occlusal rim but not through the entire width. In this way a recess for the tooth can be provided while the occlusal plane level is maintained (Fig. 79). The manner in which the anterior section of the rim is cut will help decide both labial support and appearance (Fig. 80). It will clearly show irregularities of the occlusal plane requiring correction.

Far from being of assistance, non-occluding teeth present in both jaws complicate jaw relation recordings. First of all there may well be glancing contacts in terminal hinge closure resulting in a forward thrust. Unusual wear facets are a valuable clue in this respect. Diagnosing these small glancing contacts can be more difficult than it sounds. Apart from the problems of guiding the mandible into centric relation, marking the initial contact is complicated by the fact that neither ribbon nor articulating paper is particularly effective in marking highly polished surfaces. In order to obtain accurate results the surfaces must be dry and the marking paper held in a suitable holder (Fig. 81), otherwise there is the danger of it wrinkling and giving false marks. If this problem is not readily eliminated, the centric relation record must be made at a deliberately increased vertical dimension. The second complication arises from the possible irregularities of both upper and lower arcades of teeth. Extra time and care will be required in the trimming of the rims.

Overdentures require particularly careful assessment of vertical space. There must be sufficient room for roots, copings, possibly attachments, together with an adequate thickness of denture base

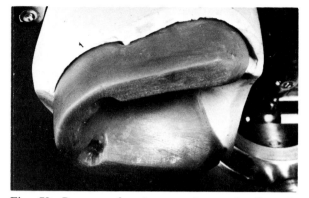

Fig. 79 Recesses for the opposing teeth allow the occlusal plane to be determined at the vertical relation of occlusion.

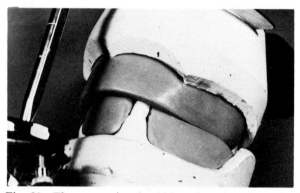

Fig. 80 The upper rim should be adapted to determine labial support.

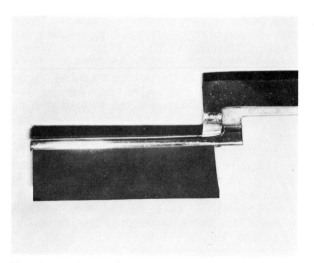

Fig. 81 A holder for ribbon or articulating paper is essential for accuracy. Without it, wrinkling of the marker is likely to give false contacts.

material and artificial teeth; all this without jeopardising the strength of the denture.

When discussing antero-posterior relations two important terms require definition: centric relation and centric occlusion. Nairn (1974) has pointed out the difficulties in terminology that stem from a reluctance to use words in the sense of their meaning only. Terms are only names for things, each can only be a name for one thing.

Centric relation is the most posterior relation of the mandible to the maxilla that can be recorded by the operator at the chosen vertical dimension. To use this term does not mean that you wish to build a dentition to this jaw relationship. This is simply a relationship of one jaw to another and can be taken as a reference point. Centric relation is usually recorded at the vertical relation of occlusion. There are, however, many circumstances where a deflective (interceptive) occlusal contact may guide the mandible forwards. Kass and Knap (1974) have explained that vertical deflective contacts close to the arc of closure make a disproportionate deflection; nevertheless, once identified, minimal adjustments are required. In these and other similar circumstances it will be necessary to record centric relation to an increased vertical relation, and to assume a hinge closure from this point.

On the other hand, *centric occlusion* is a tooth-to-tooth relationship defined as 'the relationship between opposing occlusal surfaces that results in maximum intercuspation and/or planned contact'. Once this important difference is understood, various conflicting opinions may be expressed as follows:

1. Centric occlusion (of the teeth) should coincide with centric (jaw) relation.

2. The cusp/fossa relationship of the opposing teeth should allow a small area of freedom forward and lateral to centric relation.

3. Centric occlusion should coincide with a mandibular position 2 mm anterior to centric relation.

Only the antero-posterior relations will be considered in the first part of this discussion, although the relations of the opposing teeth are, in fact, three-dimensional.

Studies with cineradiographs, cinefilms, and magnetic sensors confirm that the masticatory cycle is based on centric occlusion. The chewing cycle commences with an opening phase, followed by closure in a lateral occlusion. The teeth then slide over one another, or may be slightly separated by food, as they travel back to centric occlusion. Voluntary swallowing contacts are also based on centric occlusion; but what of involuntary swallows?

Brewer (1963) has shown that complete-denture wearers may make between 180 and 1300 non-masticatory occlusal contacts per hour. Although these contacts are transient, there is direct tooth-to-tooth contact with no intervening 'shock-absorbing' bolus. Therefore, it is important that the teeth meet evenly when these small, subconscious, non-masticatory movements are made.

Graf and Zander (1963) used minute radio transmitters built into bridge pontics to show that contacts are made only in centric relation while swallowing food and preparing to do so, but not while actually chewing. Contacts in centric occlusion occurred mainly during chewing, although some non-masticatory contacts took place as well. They suggested that some of these latter contacts were the result of an initial contact in centric relation, followed by a slide forwards.

Involuntary swallowing movements and other non-masticatory contacts appear to occur in centric relation, although this was not borne out by Glickman and co-workers (1969). These investigators pointed out that tooth contacts in swallowing were of longer duration than those in chewing, and work by Scharer et al. (1967) suggests similar conclusions.

Butler and Zander (1968) reported tooth contacts in centric relation during both chewing and swallowing, following occlusal adjustment. The chewing cycle, however, appears to centre around centric occlusion.

The centric occlusion of many young adult patients does not coincide with centric relation (Posselt 1952), and it is possible that involuntary movements may result in an initial contact followed by a forward mandibular slide of 1–2 mm. Unlike artificial teeth, however, natural teeth are supported by a periodontal ligament that incorporates extremely sensitive mechanoreceptors.

Hodge and Mahan (1967), while agreeing that occlusal slides occur, point out that most occlusal research has been carried out on dental students who tend to have a greater number of restorations than an equivalent group of patients. These authors suggest a potential iatrogenic cause for the occlusal slide. McCollum and Stuart (1955) state that people with well-formed dental arches and well-aligned and well-shaped teeth do not have a forward occlusal slide. However, the number of patients falling into this category must be comparatively small.

Care should be taken when diagnosing a discrepancy between centric occlusion and centric relation, for when the subject slowly opens his jaws, what appears to be a distinct posterior movement may be due to the fact that the teeth are moving on the arc of a circle. This movement may result in sliding contact of the inclined planes of the teeth, giving rise to a subjective feeling of posterior movement (Zola and Rothschild 1961). Aarstad (1954) described the wear facets on cusp inclines resisting retrusive forces and found that many of these facets were tangential to the posterior hinge arc of closure.

Some types of apparent forward slides result from interferences to the most posterior hinge path of closure, but do not affect the final mandibular position when the teeth meet (Zola and Rothschild 1961, Hodge and Mahan 1967). In these cases, elimination of the interferences will not alter the horizontal overlap (overjet) of the incisors. Other types of interference do, in fact, guide the mandible to a more protruded position, and in some cases there may be a lateral component to this slide.

In order to examine the occlusion a reliable method of establishing centric relation has to be found. There are, of course, many methods available. Dawson's method (1974) has been found to give consistent results.

The patient is inclined and the neck extended. The operator, seated behind the patient, stabilizes the patient's head between his forearm and ribcage. The four fingers of each hand are placed either side on the lower border of the mandible. The thumbs are placed in light contact with one another over the symphysis. With a gentle touch the jaw is moved through small arcs and manipulated into centric relation. The fingers exert upward pressure and the thumbs downwards and backwards. If there has been any tenderness in the temporo-mandibular joint regions the resistance to closure will become progressively greater as the teeth come towards each other. Slowly the closing arch allows the teeth to approximate until the initial contact is made. With the mandible held in this manner the movement is repeated. The patient is then asked to keep the jaw in that position for a second and then squeeze the teeth together. The direction in which the mandible moves is then noted. The initial contact can be marked by drying the teeth and placing ribbon between them. The ribbon should be held in a special holder to minimize the hazards of false marks.

When making a centric relation record, the wax record is placed over the occlusal surfaces of the upper teeth and the mandible manipulated by the method described. The lower teeth occlude with the wax record and are not permitted to touch their antagonists.

Mounted diagnostic casts are essential when

prosthodontic therapy is contemplated. It is, however, difficult to give hard and fast rules for the correction of forward sliding as their effects will vary. Abnormal wear facets, particularly on anterior teeth are often found. Difficulty with chewing, or temporo-mandibular pain dysfunction syndrome together with a deviation in opening and positive pterygoid sign are other possible occurrences. In many instances the cause is easily found and eliminated. However, there can be little excuse for interfering with the occlusion of the natural teeth without good reason.

Schuyler (1935) and Ramfjord and Ash (1966) suggested that a degree of freedom should be allowed in the cusp/fossae relationships of the natural teeth. At one time it was felt that movements of 1–2 mm should be allowed forward and lateral from a position corresponding with centric relation before the cusp reached an inclined plane. Problems of terminology and those of representing a three dimensional object in two have possibly contributed to the controversy these ideas still arouse. In expert hands the degree of freedom allowed seems to average 0.2 mm and often none at all. A great deal of the argument therefore seems unnecessary.

In those patients whose centric occlusion coincides with centric relation, no problem is presented. The following paragraphs are devoted to those patients who can retrude their mandibles behind the position corresponding with centric occlusion.

THE SMALL-SPAN TOOTH-SUPPORTED PROSTHESIS

Anyone who has seen the havoc wrought by well intentioned but unskilled 'prophylactic' adjustments would think twice about recommending such a procedure. However, it would be unfair to blame failings of the execution upon the technique. Suffice to say one should be aware of the hazards. Nevertheless, there can be little excuse for interfering with a natural dentition without due cause.

A short slide involving multiple even contacts seldom produces problems, while the elimination of such a slide is difficult and requires postgraduate training. Problems that do arise are often caused by single or small number of contacts. Ironically, these are usually the easiest to locate and eliminate. Common culprits are restorations, a third molar, and a slightly rotated upper first molar, or the mesial surface of the palatal cusp of the upper first premolar.

Many small restorations can therefore be made in centric occlusion, but diagnostic casts mounted in centric relation are a valuable aid in decision making. Where occlusal corrections are required, these must be completed before tooth preparation is begun.

COMPLETE DENTURES, DISTAL EXTENSION DENTURES, AND LARGE-SPAN FIXED PROSTHESES

The occlusion of any of these restorations is best made to coincide with centric relation. In an unequivocal fashion Nairn (1974) has summarised the arguments as follows: 'It is difficult to find convincing evidence for any of the views that are held, but the matter can be largely resolved on the grounds of practicability'. He goes on to point out that if you have to rebuild the occlusion, there is no practical alternative to building an even occlusion of maximum intercuspation with the mandible in its most retruded position. This is the only position which the dentist can find and repeat and this is a practical necessity. There may be a better place for the mandible in each case, but at present there is no way of finding it.

One or two of these points may be challenged today but the basis of the statement holds good.

Recording centric relation can be difficult in those patients in whom loss of posterior occlusal support has resulted in a forward mandibular posture. The apparent forward thrust of the mandible may be accentuated by a decreased vertical relation of occlusion. Nevertheless, if one fails to record centric relation, there is a danger that the patient may assume a more retruded posture after the restoration has been completed. Where a fixed prosthesis is concerned, this would involve remaking the entire restoration. Transitional restorations are particularly useful in situations like these. No matter how carefully jaw relations are made, an additional step is required for partial dentures when an altered cast technique has been employed. This usually applies to distal extension bases. Before the trial insertion of the artificial teeth, the cast of the corrected base should be related to the opposing dentition. This particular jaw relation cannot normally be made until the framework has been cast and the secondary impression made.

LATERAL AND PROTRUSIVE CONTACTS

Lateral and protrusive contacts play an important part in the efficiency of masticatory function. Studies of mastication such as those of Hildebrand (1931), Schweitzer (1961) and Adams and Zander

(1964) have shown that the normal pattern of mastication consists of small lateral and combined lateral and protrusive strokes, ending at or close to centric occlusion.

Ahlgren (1976) has divided the masticatory cycle into three components, opening phase, closing phase, and intercuspal phase. The opening movement rarely goes straight down but deviates to one side, usually the working side. He found that each individual has a characteristic pattern of mandibular movements in chewing, but there is variation between consecutive chewing cycles. Masticatory movements are influenced by subjects' occlusions as well as by the food they chew. Those with normal occlusions show simple and well co-ordinated masticatory movements, whereas those with malocclusions have an irregular and complicated pattern of movements.

Extreme vertical overlap produces an almost vertical chewing stroke. The effect of tough food is to widen the chewing cycle, so that the occurrence of tooth contact glide during the closing phase depends on the type of food and occlusion. Tooth contacts in centric occlusion are to be found in most chewing cycles, and it is at this point that maximum force is exerted for about 100 milliseconds.

The findings are corroborated if one examines masticatory function with a device like the Kinesiograph.* The anatomy of the contacting cusp sections in chewing can be mirrored in the chewing cycle. Furthermore, it is interesting to note variations in the mandibular speeds reached. Using similar foods, subjects with stable occlusions appear to reach far higher speeds than those with obvious irregularities. Maximum speed is normally reached midway through the opening and closing phases and can exceed 200 mm/sec. Matsumoto (1976) made clasp-retained and attachment-retained dentures for the same subjects. He found higher chewing speeds for attachment-retained dentures. He felt that this higher chewing speed was a result of the better retention of attachment-retained dentures.

Recent findings have therefore substantiated earlier work by Boos (1959) who felt that powerful biting was more comfortable close to centric occlusion, and Trapozzano (1960) and Woelfel (1962) who both described the influence of occlusal surfaces on the masticatory cycle.

An adjustable articulator will be required to establish the shape of the artificial occlusal surfaces. The articulator should ensure that correct separation of the teeth occurs when necessary and that desired contacts can be obtained. Adjustable articulators are often misused when attempting to copy jaw move-

* Myotronics Research Inc., Seattle, Washington.

ments. Sliding the teeth sideways or forwards from centric occlusion may be useful in establishing pathways of contact but can hardly be termed normal physiological movement. During mastication the teeth are separated when eccentric movements are made so that the timing of components of lateral movement is insignificant. The eccentric movement will have been completed before the teeth contact. Attempting to minimise masticatory movements in the reverse sense can give a misleading impression of the vectors of forces applied (Nairn 1974).

De Pietro (1977) has suggested that the Frankfort mandibular plane angle might be a useful guide in assessing the type of disclusion required in a subject's dentition. In his study of 112 subjects those with anterior guided disclusion had an FMA of 24° or less while those with group function had FMA's of 24°–40°. He has also put forward the idea that a low FMA angle and, therefore, natural disclusion is associated with higher biting forces than those with higher FMA angles and group function.

The actual requirements of lateral contacts will vary, but can be divided into the following categories.

FIXED PROSTHESIS

During protrusive movements anterior guidance should separate the remaining teeth, while throughout lateral movements the teeth on the non-working side should part. On these aspects at least there seems little disagreement.

Opinion varies as to whether there should be even sliding contact between all the cusps on the working side, or whether the canines should lift the working side cusps out of occlusion. The idea of the 'cuspid-protected occlusion' is based on the concept that the shape and size of the canine is particularly well adapted to resist lateral loads, and it should therefore lift the other working side cusps out of occlusion as the jaw is moved to one side, thereby protecting these cusps and preventing contacts on the side as well.

However, the canines could only protect the occlusion by cuspal guidance, and if this continually occurred a high rate of wear could be expected. Many patients seem to adapt to canine rise by assuming a more vertical chewing cycle, and it is in this indirect manner that the occlusion is protected. Among the applications of this type of occlusion are the situations in which porcelain covers part of the occlusal surfaces.

In several respects the anthropological and functional aspects of canine protection might be questioned. Indeed it might be argued that this concept is merely a rationalisation of a clinical procedure based on necessity (Nairn 1974). It certainly is a convenient arrangement of artificial occlusal surfaces and simplifies the elimination of non-working contacts with little evidence to show that it does any harm. On the contrary, the bulk of clinical evidence points the other way and one can look for reassurance to the fact that many natural dentitions appear to have this type of articulation. The majority of fixed prostheses appear constructed in this manner and give satisfactory service. On the other hand it would not be possible to provide this canine protection where these teeth are weak, missing, or where there was a Class III malocclusion present.

Pankey et al. (1964) felt that when the mandible was moved into a lateral position the canine and all the posterior teeth should make simultaneous contact at least until their tips were reached. This 'cuspid guidance' theory has obvious theoretical advantages and may be particularly useful when a partial denture is in opposition.

DISTAL EXTENSION DENTURES

Here a compromise must be reached between the functions the appliance can serve and the necessity to reduce to a minimum rotational loads applied to the denture base. While a narrow artificial occlusal table should limit the leverage of loads applied, it is wise to allow only 1·5–2·00 mm of working side contact of the artificial teeth, after which the guidances of the natural teeth should be allowed to take over. Where only anterior natural teeth remain, the canine teeth should normally lift the artificial teeth out of contact after about 1 mm of lateral movement. No contacts of natural or artificial teeth should take place on the non-working side. Protrusive contacts will normally be made on the anterior teeth.

A functional path recording is favoured by some operators when a distal extension denture occludes against natural teeth. The wax record on the denture base is carved by opposing cusps and a template then cast corresponding with the paths travelled by these cusps. By adjusting the denture teeth to occlude with the template, the cuspal relationships in centric relation and eccentric relations are determined. The template needs to be handled with care and made of the hardest artificial stone or it will be easily worn, or damaged and the result unsatisfactory.

COMPLETE DENTURES

The presence of a complete denture alters the situation because of the need to make it as stable as possible. There may be a complete upper and lower denture, a complete upper denture opposed to a natural dentition, or a complete upper denture opposed to a natural dentition and a partial lower denture. The requirements are similar; only the method of achieving the goal varies.

Even contact is required at centric occlusion, which in these cases must always coincide with centric relation. Lateral movements should produce even contact on the working side and simultaneous contacts on the non-working side. These non-working side contacts are required for stability of the complete denture. For a similar reason, anterior contact should be accompanied as far as possible by posterior contacts when the mandible is protruded.

These requirements can be met quite simply with complete upper and lower dentures, for the positioning and alignment of the posterior teeth is in the hands of the operator. Where natural teeth are present it becomes more difficult to incorporate them within this occlusal pattern, yet it is particularly important that it be achieved owing to the powerful displacing forces that can be exerted. For this reason, diagnostic casts should always be made, in order to assess the amount of natural tooth substance to be removed. Narrowing of the natural occlusal surfaces should accompany this grinding. The occlusal reshaping may have to be carried out in two stages, for it is difficult to determine the precise contours required until all the artificial teeth have been set up. The main occlusal reshaping should be planned on the diagnostic cast and be carried out before denture construction is begun. Further occlusal corrections may be required if it proves impossible to accommodate the natural teeth within the final occlusal pattern, in which case a new impression and jaw relation record will be subsequently required. Methods of recording jaw relationships vary; the essential factors are that the centric relation record be correct and that lateral and protrusive movements produce even contacts. To achieve this, it is imperative that occlusal corrections to the natural teeth be completed before the final jaw relation records are made and that the occlusal rims be constructed on the master cast and be stable in the mouth.

For the purpose of this discussion movements of the mandible have been described as moving laterally or forwards with the teeth in contact. Again, it must be pointed out that these types of movement are not physiological and should rarely take place. Normal movements are in the reverse sense with a separation of the teeth preceding any lateral or forward movement.

MATERIALS FOR ARTIFICIAL TEETH

Where dentures are to be constructed, thought should be given to the material of which the occlusal surfaces are to be made.

For many brought up with vacuum-fired porcelain teeth there is seldom an acceptable substitute. Porcelain teeth have an unrivalled appearance, are straightforward to arrange, and have a negligible rate of wear. Unfortunately they are prone to damage but the greatest restriction is limitation of vertical space. Owing to the need for retaining pins or the diatoric design there is a limit to the adjustment possible. This severely limits their application to partial dentures and complete dentures with space restrictions. Paffenbarger et al. (1967) described an experimental method for bonding porcelain to the acrylic resin base with a silane coupling agent. This holds promise of eliminating the need for mechanical retention but has yet to overcome problems of breaking teeth due to the stresses placed on them during processing the acrylic resin.

Considerable improvements have now been made to cross-linked acrylic resin teeth. Both from the point of appearance and wear resistance recent products have shown amazing improvements. Most partial dentures, particularly those with attachments, will require acrylic resin teeth. They are also convenient to employ for many complete dentures. If, after several years, the teeth need to be replaced this can hardly be described as catastrophic. Inserting silver alloy restorations in the occlusal surfaces of acrylic resin artificial teeth appears to reduce the rate of wear and provides good clinical results.

Acrylic resin teeth may be opposed to porcelain provided the glaze of the porcelain teeth is not disturbed. The coefficient of friction between this combination is less than that of opposed acrylic resin surfaces, so that the rate of wear should be correspondingly reduced.

Improved masticatory efficiency has always been claimed for specialised metal inserts in artificial teeth. Now that the problems of appearance, balancing the articulation, and preventing accidental tongue biting seem to have been overcome (Levin 1977), this type of metal insert is likely to prove popular.

Where natural and artificial teeth oppose each other, gold is the material of choice for the artificial occlusal surface. Acrylic resin teeth are reduced in height to allow a gold occlusal surface to be waxed up on them and covered. The wax is then removed, invested, cast and subsequently joined to the resin teeth to form the occlusal surface. The gold occlusal surface can be contoured to fine limits to provide a stable occlusion. It is appearance that limits its usefulness, although cost, weight and space must be considered as well.

OCCLUSAL SURFACES OF CROWNS

The merits of gold surfaces for denture teeth apply equally well to crowns, with considerable additional advantages. The delicate details possible with gold allow the development of an articulation that is both functional and stable. Gold produces few problems when opposed to natural teeth and is usually the material of choice.

Once again it is appearance rather than other factors that may limit the usefulness of gold. It had been felt that the hardness of porcelain might damage opposing natural teeth, and there is evidence of a degree of wear taking place. Monasky (1971) showed the rate of wear to be virtually self-limiting. The explanation rests with the production of an improved glaze on the porcelain surface and a corresponding reduction in the coefficient of friction between the two surfaces. Gold, however, had no such effect on the porcelain. Opposing gold surfaces may, therefore, be quite severely damaged in time by porcelain.

Careful treatment planning should include the occlusal surfaces of the restoration. The amount of space available, the opposing surfaces, and the loads that may be applied are all factors that need to be taken into account. A little care at an early stage makes the construction of a restoration simpler, for the amount of space available for gold, attachments, artificial teeth, and facings can be clearly seen and difficulties anticipated. Furthermore, the completed restoration will work better, require minimal adjustments, and provide the patient with the service he deserves.

REFERENCES AND FURTHER READING

AARSTAD, T. (1954) *The Capsular Ligaments of the Temporomandibular Joint and Retrusion Facets of the Dentition in Relationship to Mandibular Movements.* Akademisk Forlag, Oslo

ADAMS, S. H. and ZANDER, H. A. (1964) Functional

tooth contacts in lateral and in centric occlusion. *J. Amer. dent. Ass.*, *69*, 465

AHLGREN, J. (1976) Masticatory movements in man. In *Mastication*, by Anderson and Matthews, John Wright, Bristol

ALEXANDER, P. C. (1963) Analysis of cuspid protective occlusion. *J. prosth. Dent.*, *13*, 309

APPLEGATE, O. C. (1965) *Essentials of Removable Partial Denture Prosthesis*. 3rd edn, pp. 299–314. Saunders, Philadelphia and London

BERGMAN, B. and ERICSON, S. (1973) The effect of increasing the morphologic face height in full denture restorations on the width of the intra-articular space in the temporomandibular joint. *Acta odontol. scand.*, *31*, 75–88

BEYRON, H. L. (1954) Characteristics of functionally optimal occlusion and principles of occlusal rehabilitation. *J. Amer. dent. Ass.*, *48*, 648

BOOS, R. H. (1959) Vertical centric and functional dimensions recorded by gnathodynamics. *J. Amer. dent. Ass.*, *59*, 682

BREWER, A. A. (1963) Prosthodontic research and progress at the School of Aerospace Medicine. *J. prosth. Dent.*, *13*, 49

BRILL, N., SCHUBELER, S. and TRYDE, G. (1962) Influences of occlusal patterns on movements of the mandible. *J. prosth. Dent.*, *12*, 255

BUTLER, J. H. and ZANDER, H. A. (1968) Evaluation of two occlusal concepts. *Parodont. Acad. Rev.*, *2*, 5

CLAYTON, J. A., KOTOWITZ, W. E. and ZAHLER, J. M. (1971) Pantographic tracings of mandibular movements and occlusion. *J. prosth. Dent.*, *25*, 384.

COLMAN, A. J. (1967) Occlusal requirements for removable partial dentures. *J. prosth. Dent.*, *17*, 155

D'AMICO, A. (1958) Canine teeth – normal functional relation of the natural teeth of man. *J. S. Calif. dent. Ass.*, *26*, 6, 49, 127, 175, 194, 299

DAWSON, P. E. (1973) Temporomandibular joint pain-dysfunction problems can be solved. *J. prosth. Dent.*, *29*, 100–112

DAWSON, P. (1974) *Evaluation, Diagnosis and Treatment of Occlusal Problems*. C. V. Mosby Co. St Louis, Mo.

De PIETRO, G. J. (1977) A study of occlusion as related to the Frankfort-mandibular plane angle. *J. prosth. Dent.* *38*: 4, 452

DYER, E. H. (1973) Importance of a stable maxillomandibular relation. *J. prosth. Dent.*, *30*, 241–251

EMSLIE, R. D. (1954) Malocclusion and periodontal health. A periodontist's viewpoint. *Europ. orthodont. Soc. Trans.*, *254*

FUNAKOSHI, M., FUJITA, N. and TAKEHANA, S. (1976) Relations between occlusal interference and jaw muscle activities in response to changes in head position. *J. Dent. Res.*, *55*: 4, 684

GAZIT, E. and LIEBERMAN, M. A. (1973) The intercuspal surface contact area registration: an additional tool for evaluation of normal occlusion. *Angle Orthod.*, *43*, 96–106

GIBB, C. H., SUIT, S. R. and BENZ, S. T. (1973) Masticatory movements of the jaw measured at angles of approach to the occlusal plane. *J. prosth. Dent.*, *30*, 283–288

GILLINGS, B. R. D., GRAHAM, C. H. and DUCK-MANTON, N. A. (1973) Jaw movements in young adult men while chewing. *J. prosth. Dent.*, *29*, 616–627

GILLINGS, B. R. D., KOHL, J. T. and GRAF, G. (1961) Study of tooth patterns with the use of miniature radio transmitters. *4th Int. Conf. on Medical Electronics*, *Princeton*, 67

GILLINGS, B. R. D., KOHL, J. T. and ZANDER, H. A. (1963) Contact patterns using miniature radio transmitters. *J. dent. Res.*, *42*, 177

GLICKMAN, I., PAMEIJER, J. H. N. and ROEBER, F. (1968) Intraoral occlusal telemetry – a multifrequency transmitter for registering tooth contacts in occlusion. *J. prosth. Dent.*, *19*, 60

GLICKMAN, I., PAMEIJER, J. H. N., ROEBER, F. and BRION, M. A. M. (1969) Functional occlusion as revealed by miniaturised radio transmitters. *Dent. Clin. N. Amer.*, *13*, 667.

GRAF, H. and ZANDER, H. A. (1963) Tooth contact patterns in mastication. *J. prosth. Dent.*, *13*, 1055

HILDEBRAND, G. Y. (1931) Studies in the masticatory movements of the human lower jaw. *Skand. Arch. Physiol.*, *61*, 190

HOBO, S., SHILLINGBURG, H. T. and WHITSETT, L. D. (1976) Articulator selection for restorative dentistry. *J. prosth. Dent.*, *36*: 7, 35

HODGE, L. C. and MAHAN, P. E. (1967) A study of mandibular movement from centric occlusion to maximum intercuspation. *J. prosth. Dent.*, *18*, 19

HOFFMAN, P. G., SILVERMAN, S. and GARFINKEL, L. (1973) Comparison of condylar position in centric relation and in centric occlusion in dentulous subjects. *J. prosth. Dent.*, *30*, 582–588

JANKELSON, B. (1960). A technique for obtaining optimal functional relationship of the natural dentition. *Dent. Clin. N. Amer.*, *131*

JANKELSON, B. and HOFFMAN, C. M. (1953) Physiology of the stomatognathic system. *J. Amer. dent. Ass.*, *46*, 375

KASS, C. A. and KNAP, F. J. (1974) Analysis of occlusion before and after occlusal adjustment. *J. prosth. Dent.*, *32*: 2, 163

KINGERY, R. H. (1959) The maxillo-mandibular relationships of centric relation. *J. prosth. Dent.*, *9*, 922

KURTH, L. E. (1942) Mandibular movements in mastication. *J. Amer. dent. Ass.*, *29*, 1769

LAURITZEN, A. G. (1951) Function, prime object of restorative dentistry: a definitive procedure to obtain it. *J. Amer. dent. Ass.*, *42*, 523

LEVIN, B. (1977) A review of artificial posterior tooth forms including a preliminary report on a new posterior tooth. *J. prosth. Dent.*, *38*: 1, 3–13

LONG, J. H. (1973) Locating centric relation with a leaf gauge. *J. prosth. Dent.*, *29*, 608–610

LUCIA, V. A. (1961) *Modern Gnathological Concepts*, pp. 293–294. C. V. Mosby, St Louis, Mo.

MANN, A. W. and PANKEY, L. D. (1959) Oral rehabilitation using the Pankey–Mann instrument and functional bite technique. *Dent. Clin. N. Amer.*, 215

MANN, A. W. and PANKEY, L. D. (1960) Oral rehabilitation. I. The use of the P.M. instrument in treatment planning and in restoring the lower posterior teeth. *J. prosth. Dent.*, *10*, 135

MANN, A. W. and PANKEY, L. D. (1960) Oral rehabilitation. II. Reconstructions of the upper teeth using a functionally generated path technique. *J. prosth. Dent.*, *10*, 151

MARKOVIC, M. A. and ROSENBERG, H. M. (1973) Corrected laminagraphic evaluation of the TMJ in 100 MPD patients. *Int. Assoc. Dent. Res. Abst. No. 70*

MATSUMOTO, M. (1976) Personal Communication

McCOLLUM, B. B. (1943) Oral diagnosis. *J. Amer. dent. Ass.*, *30*, 1218

McCOLLUM, B. B. (1958) Consideration of the mouth as a functioning unit as the basis of dental diagnosis. *J. S. Calif. dent. Ass.*, *5*, 268

McCOLLUM, B. B. and STUART, C. E. (1955) *A Research Report: Basic Course for the Post-Graduate Course in Gnathology*, pp. 91–95. Scientific Press, South Pasadena

MEHRINGER, E. J. (1973) Function of steep cusps in mastication with complete dentures. *J. prosth. Dent.*, *30*, 367–372

MILLSTEIN, P. L., CLARK, R. E. and KRONMAN, J. H. (1973) Determination of the accuracy of wax interocclusal registrations. Part II. *J. prosth. Dent.*, *29*, 40–45

MÖLLER, E. (1976) Evidence that the rest position is subject to servo control. In *Mastication*, by Anderson and Matthews, John Wright, Bristol

MONASKY, G. E. (1971) Studies on the wear of porcelain, enamel and gold. *J. prosth. Dent.*, *25*, 299

NAGASAWA, T. and TSURU, H. (1973) A comparative evaluation of masticatory efficiency of fixed and removable restorations replacing mandibular first molars. *J. prosth. Dent.*, *30*, 263–273

NAIRN, R. I. (1974) Maxillomandibular relations and aspects of occlusion. *J. prosth. Dent.*, *31:4*, 361–367

NAIRN, R. I. (1976) The concept of occlusal vertical dimension and its importance in clinical practice. In *Mastication*, by Anderson and Matthews. John Wright, Bristol

PAFFENBARGER, G. C., SWEENEY, W. T. and BOWEN, R. L. (1967) Bonding porcelain teeth to acrylic resin denture bases. *J. Amer. dent. Ass.*, *74*, 1018

PAMEIJER, J. H. N., GLICKMAN, I. and ROEBER, F. E. (1968) Intraoral occlusal telemetry. II. Registration of tooth contacts in chewing and swallowing by intraoral electric telemetry. *J. prosth. Dent.*, *19*, 151

PANKEY, L. D., MANN, A. W. and SCHUYLER, C. H. (1964) The teaching manual for the P–M–S philosophy of occlusal rehabilitation. *The Occlusal Rehabilitation Seminar*

POSSELT, U. (1952) Studies in the mobility of the human mandible. *Acta odont. scand.*, *Supp. 10*, *10*, 19

POWELL, R. N. (1963) Tooth contact during sleep. *Thesis*, University of Rochester

PREISKEL, H. W. (1967) Considerations of the check record in complete denture construction. *J. prosth. Dent.*, *18*, 98

PREISKEL, H. W. (1970) Bennett's movement. A study of human lateral mandibular movement. *Brit. dent. J.*, *129*, 372

PREISKEL, H. W. (1971) The canine teeth related to Bennett's movement. *Brit. dent. J.*, *131*, 312

RAMFJORD, S. P. (1961) Bruxism, a clinical and electromyographic study. *J. Amer. dent. Ass.*, *62*, 21

RAMFJORD, S. P. and ASH, M. (1966) *Occlusion*. Saunders, Philadelphia and London

RAMFJORD, S. P., BERRY, H. M., CHARBENEAU, G. T., LEE, R. E., PAVONE, B. W. and PHILLIPS, R. W. (1974) Report of the committee on scientific investigation of the American Academy of Restorative Dentistry. *J. prosth. Dent.*, *32:2*, 198

ROTH, R. H. (1973) Temporomandibular pain-dynsfunction and occlusal relationships. *Angle Orthod.*, *43*, 136–153

SCHARER, P., STALLARD, R. E. and ZANDER, H. A. (1967) Occlusal interferences and mastication: An electromyographic study. *J. Amer. dent. Ass.*, *62*, 21

SCHUYLER, C. H. (1935) Fundamental principles in the correction of occlusal disharmony, natural and artificial. *J. Amer. dent. Ass.*, *22*, 1193

SCHUYLER, C. H. (1947) Correction of occlusal disharmony of the natural dentition. *N.Y. J. Dent.*, *13*, 445

SCHUYLER, C. H. (1961) Factors contributing to traumatic occlusion. *J. prosth. Dent.*, *11*, 708

SCHWEITZER, J. M. (1961) Masticatory function in man. *J. prosth. Dent.*, *11*, 625

SCHWEITZER, J. M. (1962) Masticatory function in man. *J. prosth. Dent.*, *12*, 262

SCHWEITZER, J. M. (1963) Concepts of occlusion: A discussion. *Dent. Clin. N. Amer.*, *649*

SHORE, N. A. (1952) Equilibrium of the occlusion of natural dentition. *J. Amer. dent. Ass.*, *44*, 414

SHORE, N. A. (1959) *Occlusal Equilibration and Temporomandibular Joint Dysfunction*, pp. 143–145. Lippincott, Philadelphia

SICHER, H. (1951) Functional anatomy of the temporomandibular joint. In *The Temporomandibular Joint*, Sarnat, B. (Ed.). C. C. Thomas, Springfield, Illinois

SICHER, H. (1949) *Oral Anatomy*, p. 171. C. V. Mosby, St Louis, Mo.

STALLARD, H. and STUART, C. E. (1961) Elementary tooth guidance in natural dentition. *J. prosth. Dent.*, *11*, 474

TALLGREN, A. (1967) The effect of denture wearing or facial morphology: a 7-year longitudinal study. *Acta odont. scand.*, *25*, 563

TRAPOZZANO, V. R. (1960) Test of balanced and non-balanced occlusions. *J. prosth. Dent.*, *10*, 476

WEINBERG, L. A. (1956) Diagnosis of facets in occlusal equilibration. *J. Amer. dent. Ass.*, *52*, 26

WEINBERG, L. A. (1973) Temporomandibular joint function and its effect on centric relation. *J. prosth. Dent.*, *30*, 176–195

WILKIE, N. D., HURST, T. L. and MITCHELL, D. L. (1974) Radiographic comparisons of condyle-fossa relationships during maxillomandibular registrations made by different methods. *J. prosth. Dent.*, *32:5*, 599

WOELFEL, J. D., HICKEY, J. C. and ALLISON, M. C. (1962) Effects of posterior tooth form on jaw and denture movement. *J. prosth. Dent.*, *12*, 922

YEMM, R. (1976) The role of tissue elasticity in the control of mandibular resting posture. In *Mastication*, by Anderson and Matthews. John Wright, Bristol

ZANDER, H. A. and HURZELER, B. (1958) Diagnosis of occlusal disharmonies. *J. S. Calif. dent. Ass.*, *26*, 382

ZIEBERT, G. J. and KNAP, F. J. (1973) Effect of jaw guidance on retruded stroke as recorded in the sagittal plane. *J. prosth. Dent.*, *29*, 262–268

ZARB, G. A., BERGMAN, B., CLAYTON, J. A. and MACKAY, H. F. (1978) *Prosthodontic Treatment for Partially Edentulous Patients.*, C. V. Mosby Company, St Louis, Mo.

ZOLA, A. and ROTHSCHILD, E. A. (1961) Condyle positions in unimpeded jaw movements. *J. prosth. Dent.*, *11*, 873

CHAPTER 4

Distal Extension Prostheses

Constructing a denture becomes more difficult when there is no distal abutment. Support and retention are among the greatest problems. However, the criteria of success include careful patient selection, evaluation and education, together with a highly trained operator supported by suitable technical resources. Compare this with the haphazard prescription and careless construction often found and it is small wonder at the disappointing results of the long term surveys carried out over the last decade or so (Carlsson et al. 1961, 1962; Rantanen et al. 1972). The conclusions of these surveys indicate that far from De Van's maxim of 'preserving what remains', the majority of removable prostheses actively contribute to the demise of their supporting structures. Considering the problems and cost of denture construction, this is an undertaking requiring planning with discretion and completion with care.

However, more optimistic results have been reported by Derry and Bertram (1970) and more recently by Schwalm, Smith and Erickson (1977). Well-made dentures provided for properly motivated and instructed patients showed remarkably good results at follow-up examination.

Levin has described 'the 28 tooth syndrome' of those operators who insist that every patient has an intact 28-tooth arch relationship irrespective of the type of occlusion or dentition. Apart from some cadaver evidence to show osteoarthritic changes in those who had lost all posterior occlusal support before death, there is little evidence to suggest that loss of one or two teeth automatically reduces masticatory efficiency to a level at which some improvement becomes necessary.

Larger spaces, of course, may require restoration for reasons that vary from appearance to the prevention of abnormal jaw postures. A surprising feature of denture construction is that having decided artificial teeth are necessary all too often they are added as an afterthought once the framework has been found to fit.

Loss of posterior occlusion may lead to a forward thrust of the mandible giving the patient a prognathic look. This apparent forward thrust may arise in two ways:

1. *Decreasing the vertical relation of occlusion* results in the mandible rotating upwards and forwards. Efforts at correcting this malocclusion by increasing the vertical relation of occlusion alone are not always successful. They may result in the problems of limited inter-occlusal space that used to be associated with the immediate post-Costen era.

2. The prognathic appearance results from an *anterior translation of the mandible* and a forward posture is assumed in an effort to provide some occluding surfaces and possibly to improve appearance as well. A prosthesis made to this prognathic posture and restoring the occlusion to this jaw relationship will cause problems when the patient, now with posterior occlusion restored, assumes centric relation. Since the condyle translates posteriorly and upwards this results in a premature posterior occlusal contact.

The new prosthesis may occlude with natural teeth, artificial teeth, or both. As a result of tooth loss, opposing natural teeth may overerupt and in extreme cases there may be little or no room between them and the edentulous ridge. Overeruption is usually accompanied by tilting so that one or two of the cusps become unduly prominent. For example, overerupted upper molars appear to tilt buccally so that the mesiopalatal cusps become prominent. Even if it were possible to find room for a denture, such a cusp would play havoc with it when the mandible was moved from side to side. It is necessary to assess the opposing dentition and decide whether or not some reshaping of the natural teeth is warranted. Occlusal reshaping may involve just reshaping a cusp; on the other hand, it may require isolated extractions, the provision of crowns, or the construction of a prosthesis. Planning the occlusal surfaces is important and cannot be carried out by guesswork.

An opposing complete denture will place comparatively little load on the denture base. It is assumed that a lower distal extension prosthesis is planned to oppose an upper complete denture since few lower dentures will survive opposed to natural upper teeth. However, there are other problems to be considered. The upper complete denture defines the occlusal plane, and this may not be satisfactory for the new lower prosthesis. Furthermore, the new lower restoration will alter the shape of the lower occlusal surface; it hardly gives the patient good service to provide him with a complex lower prosthesis that makes his existing upper denture completely unstable. It is generally wiser to remake the opposing denture. The extra time required is not great, but it simplifies the treatment and gives a far better result. The same may hold true for an opposing partial denture, since it defines the posterior section of the occlusal plane. In most situations it is quicker and better to remake an opposing denture, rather than attempt to accommodate the artificial and natural teeth of the new restoration to a prosthesis probably made by someone else under entirely different oral conditions.

The occlusal load applied to the denture base will be influenced by the shape and size of the artificial teeth on the denture saddle, the opposing dentition, and by the patient himself. It is difficult to make a quantitative assessment of this load, but it is apparent that a strong muscular man will probably apply more force to his teeth than a frail elderly woman.

Opposing natural teeth might also be expected to exert greater forces than opposing artificial teeth. By keeping the artificial occlusal table as small as possible, the bolus penetration forces necessary for mastication will be reduced. Furthermore, if the occlusal table is kept narrow and short, the leverage effects of those forces will be reduced as well (Figs. 82, 83).

There is another point to be considered when removable and fixed prosthesis are present in the same arch and possibly with natural teeth as well. It is quite possible to produce non-working interferences, by subtracting guidance from one side as well as overbuilding or overcontouring the other. For example, automatically using zero cusp teeth on every denture could result in contralateral non-working interferences if the anterior guidance were restricted. It is therefore important to relate the

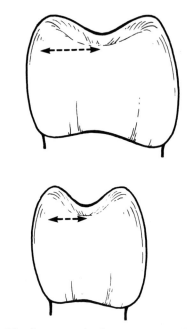

Fig. 82   The force required to penetrate a bolus of food is reduced if the occlusal table is kept narrow. The torques resulting from masticatory and non-masticatory contacts are also lessened.

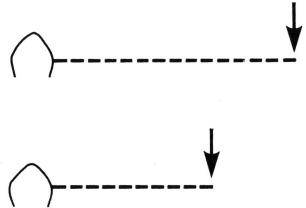

Fig. 83   A short artificial occlusal table reduces the leverages exerted by vertical and horizontal loads.

arrangement of artificial teeth and their cusp angles to the remaining dentition.

SUPPORT

Support to resist occlusal forces may be obtained entirely from the abutment teeth. The cantilevered extension from a fixed prosthesis is neat, and particularly useful where an opposing complete denture is concerned. When natural teeth are in opposition, the loads applied can be considerable. In these circumstances even a short cantilevered extension may have a limited prognosis. Lower restorations are particularly prone to dislodgement due to the lingual inclination of the displacing forces (Schweitzer et al. 1968, Henderson et al. 1970). Izikowitz (1966, 1971) and Hildebrand (1968) have described fixed prostheses for which additional support was obtained from the mucosa, but this is a method that has failed to gain wide acceptance.

Support from implants has aroused considerable interest. Johns (1976) has pointed out that support must be gained from the external surface of underlying bone or from a bony crypt within the cancellous bone. Any load that is applied will have to be transmitted across a tissue implant interface. Despite optimistic claims to the contrary, there is little evidence to suggest that intraosseous or subperiosteal designs are surrounded by anything other than fibrous tissue. However, the presence of a periodontal ligament for support may be unnecessary if loads remain within the physiological limit of the surrounding bone. Experiments with porous materials which increase the surface of the interface may result in bone deposition within the implant.

The major problem rests, naturally, with the region of transition from internal to external environment. There is little doubt that results that appear satisfactory clinically can be achieved. The bulk of evidence suggests that the epithelium will succeed in exteriorising the implant. Without meticulous plaque control the implant cannot succeed. Furthermore, unless the dentist is able to remove the prosthesis to test the implant for mobility he has little idea about whether the implant is contributing to the support, stability, and retention of the prosthesis or the situation is the other way round. While it is true that the implant could help with many awkward distal extension problems its use should be considered experimental for the time being. One can only look forward to being able to benefit from the fruits of future research.

The majority of distal extension prostheses require support from the teeth and from the mucosa. The ideal abutment might consist of all the natural teeth splinted together, but effective support from the mucosa can be obtained only by covering the largest possible area.

Compared with the natural teeth, the mucosa of the denture-bearing area is relatively displaceable. Steiger (1959) suggested that under load, the mucosa may be displaced by an amount four to twenty times

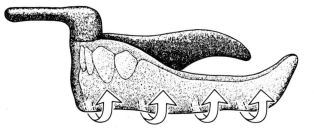

Fig. 84 Frequently overlooked is the rate at which impression material escapes around the border of the tray. A correctly adapted and extended tray is essential.

greater than a healthy natural tooth. Fortunately these are matters that can be measured. No matter how wide the mucosal coverage of the denture, on theoretical considerations it will have a tendency to rock under occlusal load. This tendency to rock is more noticeable in lower dentures due to the limited amount of mucosal coverage that is possible. The denture base tends to sink under load until the forces resisting this movement are equal to the displacing forces. Mucosal resistance will be more effective and require less movement of the denture base if its impression surface is made to correspond with the shape of the mucosa when subjected to slight displacing loads. Applegate's (1955) well-tried theory works well in practice and suitable techniques will be described.

Matsumoto (1970), following on the work of Rehm (1962), demonstrated the loads required to cause slight mucosal displacement during impression procedures. Provided the border seal is adequate, the adaptation of the tray to the mucosa is an important factor in the result. If two flat plates are brought together with a viscous material between them, the rate of flow of the material varies as the fifth power of the distance between the plates. Halve the distance between the plates and thirty two times the load is required to produce the same rate of flow. To simplify the issue, imagine that a close fitting tray is made without any space between the tray and the mucosa. If the tray is then seated in the mouth and there is subsequently impression material left in it, some displacement of the mucosa must have occurred.

A failing of some previous research has been the lack of a time-base when measuring mucosal displacement. The influence of the impression material on the mucosa depends not only on its viscosity, but at the rate at which it escapes around the border of the tray (Fig. 84). Border moulding of the tray is therefore important. Apart from the viscosity of the impression material, other factors

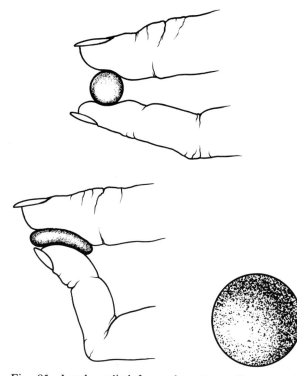

Fig. 85   Load applied for a short term allows elastic recoil.

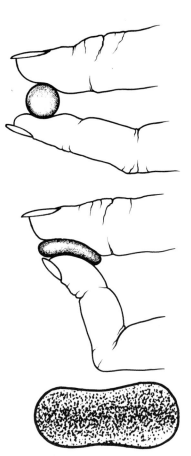

Fig. 86   Loads applied for a longer period result in plastic deformation.

involved are the rate of force application and the physical properties of the mucosa.

Recent work has clarified understanding of the mucosa's physical properties. The mucosa itself appears to behave as a visco-elastic material (Picton and Wills 1978). If a load is applied for a short time the mucosa will deform elastically; if the load is sustained the mucosa will flow-up to a point (Figs. 85, 86). Picton and Wills also demonstrated that the underlying bone behaved as an elastic material.

Waters' (1975b) theoretical analysis also lends weight to arguments favouring secondary impression techniques, or those with a closely adapted tray. He points out that under normal circumstances the tray will not be inserted parallel to the mucosa nor will the impression material be adapted to the shape of the mucosa. Flow of the impression material will occur first at any contact areas and away from those areas where pressure is highest. Only when the impression material is in contact over the whole area with mucosa, and the latter is parallel to the tray, will the flow be radial from the centre of the tray.

Trays spaced by more than 4 mm may produce completely different results, particularly when reversible hydrocolloid or alginates are used. For example, Holmes (1965) found that denture base movement ranged from 0·11 mm using a functional wax impression to 0·9 mm when an alginate impression had been employed.

One argument levelled against fluid wax is that cooling the impression from mouth temperature to room temperature might introduce significant dimensional changes. An assessment of the coefficient of expansion of Korecta Wax No. 4* yielded a figure of approximately $1·93 \times 10^{-3}/°C$. These figures were obtained in the Department of Prosthetic Dentistry, Guy's Hospital, and checked through the range 21 °C–37 °C. It seems unlikely, therefore, that this factor would produce clinically significant changes in the impression.

Distal extension prostheses gain support from their abutment teeth in a variety of ways. Henderson et al. (1970) have pointed out that fixed distal extension prostheses transmit forces inclined to the long axes of their abutments. Apart from the effects

* Korecta Wax, Kerr Mfg. Co., Michigan.

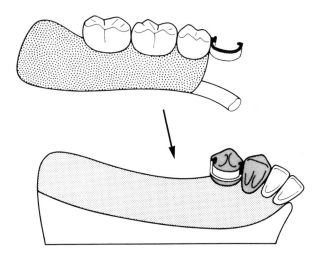

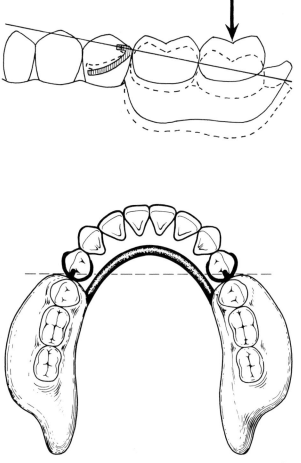

Fig. 87 A lower distal extension prosthesis should be given an inclined path of insertion.

upon the teeth, these forces may contribute to the dislodgement of one of the retaining crowns. The removable prosthesis gains support from some form of occlusal rest of attachment. The design of these structures influences the forces to which the abutment teeth will be subjected, and affects the manner in which the base may tend to move when under load.

A clasp-retained distal extension partial denture tends to rotate around its distal occlusal rests when subjected to load. Figure 87 shows a common design of this type of prosthesis. Since the vertical components of the occlusal loads are applied distal to the long axes of the teeth, there will be a marked tendency for the teeth to be tilted backwards.

The tilting effect of the distally placed loads would be accentuated with the clasp design illustrated. By engaging the mesial undercut the clasp acts on the 'bottle-opener' principle (Fig. 87).

Model experiments confirm the drawbacks associated with a distal occlusal rest. The proximity of the rest to the denture base results in the base rotating around a small radius when it is displaced towards the mucosa. Kratochvil (1963) has found a tendency for the base to move forward under load. However, the distal section of the base will tend to sink more than the mesial section and cause uneven load distribution to the mucosa. The tilting potential upon the distal abutment will be accentuated by a poorly designed clasp (Fig. 88). Another drawback is that the entire clasp unit is poorly adapted to resist posterior displacing forces (Fig. 89). When sticky foods are chewed, the posterior section of the denture base has a tendency to rotate

Fig. 88 Tilting effects on the abutment teeth are increased if rigid clasp arms are used.

around the free end of the clasp, unless an effective indirect retainer is incorporated.

The mesial occlusal rest has several worthwhile advantages (Fig. 90). Work by Nally (1963), Thompson, Kratochvil and Caputo (1977), together with other model experiments, confirms that the mesially positioned rest results in a more apical resolution of forces applied vertically to the artificial teeth. Not only is the direction of the force more favourable, but the available bone support is generally better mesially. Furthermore, the increased radius of rotation provides a more equitable load distribution. Buttressing by the anterior teeth should prevent any tendency to tilt the abutment mesially, while distal displacement of the denture is counteracted by a rigid component of the partial denture framework. The chances of tipping the abutment distally are reduced still further as the retainer will have a tendency to disengage under load.

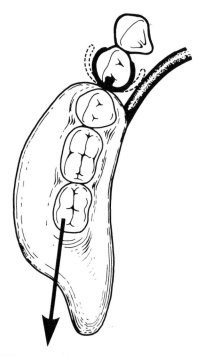

Fig. 89 Where possible, posterior displacing forces should be resisted by a rigid component of the denture framework. In this instance there will be a tendency for the clasp arms to open when distally inclined forces are applied.

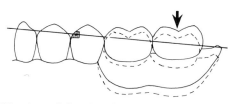

Fig. 90 A mesially placed occlusal rest showing favourable load distribution.

The mesial rest, guide plane, I-bar clasp

The mesial rest, guide plane I-bar clasp design is a particularly interesting development of the gingivally approaching clasp. Kratochvil developed the early clasp assembly while Krol modified the design and named it the R.P.I. bar clasp. When used for distal extension protheses the assembly has the following features:

1. Occlusal rest placed mesially on the most distal abutment.

2. I-shaped bar clasp engaging the mid-buccal aspect of the abutment tooth.

3. Guide planes, distal and distolingual, with abutment tooth and adjacent mucosal contact

provided by the vertical plate (and its extension) on the denture.

This comparatively simple system has obvious merit and should be considered where circumstances permit. Demer (1976) has described minor differences of design. All three clinicians place importance on potential movement of the denture base. Kratochvil constructs a full length guide plane (Fig. 91) that is subsequently relieved in the mouth to prevent torque or binding. Disclosing paste is used for this purpose. Krol (Fig. 92) has 2–3 mm of contact with the guide plane, the section below this point being relieved. The contact point is made good with the artificial tooth of the denture but a small V-shaped space is left underneath (Fig. 93). The Demer modification moves the guide plane mesiolingually so that the proximal plate contacts at the survey line only.

This ingenious and effective system requires an adequate zone of attached gingivae to be covered by the gingivally approaching retainer and a sulcus

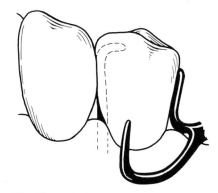

Fig. 91 The Kratochvil designed retainer with maximum contact between denture base and distal guide plane. Subsequent relief is provided at the lower extremity.

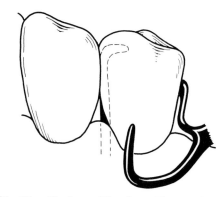

Fig. 92 The Krol modification. The occluso-gingival contact between denture base and guide plane is restricted to about 3 mm.

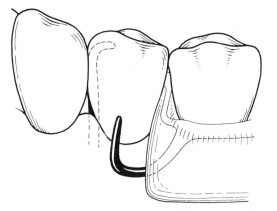

Fig. 93 The artificial denture tooth determines the contact area.

depth of about 5 mm. Individual retainers need to be identified as being in tooth supported or extension situations. Provided the jaw relations and base extension are correct, engagement of distal undercuts appears to produce no undue problems despite the warnings of the original designs. Inlays or crowns may be used with contours designed to provide the rest seats, guide planes, and undercuts that are necessary.

So far the position of the rest has been discussed; equally important is the depth of the rest seat. Cecconi (1974) analysed loads applied to a laboratory model through intracoronal precious attachments and deep (semi-precision) rests. He pointed out that many unsubstantiated claims are made for precision attachments including:–

1. Occlusal forces directed parallel to the long axes of abutment teeth.

2. Even distribution of lateral stresses.

3. Prevention of movement or tipping of the abutment teeth.

Cecconi found that the depth of the rest seat was the all important factor in prevention of abutment mobility, when distal extension situations were considered. The deeper rests significantly reduced precision units acting in a similar manner. Where they must differ is in the mechanism and effectiveness of retention.

Intracoronal attachments are usually placed distally on the abutment adjacent to the space (Fig. 94). Despite the advantage confirmed by their depth, vertical load distribution is still distal to the long axes of the teeth. This problem is accentuated with extracoronal attachments (Fig. 95). Telescopic crowns might appear to offer some advantages in this respect but these are often theoretical rather than real (Fig. 96). If the connection between fixed and

removable sections of the prosthesis were absolutely rigid, the positioning of the joint would not affect load distribution. However, not even the removable prosthesis itself can be considered absolutely rigid for clinical purposes, let alone the comparatively small junction between the two components.

The problems of off-centre vertical loads become more acute when attachments are cantilevered behind the distal abutment. Intracoronal attachments may be employed in this manner. Extracoronal

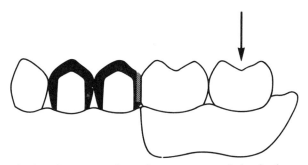

Fig. 94 Intracoronal attachments may apply loads closer to the long axes of the abutments.

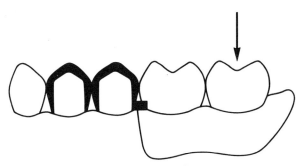

Fig. 95 Vertical loads applied through extracoronal attachments will be distal to the long axes of the abutment teeth.

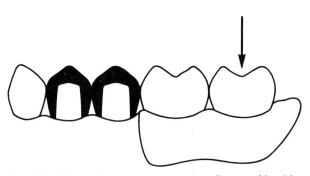

Fig. 96 Telescopic crowns appear to offer considerable advantages in vertical load distribution. In practice, these advantages may not be so clear-cut.

attachments are notorious in this respect and for this reason should not be placed distal to a cantilevered pontic.

In view of the loads that might be applied it is wise practice to employ splinted abutments of at least two connected teeth.

STRESS-BREAKING

So far the discussion has involved load distribution to the mucosa and to the teeth. Many attachments allow a certain degree of movement between the components: for this reason they are known as 'stress-breakers'. This is a misleading term for, at best, all these devices can do is to transfer load from one structure to another. 'Load distributor' is probably more descriptive, and 'stress director' would be an alternative term (Mensor 1972). If the total load is too great, no amount of 'stress-breaking' is going to help.

Another point should be considered. These devices transfer load from the teeth to the edentulous ridge. Up to a point the periodontal ligament is better able to resist these loads than the edentulous ridge.

A host of ingenious devices have been designed to allow movement between the denture base and the natural teeth. Analysis of the action of these devices is difficult, and one frequently suspects they do not achieve the results intended by their inventors – particularly after a certain amount of wear has occurred. Hinges, for example, might allow pure hinge movement while new, but are prone to wear after use in the mouth and allow lateral movement. Lateral or rotational play within an attachment may severely reduce the cross-arch support provided by the major connector.

It might be argued that on theoretical considerations, some slight movement of the denture base must occur under load, and that the tendency for the base to rotate could be eliminated by allowing movement in a vertical direction. A hypothetical attachment allowing movement in this direction alone is illustrated (Fig. 97). However, it can be seen that simple vertical movement would apply even loading only in situations where the entire mucosa were of even displaceability, and presumably, thickness; furthermore, a food bolus contacting an off-centre section of the base might jam the attachment. The spring-loaded device immediately reduces the effective support from the abutment teeth, and denture base movement relative to the papilla behind the distal abutment tooth is likely to be increased. Damage to this papilla is a common

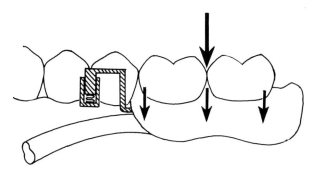

Fig. 97   A hypothetical attachment allowing movement simply in a vertical direction. Even load distribution to the mucosa occurs only when the entire mucosa is of even displaceability, while denture base movement relative to the papilla behind the distal abutment tooth may cause damage.

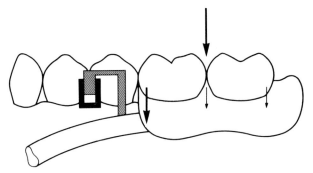

Fig. 98   Loss of the spring, or lack of resilience can remove tooth support for the denture base. Unless springs are regularly checked, damage to the gingivae and edentulous ridges may ensue.

finding among patients treated with an attachment of this type that has not been maintained regularly. Failure to change the spring regularly will result in permanent deformation of the spring that in turn leads to the denture becoming entirely mucosal borne (Fig. 98). On the other hand, if the spring is incorrectly seated, the attachment may not engage and the denture base will be lifted out of contact with the mucosa (Fig. 99).

Although a hinge in the position illustrated in Fig. 100 would not permit significant movement of the denture base adjacent to the abutment teeth, load distribution would be uneven. Some attachments allow both vertical and hinge movements, thereby combining the advantages and drawbacks that have been discussed.

The alignment of hinges will be discussed in the chapter concerned with extracoronal attachments. The distal projection, however, is likely to complicate plaque control problems. Furthermore a hinge

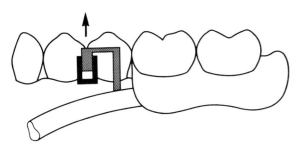

Fig. 99   An incorrect replacement spring may not permit the attachment to engage and will lift the denture base out of contact with the mucosa.

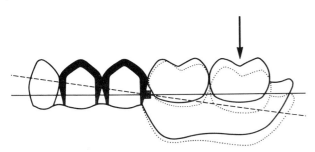

Fig. 100   A hinge may limit denture base movement adjacent to the abutments, but load distribution may be uneven.

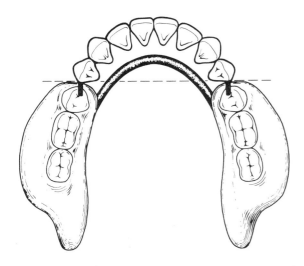

Fig. 101   The distal projection of an extracoronal attachment will complicate plaque control. When twisted out of alignment with the edentulous ridge buccolingual space requirements are increased.

out of alignment with the edentulous ridge is likely to require considerable buccolingual space (Fig. 101).

It would be too dogmatic, however, to insist that the connection between denture and abutment teeth should be rigid for every prosthesis that is made. There are situations where the number, distribution and condition of the remaining teeth cannot form a sufficiently strong abutment to withstand exceptional loads that might be applied to them by an attached distal extension prosthesis. It is here that a very slight degree of freedom of movement may be allowed between denture base and abutment teeth. This slight, potential movement should be considered as a safety valve and it must be stressed that a correctly designed and constructed denture has only the minimal tendency to move. A prosthesis that constantly moves serves little purpose apart from causing damage to the abutment teeth, their supporting structures, and possibly hastening bone resorption of the edentulous areas. Boitel,* for example, found that vertical movements of the denture base of about 0·4 mm produced significant damage to the distal gingival papillae of the abutment teeth. It is, therefore, unnecessary to introduce mechanical complexities in order to allow the denture base a large range of undesirable and potentially damaging movements.

For the majority of restorations, a comparatively straightforward and rigid connection can be used, provided the denture is stable.

There is, of course, no such thing as a rigid denture. All materials possess some inherent flexibility. Apart from major connectors, Heckneby (1969) has pointed out that the levels of transverse and sagittal flexibility of acrylic resin denture bases may well reach clinical significance.

PATH OF INSERTION

When a partial denture is in position, it may be withdrawn along its path of insertion, or it may be rocked and rotated out of place. Proximal tooth surfaces bearing a parallel relationship to one another guide the denture while it is being inserted or removed. A correctly designed clasp-retained partial denture restoring a bounded space should incorporate effective guiding planes from the abutments. If precise frictional contacts between denture base and abutment teeth are obtained, there will be no spaces into which the gingivae can proliferate

* Personal communication.

or food stagnate. The guiding planes prevent the denture being rocked or rotated out of place, for it can only move along its path of insertion. Since the tips of the retaining clasps are placed in undercuts relative to this path, removal of the denture can be achieved only by deformation of the clasp arms. The longer the guide plane the more effective it will be. Where distal extension dentures are concerned, Kratochvil (1963) and Krol (1973) have suggested that proximal guide planes be limited to about 2 mm. Where clasp retention is considered there is some advantage in the lingual surfaces of abutment teeth having surfaces parallel to the proximal guide planes. Apart from increasing the surface area of contact it may also help overcome a theoretical hazard of clasp design – unopposed lateral force application when the denture is inserted. Stern (1975) has pointed out that as the denture is inserted, the retention arm contacts the surface above the survey line and contrives to exert a lateral force until it is completely seated, when it becomes passive. If the bracing arm contacts the tooth all the time the clasp is exerting a load, no lateral components will be exerted on the abutment teeth.

Mucosal contours, as well as those of the teeth need to be considered, particularly when attachments are to be employed. Few attachments allow the partial denture to be rocked and rotated into position. A distal extension prosthesis usually requires a path of insertion approaching from the distal aspect of the abutments (Fig. 102). This path allows maximum contact between the denture base and the distal abutment, while also permitting the base to enter the retromylohyoid fossae – areas frequently undercut to an approach path at right-angles to the occlusal plane. Anterior removable prostheses often require a path of insertion with an approach from the labial aspect.

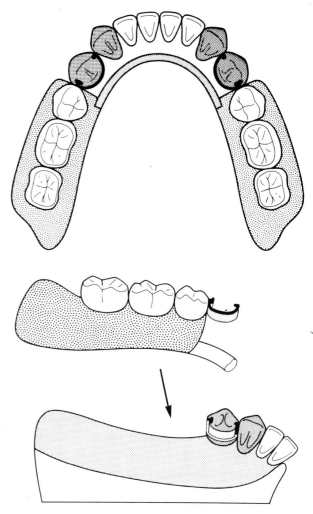

Fig. 102   The distal extension prosthesis usually requires a path of insertion approaching from the distal aspects of the abutments.

RETENTION

The retention of a denture depends on its ability to resist displacement away from its supporting structures. In this discussion retention is the degree of resistance of the prosthesis to removal in a direction opposite to that of its insertion. Retention can be provided by both clasps and attachments, but the mechanism by which they act is different.

The clasp achieves retention by means of its flexible tip placed in an undercut. This clasp tip should be passive when the prosthesis is in position although this ideal state may not always occur in practice. Nevertheless, an unseating force is required to cause deformation of the clasp before the denture can be removed, and this force is a measure of the retention provided by the clasp.

This state of affairs exists where the path of withdrawal is determined precisely. Apart from the presence of adequate guide planes, the clasp can be effective only where a suitable undercut relative to this path can be engaged. Not only the undercut depth, but its location is important. Avant (1971) has pointed out that both the undercut depth and its distance below the survey line exert important influences on retention.

Take two undercuts of the same size, one placed near the survey line, the other close to the gingivae. The work required to remove the dentures constructed would be the same. But work is the product of the force and the distance through which it acts.

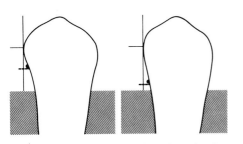

Fig. 103 Clasps in undercuts of similar depths require equal work to displace them to the survey line. Since work is the product of a force and the distance through which it acts, the clasp tip nearer the survey line will require greater force and thereby provide better retention.

The clasp near the survey line does not need to travel very far, but the force required for its movement is considerable. Retention is a measure of force, not work, and so the clasp near the survey line will provide greater retention than its counterpart closer to the gingivae (Fig. 103). The clasp near the survey line may have a bracing arm nearer the occlusal surface than the clasp close to the gingival margin.

In the majority of situations the clasp will be the retainer of choice. Recent developments with the bar (gingivally approaching) retainer makes possible a neat and effective unit. An adequate guide plane, undercut, and sulcus depth is required. Whether or not the guide plane should reach the gingival margin is a point at issue. However, as a matter of principle the less effective the guide plane the more cumbersome the retaining arm must be. Occlusally approaching clasp arms are more rigid, simpler to make, but may interfere with appearance. For a detailed examination of clasp retainers the reader is referred to McCraken's *Removable Partial Prosthodontics* (Henderson and Steffel 1977) or Neill and Walter (1977).

Unlike clasps, attachments provide their retention by frictional contrasts or by mechanical locks. Some units employ both. The retention provided is usually extremely effective and achieved irrespective of the contours of the natural teeth.

INDIRECT RETENTION

Movement of a distal extension base away from its supporting tissues may occur as a rotation about an axis, or as a displacement of the entire denture along its path of insertion. Movement along the path of insertion should be prevented by the direct retainers, but rotational movements present a problem.

When the denture base is tilted away from the mucosa, the denture tends to rotate around the direct

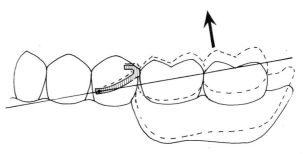

Fig. 104 Unless an effective indirect retainer is incorporated, there is little to prevent the posterior sections of the denture bases rotating around the free ends of the clasps.

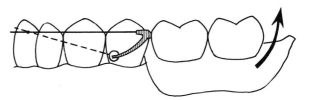

Fig. 105 The indirect retainer replaces the clasp tip as the centre of rotational movements of the saddle away from the mucosa. The clasp tip is thereby placed in an undercut relative to the movement which it can then prevent.

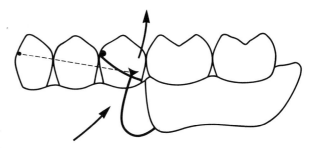

Fig. 106 Clasps placed in some distal undercuts might be ineffective when used in conjunction with indirect retainers as they might not be in undercuts relative to rotational movements around the indirect retainer. This problem should not arise if the cast is surveyed with a 'nose-down' tilt.

retainers (Fig. 104). It tends to rotate, in fact, about an axis passing through the tips of the distal retaining clasps which are, therefore, virtually powerless to prevent this movement. However, this rotational movement can be prevented by rigid components of the denture base placed anterior to the axis or rotation, on the principle of the Class 2 lever (Fig. 105). The indirect retainer replaces the clasp tip as the centre of rotation and the clasp tip is thereby placed in an undercut relative to this movement which it can then prevent. Nairn (1966) felt that clasps placed in distal undercuts of abutment teeth might be ineffective when used in conjunction with indirect retainers, as they might not be in undercuts relative to rotational movements around the indirect retainer (Fig. 106). However, if the cast was surveyed with a nose-down tilt, as should normally be the case for distal extension prostheses, the clasp should well be able to resist this movement.

An indirect retainer can be effective only if it is placed some considerable distance anterior to the direct retainers. When only anterior teeth remain, the distance between direct and indirect retainers must be small and thus there is little to prevent the denture base separating from the mucosa. A clasp-retained denture in the situation illustrated (Fig. 107) would have a tendency to drop away from the mucosa posteriorly. For this reason many prosthodontists have, in the past, preferred to construct complete immediate replacement dentures for similar situations.

Attachments have great advantages with respect to indirect retention. Intracoronal units possess such a precise path of insertion that there is little opportunity for the denture base to rotate. Some extracoronal attachments incorporate effective tilt-stopping devices, but with others additional components need to be added to the denture framework.

Attachments normally require splinted abutments and involve additional complications compared with clasps. Nevertheless, their invisible and most effective retention together with their ability to resist tilting and other displacing forces make attachments useful where the clasp might be ugly and inoperative.

CONNECTORS

If the distal extension base is to resist forces applied in all directions, as indeed it must, additional support from other quadrants of the mouth is nearly always necessary. By distributing lateral loads the major connector prevents any tendency for the denture base to whip (Fig. 108). Another example of how the major connector functions concerns forces applied through the buccal cusps of the artificial teeth. These forces may cause the entire prosthesis to rotate (Fig. 109). Attachments or clasps on the side of the applied force resist with a poor mechanical advantage. Direct retainers on the opposite side of the arch can resist these forces with an appreciable mechanical advantage.

The major connector can only serve these

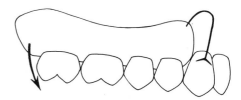

Fig. 107   As a result of lack of indirect retention, a clasp-retained denture has a tendency to drop away from the mucosa posteriorly.

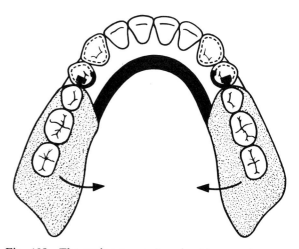

Fig. 108   The major connector should prevent any tendency for the denture bases to whip.

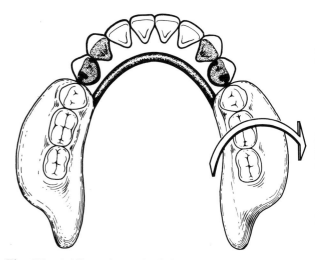

Fig. 109   A bilateral prosthesis is able to resist horizontal loads with the teeth and mucosa of both sides of the jaw. Rotational loads applied to one side are resisted by the retainers of the opposite side acting with a considerable mechanical advantage.

functions if it is comparatively rigid. Space limitations of the mouth and the restricted stiffness of the materials available today make it virtually impossible to construct the major connector of a lower distal extension prosthesis that will not flex by at least 0·3 mm when subjected to loads of 10 kg. For example, Bates (1966) reported base deflections of 0·65 mm when subjected to 1·2 kg. In practice it is extremely difficult to evaluate the stiffness or load/deflection characteristics of a cast lingual bar, with an irregular and variable cross-section and whose geometrical shape is determined by the characteristics of the patient's jaw. Since any significant flexing of the connector will degrade the benefit of cross arch support, the major effort should be directed at producing a connector of adequate stiffness, not the reverse.

Lingual bars are popular lower connectors when attachments are employed as there is seldom need for additional indirect retainers. Unfortunately, the space available for the bar is often limited. Short lingual sulcus depth can be overcome by spacing the bar lingually from the mucosa (Fig. 110). Within the limitations of patient tolerance this has the additional advantage of reducing the length of the major connector and decreasing the radius of curvature, factors that contribute to its tortional rigidity. Where space restrictions apply the higher modulus of elasticity (stiffness) of chrome compared with gold has obvious advantage.

The design of upper major connectors generally poses less of a problem. The strength inherent in a ring type of connector is to be preferred (Fig. 111). Where patient tolerance dictates a posterior palatal strap, the design is weakened (Fig. 112). Choice of materials and the cross-section of components becomes critical in this situation. The anterior palatal bar or horseshoe manages to combine most of the drawbacks of the rings and bars with few advantages save where an inoperable torus exists.

Chrome cobalt alloys have obvious advantages where spans are long and space is restricted. There are, however, drawbacks some of which are peculiar to attachment retained restorations.

Whereas a good connector can be cast in any laboratory capable of constructing the abutment crowns, chrome cobalt alloys require special facilities. It is also extremely difficult to produce a chrome casting that will fit the intricacies of milled bracing arms or other prepared components. Problems arising from differential hardness of gold and chrome cobalt are frequently overrated; it is the adaptation that is so hard to produce. Soldering chrome cobalt alloys to precious metal components

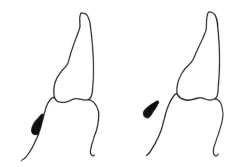

Fig. 110 Where vertical space restrictions are present it may be possible to space the lingual bar from the mucosa.

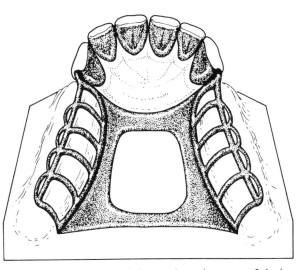

Fig. 111 The strength inherent in a ring type of design is to be preferred.

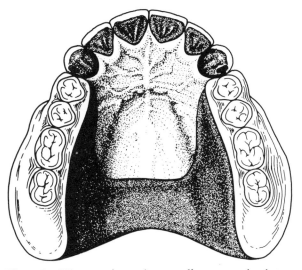

Fig. 112 Where patient tolerance dictates a palatal strap the design is weakened.

is not impossible, but requires great skill as the attachments are easily damaged in the process. On the other hand certain extracoronal attachments, like the Dalbo, can be buried in the denture base acrylic resin and require no bracing arm. Chrome cobalt alloys produce no problems with these types of unit. The lower stiffness of a hard yellow gold alloy requires the cross section of the connector to be about twenty five per cent thicker than one made in chrome cobalt. There is one final point. In considering technical problems it is all too easy to forget the patient. There are still many patients who, despite the extra bulk required, prefer gold.

Even supposing that a rigid major connector could be constructed, heat cured acrylic resin has only about one seventieth the stiffness of chrome cobalt. Heckneby (1969) has shown that the denture base itself is quite capable of flexing by 0·3 mm under occlusal load.

For practical purposes it is therefore almost impossible to produce a denture that will resist occlusal and masticatory forces without these slight movements that should be all that is required – under normal circumstances at least. There seems little point in weakening the structure to allow a range of uncontrolled, unnecessary, and potentially damaging movements that complicate construction and maintenance of the restoration.

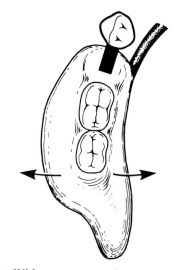

Fig. 113   Without cross arch support the prosthesis stands little chance of resisting the forces causing the base to whip.

THE UNILATERAL DISTAL SPACE

A removable prosthesis restoring such a space normally requires support from the teeth of both sides of the arch. Without this support, the denture and its abutments stand little chance of resisting forces causing the base to whip (Fig. 113), or those tending to rotate it around a sagittal axis (Fig. 114). Support from the other side of the arch makes the base stable, and damaging torques on the abutments will be eliminated.

Joining the two sides of the arch make it tooth-supported on one side and tooth- and mucosal-supported on the other. It used to be argued that under occlusal load the tooth- and mucosal-supported part of the prosthesis might be displaced more than the tooth-supported section, thereby introducing unfavourable forces on the abutments. Ingenious attachments were, in fact, developed that allowed different movements on the two sides of the prosthesis. Many dentures are still made in this way. However, one must not forget that movement occurring between the denture base and the major connector, or between the abutment crowns and

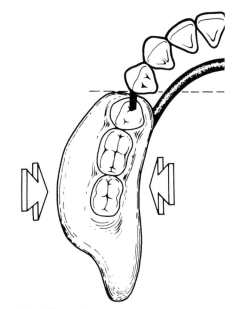

Fig. 114   The major connector will prevent the base rotating around a sagittal axis.

bases, reduce support from the teeth and the effectiveness of cross-arch bracing. Impression techniques, jaw relations and maintenance therapy are more difficult when a movement potential exists. For these reasons, prostheses restoring unilateral spaces are usually best made with comparatively rigid attachments, if indeed attachments are indicated.

The clasp-retained prosthesis is usually to be recommended where there is no missing tooth on the

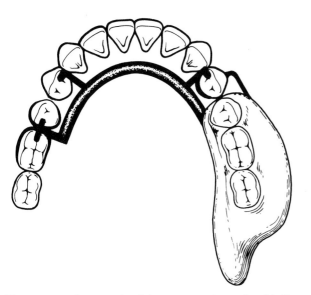

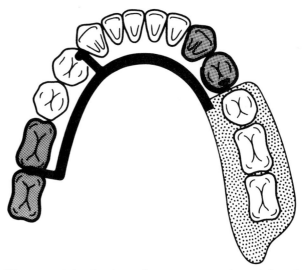

Fig. 116 Joined telescopic crowns may be employed where no space exists on one side of the arch.

Fig. 115 A clasp-retained denture may be preferable for some unilateral spaces. The extensive tooth preparation required for an attachment-retained prosthesis may not be offset by its marginal advantages in retention and stability.

opposite side of the arch to the distal space. Adequate guiding planes can be provided, usually producing effective clasp retainers that are economical, neat, and require little or no preparation of the abutments (Fig. 115).

Where the abutment teeth in any case require large restorations, attachments have much to offer. If no space is present on one side of the arch it might be tempting to place an attachment between two adjacent splinted crowns, but this is not recommended as it almost invariably necessitates an encroachment on the proximal space. Joined telescopic crowns are usually recommended in these situations (Figs. 116–118). A minimum of two splinted crowns is normally required on this side of the mouth and these may need to be devitalised if lingually inclined. The walls of the inner copings must be aligned with attachments on the side of the arch.

Intracoronal attachments can be employed when teeth are missing on both sides of the arch. It might then be tempting to design a prosthesis with attachments in the teeth adjacent to the spaces. However, intracoronal attachments require box preparations in the abutments. Since the intracoronal units need to be aligned with one another, a path of insertion virtually at right angles to the occlusal plane may need to be selected. This path of insertion may prevent the extension of the denture base to gain the mucosal support it needs (Fig. 119).

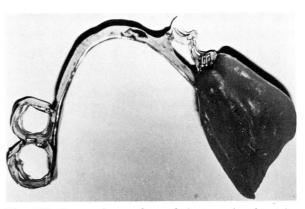

Fig. 117 Impression surface of denture showing telescopic crowns.

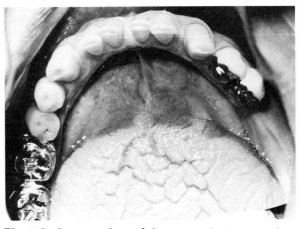

Fig. 118 Inner sections of the crowns in the mouth.

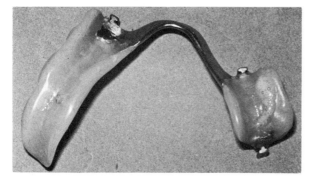

Fig. 119 Inadequate extension of the denture base resulting from a path of insertion at right-angles to the occlusal plane.

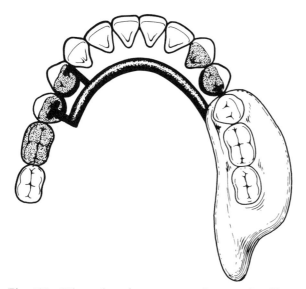

Fig. 120   Where there is a space on the opposite side to the distal extension, the denture can gain support from an attachment placed bucco-lingually in a bridge restoring the gap.

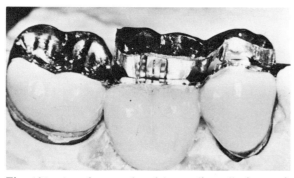

Fig. 121   Attachment placed bucco-lingually in pontic. Note the indirect retainer that also acts as an additional handling point.

A modification of this technique, and one to be preferred, is to construct a fixed prosthesis across the bounded space (Figs. 120, 121). An intracoronal unit can then be placed bucco-lingually within this prosthesis. Neither the size nor the alignment of the attachment is limited by pulpal considerations, and the distal abutment is permanently splinted.

An intracoronal retainer within a pontic can be difficult for the patient to remove. An additional handling point should be combined with an indirect retainer. The indirect retainer is necessary to reduce loads falling on the lateral surface of the attachment, and to contribute to the stability of the denture.

A neat and simple indirect retainer would take the form of an occlusal rest attached to a minor connector and recessed within the contour of one of the mesial abutment crowns. Lingual bracing arms can be milled and modified to carry out similar roles.

The fixed prosthesis restoring the bounded space may take the form of a bar unit. The bar unit becomes more valuable when the bounded space is long, for some mucosal support can be gained for the prosthesis (Fig. 122).

MISSING ANTERIOR TEETH

As a general rule anterior teeth should not be added to bilateral distal extension dentures. No matter how well the prosthesis is made there is always a tendency for it to rotate around the abutments (Fig. 123). Where possible, the anterior space should be restored by a fixed prosthesis. Alternatively, a bar can be used to span the anterior edentulous gap, thereby splinting the abutments either side.

THE CHECK RECORD

The importance of accurate jaw relations has been stressed throughout the text. When a distal extension denture opposes a complete denture there are apparent practical difficulties in making a check record, yet it is particularly important that this be carried out.

A remount cast is made for the upper denture and a new facebow record taken. The upper denture and its remount cast can now be mounted on the articulator. A record rim of extra hard wax is then applied to the upper denture and after suitable warming, the centric relation record made, with the teeth just failing to contact. By dampening the lower natural and artificial teeth one can ensure that the rim stays adhered to the upper denture.

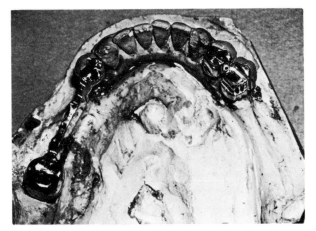

Fig. 122 The fixed prosthesis may take the form of a bar unit.

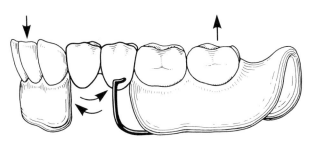

Fig. 123 An anterior base results in a tendency for the prosthesis to rotate around its abutments. Where possible an anterior fixed prosthesis should be constructed, or the abutments connected by a bar.

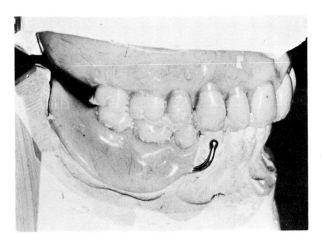

Fig. 124 Lower partial denture remounted on articulator by means of a check record.

If the lower master cast has been destroyed, an impression of the entire lower dentition is made removing the denture in the impression. The cast of this impression is subsequently mounted on the articulator using the centric relation record (Fig. 124). It is then possible to perfect the occlusion and articulation without the possible complication of denture base movement.

To summarise, the clasp retainer is still the retainer of choice for the majority of removable prostheses, being comparatively cheap, effective, straightforward to use, and requiring the minimum of preparation of the abutment teeth. However, the shape, number, or distribution of the natural teeth does not always allow the effective use of clasps, and it is here that attachments are particularly valuable. For the intermediate situations, the practitioner must weigh carefully the mechanical advantages of attachments and the better appearance against the tooth preparation required and the extra cost involved. The need to provide better distal extension prostheses has been recognised, and attachments have much to contribute to this end.

REFERENCES AND FURTHER READING

APPLEGATE, O. C. (1955) The partial denture base. *J. prosth. Dent.*, *5*, 636

APPLEGATE, O. C. (1959) *Essentials of Removable Partial Denture Prosthesis.* 2nd ed. Saunders, Philadelphia

ATWOOD, D. A. (1962) Some clinical factors related to rate of resorption of residual ridge. *J. prosth. Dent.*, *12*, 411–450

AVANT, W. E. (1971) Factors that influence retention of removable partial dentures. *J. prosth. Dent.*, *25*, 265

BATES, J. F. (1963) Cast clasps for partial dentures. *Int. dent. J.*, *13*, 610

BATES, J. F. (1963) Retention of cobalt–chromium partial dentures. *Dent. Practit.*, *14*, 168

BATES, J. F. (1966) Studies related to the function of partial dentures. The functional strain in cobalt-chromium dentures: a preliminary report. *Brit. dent. J.*, *5*, 120:79

BATES, J. F. (1970) *Partial Denture Construction: A Laboratory Manual.* John Wright, Bristol

BRADEN, M. (1976) Personal communication

CARLSSON, G. E., HEDEGÅRD, B. and KOIVUMAA, K. K. (1961) Studies in partial dental prosthesis. II. An investigation of mandibular partial dentures with double extension saddles. *Acta odont. scand.*, *19*, 215–237

CARLSSON, G. E., HEDEGÅRD, B. and KOIVUMAA, K. K. (1962) Studies in partial dental prosthesis. III. A longitudinal study of mandibular partial dentures with double extension saddles. *Acta odont. scand.*, *20*, 95–119

CARLSSON, G. E., HEDEGÅRD, B. and KOIVUMAA, K. K. (1965) Studies in partial dental prosthesis. IV. Final results of a 4-year longitudinal investigation of dentogingivally supported partial dentures. *Acta odont. scand.*, *23*, 443–472

CARLSSON, G. E. and PERSON, G. (1967) Morphologic changes of the mandible after extraction and wearing dentures. *Odontologisk Revy*, *18*, 27–54

CECCONI, B. T. (1974) Effect of rest design on transmission of forces to abutment teeth. *J. prosth. Dent.*, *32:2*, 141

CECCONI, B., ASGAR, K. and DORTZ, E. (1972) Cusp assembly modifications and their effect on abutment tooth movement. *J. prosth. Dent.*, *27*, 160–167

CECCONI, B. T., ASGAR, K. and DORTZ, E. (1971) The effect of partial denture clasp design on abutment tooth movement. *J. prosth. Dent.*, *25*, 44

CHRISTENSEN, F. T. (1962) Mandibular free-end denture. *J. prosth. Dent.*, *12*, 111

CLAYTON, J. A. and JASLOS, C. (1971) A measurement of clasp forces on teeth. *J. prosth. Dent.*, *25*, 21

COOPER, H. (1967) Precision attachment bridgework. *Postgrad. Course Univ. Michigan*

DAHL, G. (1963) Mechanical principles of superplants. *Acta odont. scand.*, *21*, 515

DEMER, W. J. (1976) An analysis of mesial rest-1-bar clasp designs. *J. prosth. Dent.*, *36:3*, 243

DERRY, A. and BERTRAM, U. (1970) Clinical survey of removable partial dentures after 2 years usage. *Acta. odont. scand.* 28. 581–598

ELLINGER, C. W., RAYSON, J. H. and HENDERSON, D. (1971) Single complete dentures opposed to natural teeth. *J. prosth. Dent.*, *26*, 4

FAUST, H. E. (1967) Precision attachment bridgework. *Postgrad. Course Univ. Michigan*

FRANK, R. P. and NICHOLLS, J. I. (1977) An investigation of the effectiveness of indirect retainers. *J. prosth. Dent.*, *38:5*, 494–506

FRECHETTE, A. R. (1956) The influence of partial denture design on the distribution of force to abutment teeth. *J. prosth. Dent.*, *6*, 195

HECKNEBY, M. (1969) Distribution of load with the lower free-end partial denture. *Acta odont. scand.*, *27* (Supp. 52), 140

HENDERSON, D. and SEWARD, T. E. (1967) Design and force distribution with removable partial dentures. A progress report. *J. prosth. Dent.*, *17*, 350–363

HENDERSON, D. and STEFFEL, V. L. (1977) *McCracken's Removable Partial Prosthodonties*. 5th edn. C. V. Mosby, St Louis, Mo.

HENDERSON, D., BLEVINS, W. R., WESLEY, R. C. and SEWARD, T. (1970) The cantilever type of posterior fixed partial dentures: a laboratory study. *J. prosth. Dent.*, *24*, 47

HILDEBRAND, G. Y. (1968) Fixed saddle bridges. *Acta odont. scand.*, *26*, 435

HOLMES, J. B. (1965) Influence of impression procedures and occlusal loading on partial denture movement. *J. prosth. Dent.*, *15*, 474

IZIKOWITZ, L. (1966) The superplant. *Acta odont. scand.*, *24*, Suppl. 47

IZIKOWITZ, L., MOLIN, C. and SUNDBERG, C. (1971) The fixed saddle-bridge – the superplant. *Svensk tandläk. T.*, *64*, 719

JOHNS, R. B. (1976) *Implants as Abutments: Proceedings of the British Society for Restorative Dentistry*. J. Wright, Bristol

KAIRES, A. K. (1958) A study of partial denture design and masticatory pressures in a mandibular bilateral distal extension case. *J. prosth. Dent.*, *8*, 340

KASS, C. A. and KNAP, F. J. (1974) Analysis of occlusion before and after occlusal adjustment. *J. prosth. Dent.*, *32:2*, 163

KRATOCHVIL, F. J. (1963) Influence of occlusal rest position and clasp design on movement of abutment teeth. *J. prosth. Dent.*, *13*, 114–124

KRATOCHVIL, F. J. and CAPUTO, A. A. (1974) Photoelastic analysis of pressure on teeth and bone supporting removable partial dentures. *J. prosth. Dent.*, *32:1*, 52

KROL, A. J. (1973) Clasp design for extension–base removable partial dentures. *J. prosth. Dent.*, *29*, 408

LAMMIE, G. A. and OSBORNE, J. (1954) The bilateral free-end saddle lower denture. *J. prosth. Dent.*, *4*, 640

LEE, J. B. (1955) The advantages of an oblique path of insertion in tissue-borne nonmetallic partial dentures. *Brit. dent. J.*, *99*, 191

LUBESPERE, A. and ROTENBERG, A. (1976) *Attachments et Prothèse Combinées*. Ed. Julien Prélat Paris

MATSUMOTO, M. (1963) Morphological changes in the human mandible following the loss of molars and premolars. IV (in Japanese). *J.J.P.S.*, *7*, 183–189

MATSUMOTO, M. (1970) An experimental investigation of analysing the influence of impression procedures in clinical techniques. *Bull. Tokyo Med. Dent. Univ.*, *17*, 4

MENSOR, M. C. (1972) Personal communication

MUHLEMANN, H. R. (1960) 10 years of tooth mobility measurement. *J. Periodont.*, *31*, 110

NAIRN, R. I. (1966) The problem of free-end denture bases. *J. prosth. Dent.*, *16*, 522

NALLY, N. N. (1963) Methods of handling abutment teeth in Class I partial dentures. *J. prosth. Dent.*, *30*, 561–566

NEILL, D. J. (1958) The problem of the lower free-end removable partial denture. *J. prosth. Dent.*, *8*, 623

NEILL, D. J. and WALTER, J. D. (1977) *Partial Denture Prosthetics*. Blackwell Scientific, London

NEUFELD, J. O. (1958) Changes in the trabecular pattern of mandible following the loss of teeth. *J. prosth. Dent.*, *8*, 685–697

PICTON, D. C. A. and WILLS, J. (1978) Viscoelastic properties of the periodontal ligament and mucous membrane. *J. prosth. Dent.*, *40:3*, 263

PREISKEL, H. W. (1971) Impression techniques for attachment-retained distal extension removable partial dentures. *J. prosth. Dent.*, *25*, 620

RANTANEN, T., MÄKILA, E. and YHI-URPO, A.

(1972) Investigations of the therapeutic success with dentures retained by precision attachments. II. Partial Dentures. *Suom. hammaslaak. toim.*, *68*, 73

REHM, H., KÖRBER, E. and KÖRBER, K. H. (1962) Biophysikalischer Beitrag zur Problematik starr abgestützter Freiendprothesen. *Dtsch Zähnarztl.*, *17*, 963–975

SCHUYLER, C. H. (1953) An analysis of the use and relative value of precision attachment and the clasp in partial denture planning. *J. prosth. Dent.*, *3*, 711–714

SCHWALM, C. A., SMITH, D. E. and ERICKSON, J. D. (1977) A clinical study of patients 1 to 2 years after placement of removable partial dentures. *J. prosth. Dent.*, *38:4*, 380–391

SCHWEITZER, J. M., SCHWEITZER, R. D. and SCHWEITZER, J. (1968) Free-end pontics used on fixed partial dentures. *J. prosth. Dent.*, *20*, 120

STEFFEL, V. L. (1963) Clasp partial dentures. *J. Amer. dent. Ass.*, *66*, 803

STEIGER, A. and BOITEL, R. (1959) *Precision Work for Partial Dentures.* Stebo, Zürich

STERN, W. J. (1975) Guiding planes in clasp reciprocation and retention. *J. prosth. Dent.*, *34:4*, 408

THOMPSON, W. D., KRATOCHVIL, F. S. and CAPUTO, A. A. (1977) Evaluation of photoelastic stress patterns produced by bilateral distal-extension removable partial dentures. *J. prosth. Dent.*, *38*, 261

WARREN, A. B. and CAPUTO, A. A. (1975) Load transfer to alveolar bone as influenced by abutment designs for tooth-supported dentures. *J. prosth. Dent.*, *33:2*, 137

WATERS, N. E. (1975a) Aspects of dental biomechanics. In *Scientific Aspect of Dental Materials*, by Von Fraunhauf. J. A. Butterworths, London

WATERS, N. E. (1975b) Denture foundation. A consideration of certain aspects of the displacement of, and the pressure distribution within, the mucoperiosteum. *J. Dent.*, *3:2*, 83

WEAVER, S. M. (1938) Precision attachments and their advantages in respect to underlying tissues. *J. Amer. Dent. Soc.*, *25*, 1250

ZACH, G. A. (1975) Advantages of mesial rests for removable partial dentures. *J. prosth. Dent.*, *33:1*, 32–35

ZARB, G. A., BERGMAN, B., CLAYTON, J. A. and MACKAY, H. F. (1978) *Prosthodontic treatment for partially edentulous patients.* C. V. Mosby Company, St. Louis, Mo

ZOELLER, G. N. and KELLY, W. J. (1971) Block form stability in removable partial prosthodontics. *J. prosth. Dent.*, *26*, 141

CHAPTER 5

Prefabricated Attachments

Prefabricated attachments usually consist of two matched precious metal components. Since the functions served by an attachment vary with the manner in which it is used, the classification employed in this book is based upon attachment shape. The purposes for which an attachment can be used are discussed in the relevant chapters.

1. INTRACORONAL ATTACHMENTS

The two parts of an intracoronal attachment consist of a flange and a slot. The flange is joined to one section of the prosthesis and the slot unit embedded in a restoration forming part of another section of the prosthesis. Two types of intracoronal attachments are available:

(a) Those whose retention is entirely frictional (Fig. 125).

(b) Those whose retention is augmented by a mechanical lock (Fig. 126).

These attachments usually provide a rigid connection between the two sections of the prosthesis.

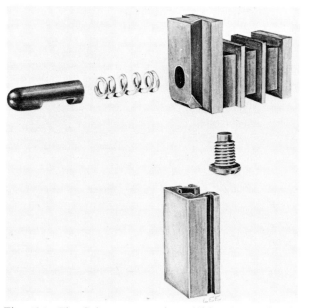

Fig. 126   The Schatzmann unit. Additional retention is provided by a spring-loaded plunger.

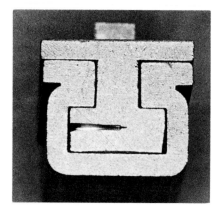

Fig. 125   The McCollum intracoronal unit. A well tried example of a unit with entirely frictional retention.

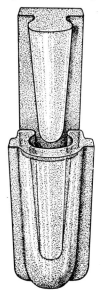

Fig. 127   Pattern for a semi-precision (tapered) intracornal attachment.

2. EXTRACORONAL ATTACHMENTS

These attachments have part or all of their mechanism outside the crown of a tooth. Many of these units allow a certain amount of movement between the two sections of the prosthesis. Extracoronal attachments can be subdivided into the following groups:

(a) Projection units

The units are attached to the proximal surface of a crown. These groups can be divided in turn into:

1. Those that provide a rigid connection (Fig. 128).

2. Those that allow play between the components (Figs. 129–131).

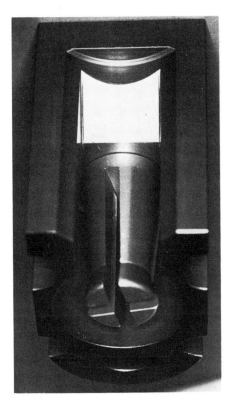

Fig. 128 Removable section of the Conex attachment. Note the parallel walls that provide a precise path of insertion.

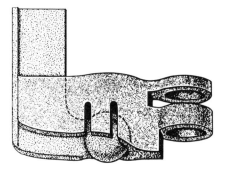

Fig. 130 Miniaturized version of the Dalbo extracoronal projection unit.

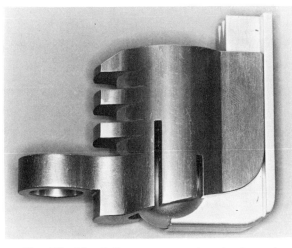

Fig. 129 The Dalbo extracoronal projection unit.

Semi-precision intracoronal attachments feature significant taper (Fig. 127). They may be cast from patterns or entirely laboratory produced. Unlike precision attachments an additional retentive element is essential.

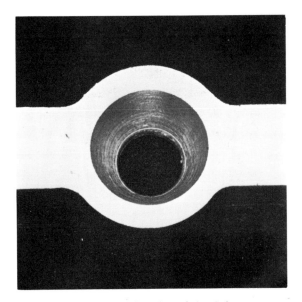

Fig. 131 The retaining ring of the Ceka system.

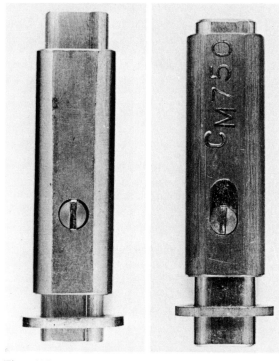

Fig. 132 Rotation Joint providing predetermined hinge movement.

Fig. 133 Axial Rotation Joint providing restricted vertical travel together with predetermined hinge movement.

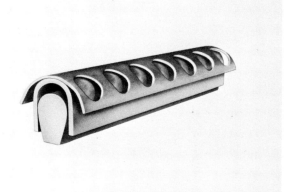

Fig. 135 The Dolder Bar Joint. A well tested example of a single sleeve joint allowing vertical and rotational units.

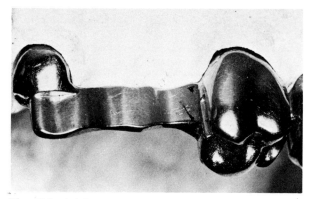

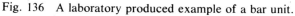

Fig. 136 A laboratory produced example of a bar unit.

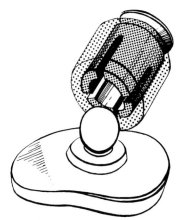

Fig. 134 The Dalbo stud unit. A small yet sturdy attachment, particularly useful for joining a complete overdenture to root diaphragms.

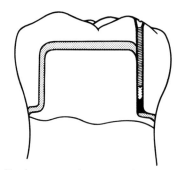

Fig. 137 By incorporating a precious metal threaded sleeve within the inner coping, the outer section can be retained with a screw.

(b) Connectors

These units connect two sections of a removable prosthesis and allow a certain degree of play (Figs. 132, 133).

(c) Combined units

The attachments are an extracoronally placed hinge-type unit connected to an intracoronal attachment.

3. STUD ATTACHMENTS (Fig. 134)

These attachments are so called because of the shape of the male units that are usually soldered to the diaphragm of a post crown. Some of these units provide a comparatively rigid connection; others allow movement between the two sections.

4. BAR ATTACHMENTS

Bar attachments consist of a bar spanning an edentulous area joining together teeth or roots. The denture fits over the bar and is connected to it with one or more sleeves. Bar attachments fall into two categories:

(a) Bar joints (Fig. 135)

These units allow play between the denture and bar.

(b) Bar units (Fig. 136)

With these attachments the sleeve/bar junction is rigid. Single or multiple sleeves may be used with either category.

5. AUXILIARY ATTACHMENTS

This miscellaneous group consists basically of:

(a) Screw units (Fig. 137)

These devices are useful for securing and dismantling parts of a prosthesis in the mouth, when there is no common line of insertion of the whole. They are particularly useful for joining the two components of a telescopic crown.

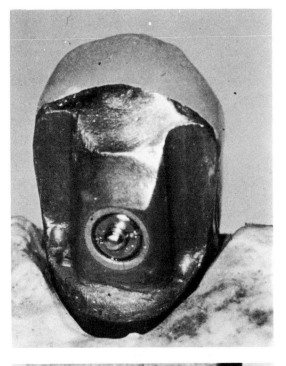

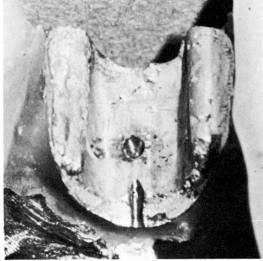

Fig. 138 Plunger unit employed to increase retention between the fixed and removable sections of a telescopic prosthesis.

(b) Friction devices

Spring-loaded plungers are commonly employed to increase retention between the two sections of a telescopic prosthesis (Fig. 138).

Split posts (Fig. 139) can be used in conjunction with sectional dentures.

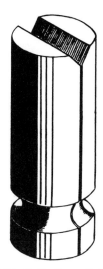

Fig. 139 The P.W. Split Post. Split posts have useful applications in sectional denture construction.

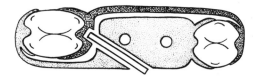

Fig. 140 Diagram of a bolt assembly to illustrate how two sections of a removable prosthesis with different paths of insertion are joined in the mouth.

(c) Bolts (Fig. 140)

Bolt units are used to connect the two parts of a sectional denture in the mouth. Each part of the denture is inserted separately and the patient locks them together with the bolt.

(d) Hinged flanges (Fig. 141)

This type of device allows mucosal undercuts and interdental spaces to be used for retentive purposes.

Although components of prefabricated attachments are carefully matched, they are not only produced in identical metals. For example, sections of attachments to be joined to the fixed section of the prosthesis are available in platinised golds, compatible with abutments of similar alloys; the removable section of the attachment is likely to be made of a yellow gold. Apart from the vital difference in melting ranges, minor design differences are often to be found between components for use with yellow golds and those to be employed with bonded porcelain to gold techniques. Continued research with non-precious alloys holds promise of reduced component size in the future.

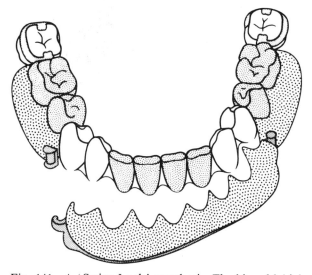

Fig. 141 A 'Swing-Lock' prosthesis. The hinged labial flange allows proximal spaces to be used for retention.

CHAPTER 6

Intracoronal Attachments

Intracoronal attachments consist of two parts, a slot and a flange. The flange is joined to one section of the prosthesis and the slot unit, embedded in a restoration, forms part of another section of the prosthesis. In this way the two units can be joined in the mouth, the connection taking place within the contour of a tooth crown. Precision attachments have parallel-sided flanges; the flanges of semi-precision units are slightly tapered.

Towards the end of the last century, Carr, Peeso, Parr, Alexander and Morgan had all designed and used simple intracoronal attachments (Figs. 142, 143). Griswald had designed not only his own attachment, but also an ingenious paralleling device for alignment. In 1906 Herman Chayes designed the attachment which, with modification, is still in production and carries his name (Fig. 144). His original idea was to position the attachment lingually, but subsequently a mesiodistal position was suggested.

Intracoronal attachments serve retentive and supportive functions, as do clasp units. The retention provided by the attachment mainly depends on the frictional surface area of contact between the two parts. The bracing action is provided by the laterally facing surfaces of the attachment when used conventionally. In view of the excellent retention and stability provided by intracoronal attachments, they have applications in both fixed and removable partial prostheses.

Since the retention provided by the attachment depends largely on friction between the two components, it is desirable to provide as much frictional surface area as possible. The surface area available for friction is a product of the cross-section of the male part and its length. The length of the attachment is governed by the height of the clinical crown of the tooth and is a most important factor in attachment retention and stability. The attachment cross-section is limited because it is necessary to recess the female part within the circumference of the tooth.

If the female part of the attachment is not recessed, the contour of the tooth is altered, a permanent projection is left at the gingival margin of the restoration, and the length of the attachment is limited both by the gingival tissues and by the fact that it may intrude on the area where the tip of the opposing cusp occludes (Fig. 145).

Cross-sections of several attachment types are illustrated and it can be seen that the H-shaped flange of the modern attachments has great advantages over earlier T-shaped flanges (Fig. 146). The external frictional flange of the H-shaped unit virtually doubles the frictional surface area and strengthens the attachment, without increasing the size of the female part. With some attachments, an external frictional flange can be cast onto the removable section. However, one cannot quite expect the accuracy of adaptation to match that of a precision engineered flange integral to the attachment.

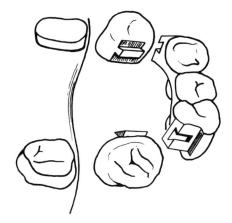

Fig. 142 An attachment system designed by Alexander at the end of the 19th century. The male sections were joined to the crowns, the attachments were tapered and used with a buccolingual path of insertion for the prosthesis.

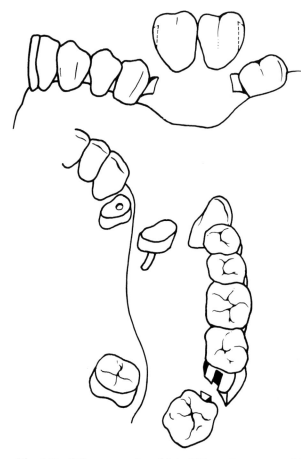

Fig. 143 Other examples of late 19th century removable bridgework. Note that the male sections were placed in the fixed prostheses.

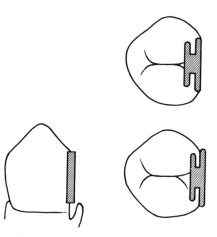

Fig. 145 The female part of the attachment should be recessed within the contour of the abutment crown (above). If this is not done, the contour of the tooth is completely altered and a permanent projection is left at the gingival margin.

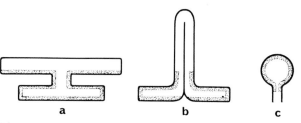

Fig. 146 Cross-sections of several types of attachment. The H-shaped flanges of the modern attachments are stronger and have nearly double the frictional surface area of the earlier T-shaped flanges. Attachments with a circular cross-section are suitable only for joining two sections of a fixed prosthesis.

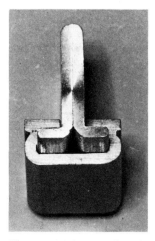

Fig. 144 The Chayes attachment, described in 1906. This T-shaped unit is still in production today.

FRICTION FIT INTRACORONAL ATTACHMENTS WITH ADJUSTMENT POTENTIAL

Constant insertion and removal of the prosthesis will cause the attachments to wear, so that some form of adjustment is desirable. While comparatively simple attachments such as the Chayes unit can be adjusted by opening the two halves with a razor blade or scalpel, the more complicated units require careful handling and strict adherence to the manufacturer's instructions. At one time, the male sections of some of the attachments were manufactured in two halves which were then soldered together. The soldered junction was comparatively weak and adjustment of the male part could lead to fracture.

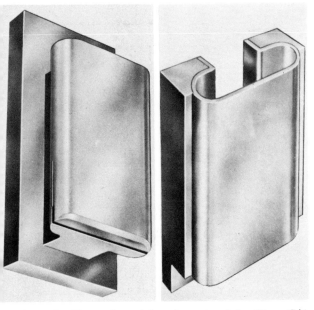

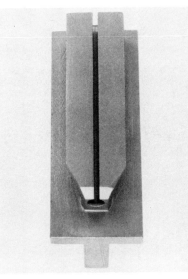

Fig. 147 The male and female parts of the Stern G/A attachment. These robust well-tried units are available in several sizes.

Fig. 149 The male section of the Crismani Unit. Note the chamfer and taper of the gingival section of the unit to facilitate insertion.

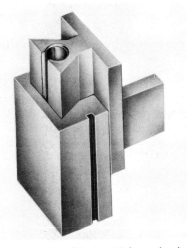

Fig. 148 The narrower of the two Crismani units features a central groove for adjustment.

Numerous prefabricated attachments are produced by manufacturers in Europe and in the United States. The choice of attachment is usually governed by its shape and size rather than any mechanical attribute claimed for it. Several examples of modern, well tried attachments are illustrated. The Stern G/A (Fig. 147) unit is produced in the United States, the others in Europe.

The Crismani series of intracoronal attachments are available in two basic configurations. The narrower version (2·8 mm) features an adjustable central groove (Fig. 148). Refined over the years, this attachment now incorporates a chamfer and tapered gingival male section to facilitate insertion (Fig. 149). The unit is 7 mm tall but can be shortened by up to 2 mm.

The McCollum attachment has now been re-designed for additional strength (Fig. 150). The adjustment split runs part way through the attachment from one side. Imagine a lower distal extension restoration viewed from above. Since the splits should face laterally it is necessary to produce left and right sided attachments. The manufacturers have selected the lower restoration for their terminology. Rather confusing is the fact that when an upper denture is constructed a left sided attachment should be placed on the right side and vice versa if the slots are to face laterally.

The McCollum units are now among the most robust of those made. As with most intracoronal attachments, the units are available in metals compatible with bonded porcelain to gold techniques as well as with conventional yellow golds. A combination is also produced in which the female element is to be employed with porcelain to gold while the male is to be incorporated with yellow gold alloys.

The Ancra is a well established intracoronal attachment. This unit features an 'H' shaped profile with external frictional flange while the male unit incorporates slots either side to allow for modification

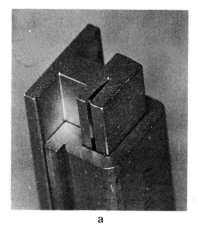

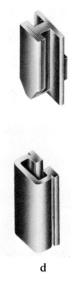

d

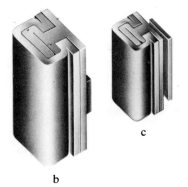

c

b

Fig. 150(a) The redesigned McCollum attachment.
(b) The McCollum for use with conventional yellow golds.
(c) The McCollum for use with bonded gold to porcelain techniques.
(d) Note the taper of the gingival section of the male unit to aid insertion.

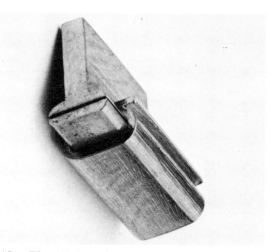

Fig. 151 The 'T-Geschiebe 123' intracoronal attachment.

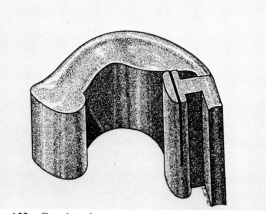

Fig. 152 Cast bracing arm and external frictional flange.

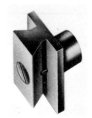

Fig. 153 The wider Crismani units incorporate a wire retaining clip for additional retention.

of retention. Two sizes of attachment are available and the female unit may be obtained in either high heat or conventional yellow gold alloys.

The T-Geschiebe 123 (Fig. 151) represents another approach to the problem. When used to retain removable prostheses, an external frictional flange is cast, together with a bracing arm (Fig. 152).

Auxiliary retentive features

Since the shape and size of the tooth governs both the cross-section and length of an intracoronal attachment, there exists a definite limit to the retention available. Auxiliary retentive features are incorporated in some attachments in an effort to provide more retention for a given frictional area,

although no extra stability is provided. A minimum of 4 mm vertical space is still usually necessary.

The wider Crismani units incorporate a wire clip to increase retention (Fig. 153). Access to the clip is obtained by removing the screw in the male unit.

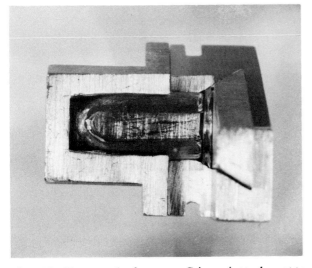

Fig. 154 Photograph of cutaway Crismani attachment to show the retaining clip.

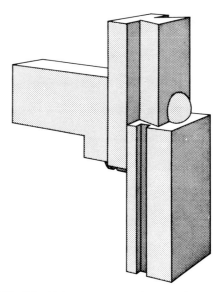

Fig. 156 The Schatzmann attachment, the retention of which is increased by a spring-loaded plunger assembly. The male section illustrated is designed to be soldered to a metal framework.

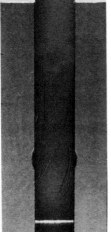

Fig. 155 External surface of the Crismani female unit to show the retaining slot.

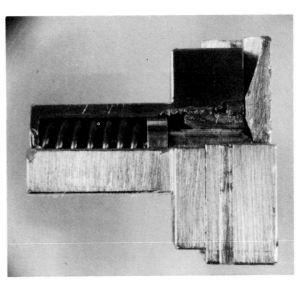

Fig. 157 Photograph of a partly cutaway Schatzmann attachment to show the plunger mechanism. The applications of this robust unit are limited by its bulk.

Failure to tighten the screw correctly will prevent the male unit sliding into place (Fig. 154). The female unit contains two depressions for the retaining wire (Fig. 155), and is 7·0 mm tall. No significant shortening should be carried out.

Other devices consist basically of a spring-loaded piston on the male part engaging a socket within the female element – rather like a simple cupboard door catch. The Schatzmann is a good example of this type of unit (Fig. 156). The applications of this robust unit are limited by its bulk. Apart from the choice of female units compatible with bonded gold to porcelain techniques or with yellow golds, there is also a choice of male sections for soldering to a metal framework (Fig. 157), or for burying in acrylic resin (Fig. 158).

The Stern gingival latch attachment (Fig. 159) offers a novel method of additional retention. The

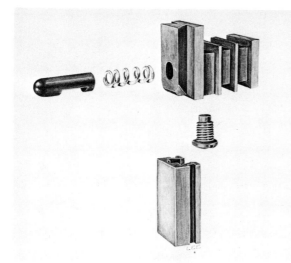

Fig. 158   The Schatzmann attachment incorporating a male section that can be retained by acrylic resin in the denture base.

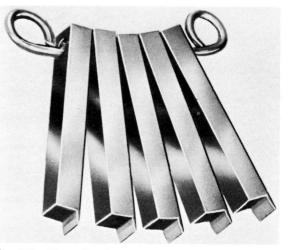

Fig. 160   The adjusting instrument for the Stern G/L attachment. The free ends are of varying thickness, and the male unit is adjusted by inserting the adjusting instruments in sequence until the retention desired is achieved.

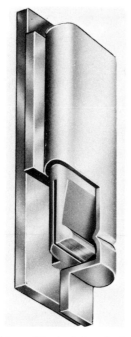

Fig. 159   The Stern Gingival Latch Attachment. The retention is adjusted by opening out the base of the male unit with a special instrument.

base of the male unit is split and formed in the shape of a door latch. The result is to provide a lock as the male slide is engaged. Adjustments for retention are made with a purpose-built tool (Fig. 160).

Two sizes of unit are produced, standard and miniature. One of the factors limiting the extent to which the male unit can be shortened is the height of the split. On the standard unit the split is 2·5 mm high, on the miniature unit only 1·5 mm high. The manufacturers claim this allows the standard unit to be shortened to 3·6 mm and the miniature unit to 2·62 mm. From the point of view of the retention mechanism this is obviously possible. However, the resistance to rotational forces is borne by the lateral surfaces of the attachment. Operators are therefore cautioned to think twice before reducing any intra-coronal attachment below 4 mm if unacceptable movement is to be avoided at a later date.

Other modifications of the G/L system include a unit with squared lateral surfaces thereby allowing the bucco-lingual dimensions to be reduced. This unit, known as the Micro, is among the smallest of intracoronal attachments with auxiliary retention.

The 'dovetail' and ES1 versions are modifications of the tagging of the male unit. The dovetail design simplifies soldering and is useful when the attachment is used in a 'split-pontic' mode. The ES1 features a long extension plate that simplifies electro-soldering the male to the denture framework. Alternatively the extension can be roughened to permit retention by the acrylic resin.

Before choosing an attachment with auxiliary retentive devices the following factors should be considered.

Bulk

Any retentive device requiring a larger female element is defeating its own purpose. The purpose of the device is to increase the retention available from a given box size. If a larger box is necessary a larger attachment would give better results; it would not only give more retention because of the greater frictional area, but it would also be stronger and provide greater stability to horizontal and rotational loads. The best retention devices are the simple ones, and generally their female elements are practically identical with a simple intracoronal attachment, except for a small recess. It should be remembered that these devices usually increase the retention, but seldom the bracing action, of the attachment.

The plunger or spring mechanism has to be incorporated within the male element. In a well-designed attachment the retention mechanism should not affect the cross-sectional size of the part engaging the female element.

Adjustment

The adjustment of any retentive device must be straightforward. Many retention devices are spring-activated and since it will be necessary to replace the springs at six-monthly or yearly intervals, easy access to the spring should be provided.

Retention mechanism

Most attachment breakages occur while they are being adjusted. Incorrect heat treatment during construction of the prosthesis may play a part, as may incorrect adjustment by the dental surgeon. However, it is also important to select a sturdy attachment and reduce even further the chances of accidental breakages. Any springs incorporated in the mechanism should be protected from impaction of food.

Trimming the attachment

It is sometimes necessary to shorten an attachment to accommodate it within a tooth. The retention device should work at least halfway down the attachment. If it engages near the occlusal surface it will be damaged as soon as the attachment is shortened.

Plaque control

The retentive mechanism should be straightforward to clean without nooks and crannies to complicate plaque removal.

FRICTION FIT INTRACORONAL ATTACHMENTS WITHOUT ADJUSTMENT POTENTIAL

Lack of adjustment potential renders this type of unit unsuitable for removable prostheses, as repeated insertion and removal will cause the attachment to wear. They are, however, useful for joining a series of crowns without a common path of insertion. Round profiles are useful where anterior teeth are concerned (Fig. 161), whereas the Beyeler attachment offers more frictional surface area (Fig. 162). Note that both units feature an external frictional flange.

APPLICATIONS OF INTRACORONAL ATTACHMENTS

Intracoronal attachments are among the most commonly used of all prefabricated attachments. A minimum of 4 mm vertical space is normally required and preferably 5 mm. Furthermore, almost as much bucco-lingual space is needed, while pulpal and anatomical considerations must allow the female section to be accommodated within the crown contour. Careful analysis of diagnostic casts is indicated as mistakes with space requirements can be extremely expensive to correct at later stages. The small tolerances of the attachments dictate precise clinical techniques and technical skill. Frequently overlooked is that they require a degree of manual dexterity on the part of the patient, as well. Intracoronal attachments are easily damaged by clumsy or careless patients. With these provisos, their many valuable applications can be considered under two headings.

1. Retainers

Intracoronal attachments are effective and almost invisible retainers for bilateral and unilateral prostheses.

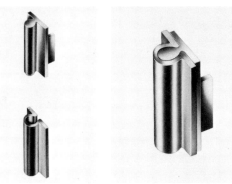

Fig. 161   The Interlock Attachment, useful for connecting anterior crowns.

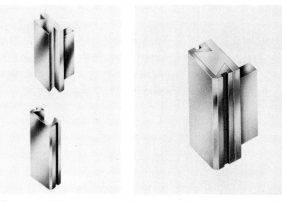

Fig. 162   The Beyeler Attachment, for use in posterior quadrants.

2. Connectors

Sections of a fixed prosthesis may be joined with intracoronal attachments. This possibility can be useful where:

(a) Prostheses do not share a common path of insertion yet can be connected rigidly in the mouth.

(b) The operator prefers to limit the length of individual castings while making a large span fixed prosthesis.

(c) The prognosis of a distal abutment is dubious. Connecting the posterior segment with an attachment allows its subsequent removal without damage to the main restoration. The attachment slot can be used for later construction of an attachment-retained denture.

REMOVABLE PARTIAL DENTURES FOR BOUNDED SPACES

Intracoronal attachments may be used to retain unilateral and bilateral dentures. For the purposes of description the two types of restoration will be discussed separately.

1. The bilateral denture

The major connector provides cross-arch support that contributes to the stability of the prosthesis. Horizontal displacing forces are resisted by the retainers of the opposite side, acting with a considerable mechanical advantage (Fig. 163).

When used for this type of prosthesis, an intracoronal attachment serves the functions of a clasp arm, occlusal rest, and bracing arm (Fig. 164). The relative merits of the two types of retainer should therefore be considered. The intracoronal attachment has the following advantages over the clasp retainer:

(a) Appearance

Since there is no need for buccal or labial clasp arms, the appearance is far better. This factor becomes particularly important in anterior parts of the mouth.

(b) Retention unaffected by crown contour

The intracoronal attachment provides excellent retention irrespective of the crown contour; a clasp arm can only provide retention if its free end is able to engage an area undercut to the path of insertion of the denture. The clinical crowns of canines and premolars in young patients may be virtually free of undercut, while aesthetic problems may preclude positioning a clasp arm to engage what little undercut may be present.

(c) Reduced bulk

Since an intracoronal attachment fits within the contour of a tooth crown yet serves the functions of an occlusal rest, clasp arm, and bracing arm, there is a considerable reduction in the bulk of the prosthesis.

(d) Stability

Intracoronal attachments provide good resistance to horizontally inclined or rotational displacing forces. This stability can be augmented by a palatal bracing

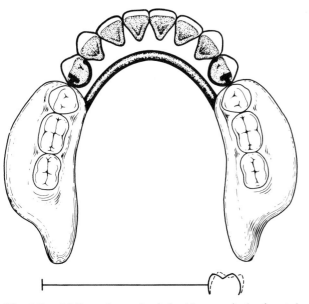

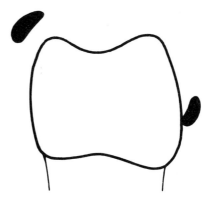

Fig. 165 When a clasp-retained partial denture is inserted, the clasps have to be deformed before they engage the undercut. If this occurs before the bracing arm engages the tooth, lateral tilting loads will be applied.

Fig. 163 A bilateral prosthesis is able to resist horizontal loads between the teeth and mucosa of both sides, while rotational loads applied to one side are resisted by the retainers of the opposite side acting with the mechanical advantage of the width of the arch.

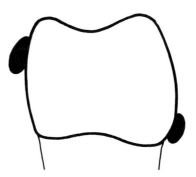

Fig. 166 In theory, tilting of the abutment teeth could be caused by a badly made clasp retainer, as the bracing arm is seldom at the same height as the clasp arm.

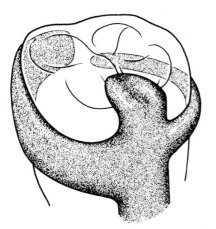

Fig. 164 An intracoronal attachment serves the function of a retaining arm, occlusal rest, and bracing arm.

arm constructed to fit within the contour of a tooth. In comparison, rigid bracing arms of a partial denture would be bulky.

(e) Elimination of food stagnation

Complex designs of clasps, especially those used on posterior teeth, may lead to food stagnation, gingival irritation, and caries. The elimination of this potential source of trouble is a major advantage.

(f) Stresses on abutment teeth minimised

When a clasp-retained partial denture is inserted, the clasps have to be deformed until they engage the undercut (Fig. 165). During deformation they apply lateral loads to the clasped teeth, whereas an attachment should slide into place without this lateral stress. Provided the clasp has been correctly designed and constructed the advantage possessed by an attachment in this respect is theoretical rather than real.

Some authorities feel that a clasp may cause rotation of the teeth, since it is not always possible to apply a 'reciprocal' at the same level as the clasp (Fig. 166). The term 'reciprocal' is misleading, since the clasp should be passive while at rest and should only become active when the denture is displaced. Convincing clinical evidence of this type of mishap has not been presented, but there is no possibility of it occurring if an intracoronal attachment has been used.

To summarise, intracoronal attachments can be used to provide a well-retained and stable partial denture with the minimum of bulk and with no clasp arms to mar appearance. However, the use of these attachments has some drawbacks and these should be considered as well.

(a) Extensive preparation of abutment teeth required

Intracoronal attachments require extensive preparation of all the abutment teeth and their neighbours. This is probably their greatest disadvantage. Most clasp-retained partial dentures require only reshaping of the occlusal surfaces or recontouring of proximal surfaces.

(b) Cost and time

It takes considerable chairside time to carry out the procedures involved in making an appliance with intracoronal attachments, and even more laboratory time. This extra expenditure of time and materials must be reflected in the cost; the cost of the actual attachments themselves is comparatively small.

(c) Crown length and pulp size

Intracoronal attachments require a minimum of 4 mm vertical space. Since they need to be recessed within the crown contour, extensive preparation of the abutment tooth is required. Where bucco-lingual room is restricted, or the pulps are large, there may be inadequate space available for the attachment. Occasionally, a cantilevered pontic can be employed, but the occlusal load and its distribution then requires considerable attention.

(d) Difficulty

Constructing an attachment-retained denture requires no skills other than those employed in the fields of fixed and removable partial prostheses; however, it does show up small errors and requires careful planning of the treatment.

(e) Handling by the patient

Prostheses retained by intracoronal attachments require some manual dexterity by the patient. Arthritic patients with restricted finger movements would find them difficult to manipulate. Neither are they suitable for patients suspected of being clumsy or careless.

Intracoronal attachments are by no means substitutes for all conventional clasp units. If employed carefully, they can provide a prosthesis combining many of the advantages of a fixed and of a removable prosthesis.

2. The unilateral denture

A unilateral denture can be made when the teeth on either side of the space can be made into sufficiently strong abutments. The problem then resolves itself into one of anchoring the prosthesis to the teeth.

The unilateral, clasp-retained 'side-plate' partial denture requires undercut on both lingual and buccal aspects of the teeth. The retention and stability of this type of prosthesis frequently cannot resist the displacing forces to which it will be subjected, so that the hazard of the patient inhaling or swallowing the denture must be taken into account. If a clasp-retained denture is to be made, it usually requires support from more than one quadrant of the mouth; a major connector should therefore be incorporated.

The fixed prosthesis is usually the restoration of choice for restoring small gaps. However, where a flange is necessary for appearance or support, a removable prosthesis has much to offer. It is here that intracoronal attachments are useful, allowing the construction of a small, rigid and well-retained prosthesis removable by the patient (Fig. 167).

Although the attachment-retained prosthesis has a superficial resemblance to the fixed prosthesis, the principles involved in the construction differ. A fixed bridge is one solid structure and requires all the abutment preparations to be mutually aligned. It may be necessary to devitalise teeth and use telescopic crown procedures, but once inserted it locks all the abutments together and has only to resist the occlusal loads applied to the structure.

An apparently similar attachment-retained prosthesis consists of three basic units; a removable section, and the two groups of abutments on either side (Fig. 168). While the attachments must be aligned with precision, the paths of insertion of the two groups of crowns and that of the removable prosthesis may differ. A slight divergence between the various paths of insertion can be helpful, in fact, for the abutment crowns have to resist not only the occlusal forces, but the considerable displacing forces exerted when the prosthesis is removed. The retention available for the prosthesis is governed in the end by the retention of the abutment preparations, while the size of the attachments is determined by the size of the boxes that can be cut into the abutments adjacent to the gap.

Once the prosthesis is made removable, the

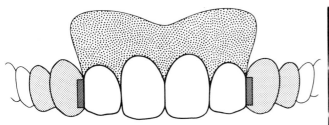

Fig. 167 Where bone loss needs to be replaced with artificial mucosa, intracoronal attachments allow the construction of a small, rigid, and well-retained prosthesis.

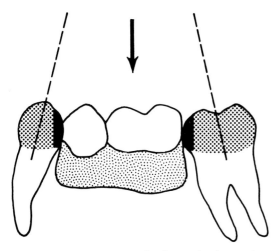

Fig. 168 An attachment-retained prosthesis consists of three basic units; a removable section and the two groups of abutments either side.

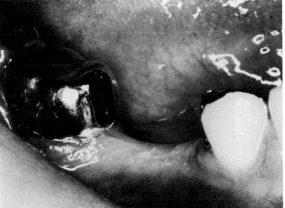

Fig. 169 An example of poor treatment planning. The prosthesis was loose due to lack of retention from the short anterior attachment. Furthermore, the projection of the attachment led to considerable gingival damage.

mucosal coverage can be treated as a partial denture flange. The flange may contribute to the support of the prosthesis and can be rebased should further resorption occur. The ability to remove the prosthesis naturally simplifies plaque control.

The main problem posed by intracoronal attachments in the anterior quadrant of the mouth is that of finding space for the female section within the contour of the abutment teeth. Devitalisation may help, but not always. For example some lateral incisors cannot accommodate the bulk of an intracoronal attachment even when devitalized. An intracoronal attachment may be placed closer to the centre of a non-vital tooth, but if the crown has insufficient buccolingual space the attachment still cannot be employed. Over-contouring crowns, or leaving the female section projecting, results in several problems (Fig. 169). The appearance will be poor, and the attachment may be shortened to such an extent that the retention may then be unsatis-

factory. The projection at the gingival margin, together with the poor gingival contour, is likely to lead to periodontal damage.

Where adequate crown bulk exists, intracoronal attachments are neat and effective retainers. They are usually simpler to employ with older patients whose clinical crowns are longer and whose pulps are smaller.

Posteriorly, it is easier to find room for the attachments. As with anterior restorations, the great advantage of the attachment-retained prosthesis rests with the fact that the removable part can be treated as a partial denture. Wide mucosal coverage is, therefore, possible; it has considerable hygiene advantages, and facings on artificial teeth can be replaced in the laboratory. On the other hand, the splinting action between the two groups of abutments is never quite as effective as that exerted by a one-piece restoration.

Unilateral attachment-retained prostheses may be employed to restore many types of gaps (Figs. 170–172). However, there must be a definite reason for making a restoration removable, and every advantage then taken of this facility.

REMOVABLE DISTAL EXTENSION PARTIAL DENTURES

The relative merits of intracoronal attachments and clasp arms as retainers have already been discussed. The excellent retention and stability provided by the precise path of insertion of the attachment is particularly valuable in the case of distal extension prostheses. Intracoronal attachments provide a neat

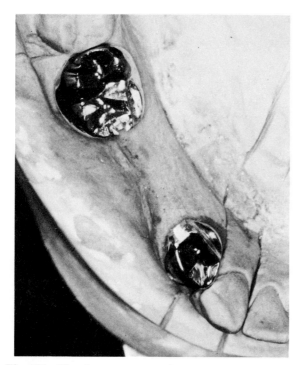

Fig. 170   The abutment restorations remade. Note lingual steps in the crowns, prepared for bracing arms of the removable section.

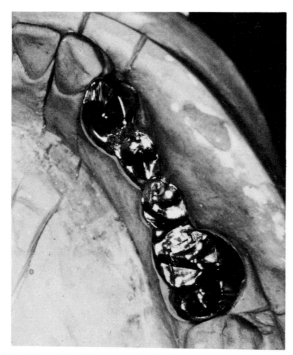

Fig. 171   Metal framework of the removable section in place.

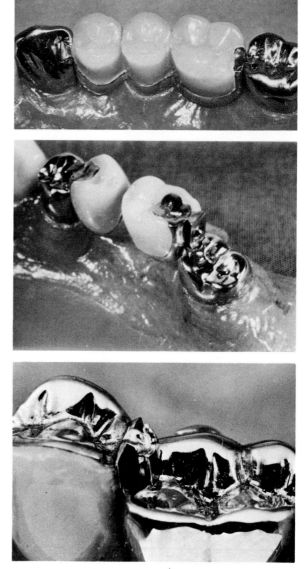

Fig. 172   Three examples of unilateral attachment-retained prostheses.

and rigid junction between the denture and abutment crowns. They are the attachment of choice whenever they can be used. It is essential, however, that the design and construction of the denture reduces to a minimum forces applied to the attachment and to the abutment teeth.

No matter how carefully the denture is designed, intracoronal attachments used to retain distal extension dentures are subjected to considerable forces. Strong attachments should be selected and used in conjunction with lingual bracing arms (Figs. 173,

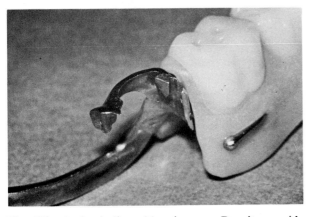

Fig. 173 A simple lingual bracing arm. Despite considerable wear of the home-made attachment the denture remained stable and well-retained.

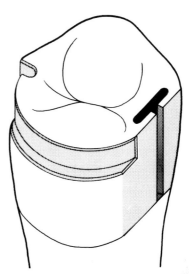

Fig. 176 Lingual space requirements can be reduced by making the step near to the occlusal surface and carrying a skirt of metal to the full depth of the attachment.

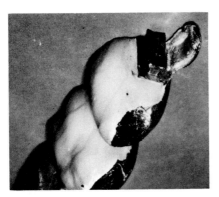

Fig. 174 A lingual bracing arm with its vertical wall aligned with the lateral surfaces of the attachment. The example illustrated is connecting two sections of a fixed prosthesis.

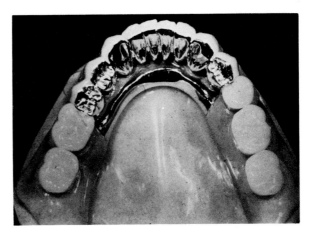

Fig. 177 Splinting all the remaining teeth forms a rigid abutment. This arrangement is usually necessary where seven or fewer anterior teeth remain.

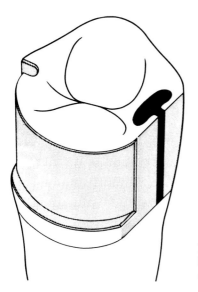

Fig. 175 The lingual bracing arm should be the same height as the attachment and carried around to the opposite proximal space.

174). The lingual bracing arm reduces the loads to which the attachment is subjected, thereby minimising wear. Where possible the arm should be the same height as the attachment and carried around to the opposite proximal space (Fig. 175). This arm not only adds to the stability of the prosthesis but also provides the patient with a handling point to aid removal and insertion of the denture. Additional lingual tooth reduction is necessary to accommodate this arm. Where lingual space is restricted, the step can be placed near the occlusal surface and a narrow skirt of metal carried down the lingual surface of the crown (Fig. 176).

Distal extension prostheses require a minimum of two splinted abutment teeth on either side. Where there are seven or fewer anterior teeth remaining it is necessary to splint them all together to form one rigid abutment (Fig. 177).

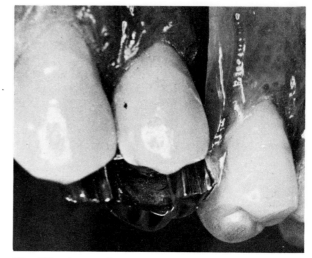

Fig. 178   An attachment-retained denture being inserted.

PROSTHESES FOR BILATERAL DISTAL EXTENSION SPACES

Intracoronal attachments may be used to provide a well-retained and stable prosthesis without visible buccal or labial retainers. They are particularly useful where several anterior teeth as clasp retainers might be ineffective and unsightly in these situations. The additional space normally available in upper teeth makes them more useful intracoronal abutments (Fig. 178). Devitalising canines, or other teeth for that matter, may allow the attachment to be placed closer to the centre of the tooth but will be of no avail if there is inadequate labio-lingual space. While intracoronal attachments can be employed to retain many different types of bilateral distal extension prostheses, the limiting factor must always be the provision of adequate abutments with sufficient vertical and bucco-lingual space (Fig. 179).

Where there is insufficient room within the most distal abutment for the attachment, an artificial tooth can be cantilevered from it to carry the attachment (Fig. 180). This arrangement has considerable advantages, for the attachment does not interfere with the contour of the abutment crowns, no box preparation is required in the abutment teeth, and the maximum length and size of attachment can be used (Fig. 181). For these reasons, many experienced operators prefer the method, especially as there can be no question of the denture or attachment damaging the distal gingival papilla of the abutment tooth.

The cantilevered extension can result in considerable torques falling upon the abutments so that the

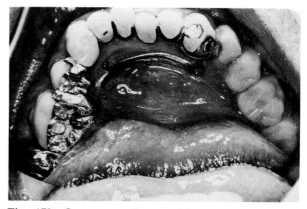

Fig. 179   Over-contouring resulting from attempts to employ intracoronal attachments where inadequate buccolingual space exists.

total load and its distribution requires careful assessment. The hazards of damaging forces applied to the abutments are increased if the prosthesis is opposed by natural teeth.

The loads applied by the denture to the teeth are transmitted through the attachments now positioned at right angles to the way in which many were designed to function. Most prefabricated attachments work perfectly well in this position, but it is wise practice to protect their lateral surfaces with a component of the denture framework.

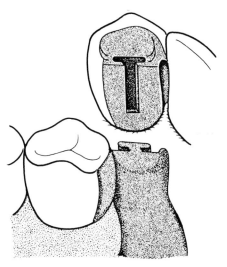

Fig. 180 Where there is insufficient space for an attachment within an abutment tooth, an artificial tooth can be cantilevered from the splinted abutments.

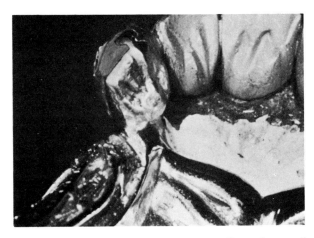

Fig. 181 This cantilevered arrangement allows the use of maximum length and size of attachment, and yet does not interfere with the contour and gingival margins of the distal abutment tooth.

PROSTHESES FOR UNILATERAL DISTAL EXTENSION SPACES

A distal extension prosthesis requires support from both sides of the jaw, even if the gap to be restored is only on one side. In view of the extensive tooth preparation required for attachment prostheses, the relative merits of a clasp-retained denture should be considered. An attachment-retained denture to replace the gaps shown in Fig. 182 would require

crown preparations on a minimum of four teeth, and probably more. It is doubtful, in this instance, if the retention and stability achieved for the prosthesis would be significantly greater than that for a correctly designed clasp-retained denture.

On the other hand, advantage can be taken of attachments when extensive restoration of the abutments is necessary. Where there is a space on the opposite side, the denture can gain support from an attachment placed bucco-lingually in a fixed prosthesis restoring the gap (Fig. 183).

The advantages of restoring the jaw in this way, compared with the alternative method of replacing the spaces either side with the denture have been discussed in a previous chapter. The fixed prosthesis unites its mesial and distal abutments, allowing the positioning of a generous sized attachment in the pontic (Figs. 184–187). Only two attachments need to be aligned, and box or wide shoulder preparations are necessary on the side to be restored with the fixed restoration.

The attachment and associated bracing components forms an extremely neat and effective retainer (Figs. 188, 189). Since intracoronal attachments cannot be rocked or rotated out of place, removal of the denture could be extremely difficult as there is so little purchase available. An additional handling point should be provided, preferably in line with the attachment (Fig. 190).

It might be tempting to shorten the major connector by connecting it to the mesial section of the bracing components, rather than to the attachment itself. Unfortunately, this results in an increased bucco-lingual bulk of the restoration while the handling aid for the patient is malaligned with the attachment (Fig. 191).

Lower anterior teeth seldom possess adequate labio-lingual space for intracoronal attachments. In order to accommodate such a unit, even a non-vital lower canine may need to be overcontoured to resemble a premolar together with lingual cusp (Fig. 192). This arrangement is obviously far from satisfactory. Where sufficient abutments and vertical space are present a cantilevered extension may be used, otherwise another retaining system should be selected.

Where no space exists on the opposite side of the jaw, the denture may be joined to the teeth of that side by means of telescopic crowns (Figs. 193–196). Some form of indirect retainer should be incorporated where possible. Intracoronal attachments placed between the teeth are seldom satisfactory as they encroach upon the gingivae, while clasps placed around the teeth and used in conjunction with

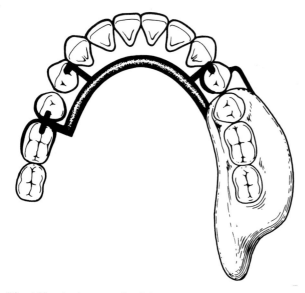

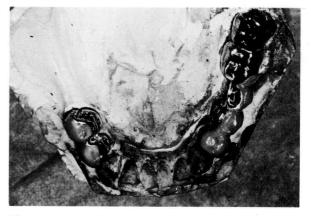

Fig. 184 Bucco-lingual positioning of the attachment in the pontic allows the use of a generous sized attachment and simplifies alignment of the retainers.

Fig. 182 A clasp-retained denture may be preferable for some unilateral spaces. The extensive tooth preparation required for an attachment-retained prosthesis may not be offset by its marginal advantages in retention and stability.

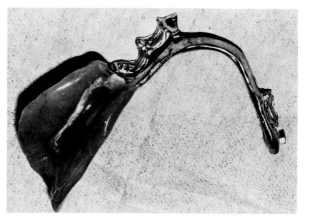

Fig. 185 The removable section of the prosthesis. Note the attachment and additional bracing component.

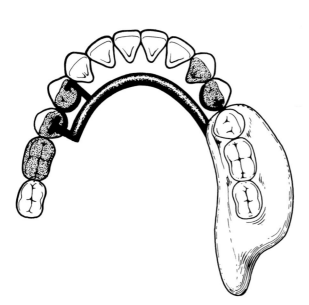

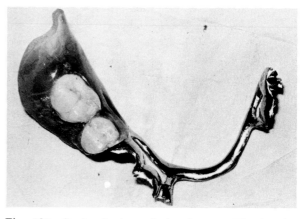

Fig. 183 Where there is a space on the opposite side to the distal extension base, the denture can gain support from an attachment placed bucco-lingually in a bridge restoring the gap.

Fig. 186 Occlusal view of the denture. The bracing components act as handling points to aid removal and insertion of the prosthesis.

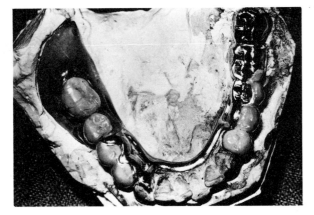

Fig. 187 The assembled prosthesis on the master cast.

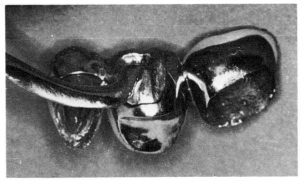

Fig. 190 Attachment seated. Note depression above the attachment to facilitate withdrawal along its path of insertion.

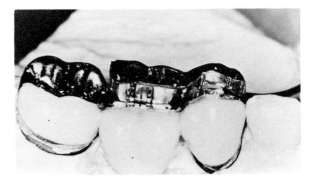

Fig. 188 Crismani attachment and associated bracing components being inserted into the pontic.

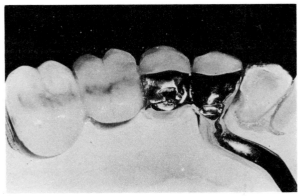

Fig. 191 Joining the major connector to the bracing components, rather than to the attachment, increases the bucco-lingual bulk of the restoration and places the handling aid out of alignment with the attachment.

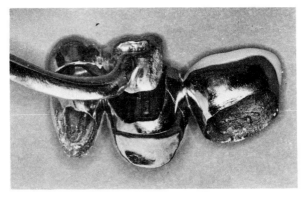

Fig. 189 Lingual view.

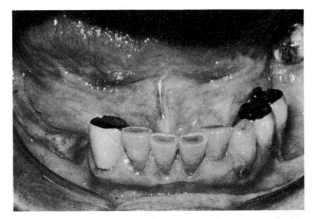

Fig. 192 The lower canine is usually an unsuitable abutment tooth for an intracoronal attachment. To gain sufficient room for the attachment it is frequently necessary to build up the crown to resemble a premolar.

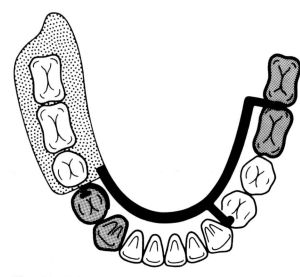

Fig. 193   Where no space exists on the opposite side of the jaw to the distal extension space, telescopic crowns may be employed to join the denture to these teeth.

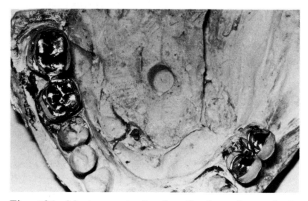

Fig. 194   Master cast showing fixed sections of the prosthesis.

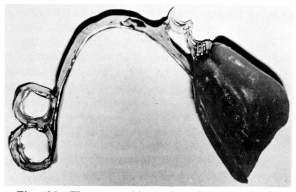

Fig. 195   The removable section of the prosthesis.

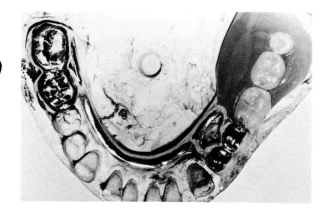

Fig. 196   The assembled restoration on the master cast.

attachments on the other side of the jaw frequently lead to unfavourable load distribution and damage.

The principles involved in the construction of a distal extension denture are the same, be it retained by clasps or by an attachment system. The clinical application of these principles may differ slightly, and they are described in the relevant sections.

CONNECTORS

Intracoronal attachments can be employed to join sections of a fixed prosthesis. A distinction must be made between instances where the operator employs attachments to limit the length of individual castings or connect abutments without a common path of insertion and those in which he may be faced with constructing a partial denture at a later date.

Where the restoration is to remain fixed, the attachments will not be subjected to the constant wear and tear of removal and insertion. Comparatively small units can be selected as subsequent adjustments will be unnecessary. If there is a possibility of replacing a distal section with a partial denture, provision should be made for an attachment of adequate strength and a bracing arm.

Suppose a misalignment of abutments on the master cast is discovered in the laboratory. Splitting the casting and connecting the two sections in the mouth with an attachment might save the day. But where is the attachment to be placed? Long clinical crowns and good fortune might provide adequate space. Otherwise one is faced with repreparing several of the teeth and a new impression. It is obviously far better to plan the restoration on diagnostic casts, assess the alignment of teeth and

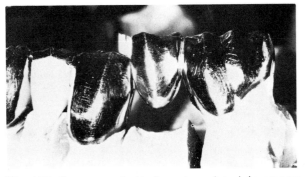

Fig. 197 Intracoronal attachment used to join crowns without a common path of insertion.

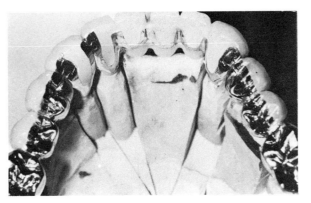

Fig. 200 Prosthesis assembled on the master cast.

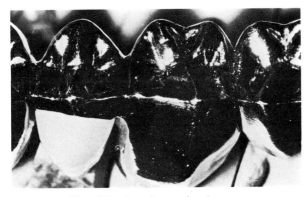

Fig. 198 Attachment in place.

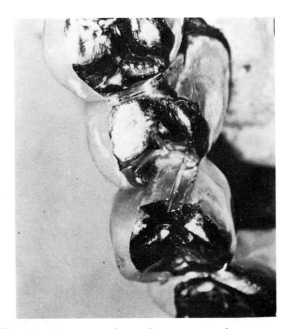

Fig. 201 Intracoronal attachment connecting two sections of the prosthesis. Parallel-sided units of adequate size must be employed to prevent play.

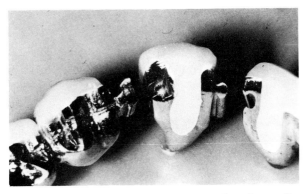

Fig. 199 Intracoronal attachments employed to split a large bonded porcelain to gold restoration into small sections.

design the preparation to include sufficient vertical and adjacent proximal space for the attachment, the neck of which will cross this proximal area. There must be adequate room for plaque control. Where teeth are missing it is possible to place the connection in a pontic.

If attachments are employed, the crown preparations can be aligned in groups, and these groups of crowns then joined with intracoronal attachments. Ideally, the attachments should be sited distally in teeth. The groups of crowns are inserted separately and interlock in the mouth with intracoronal attachments (Figs. 197, 198). Assembling the prosthesis in this manner may avoid devitalisation of several teeth. It allows a large prosthesis to be assembled from comparatively small castings, preferred by some when porcelain fused to gold is employed (Figs. 199, 200). Others claim that there is some physiological advantage in constructions of this

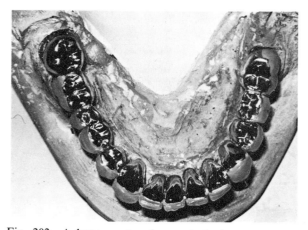

Fig. 202   A lower restoration made in four connected sections due to malalignment of the abutments.

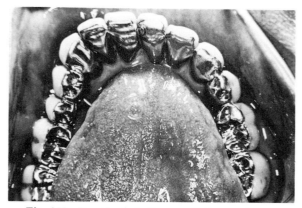

Fig. 203   Prosthesis in the mouth 9 years later.

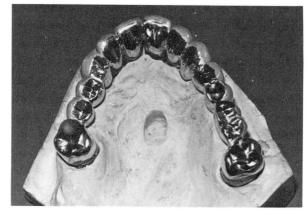

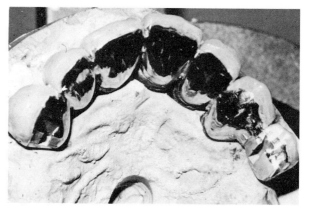

Fig. 204   The anterior teeth are splinted and joined to the posterior sections with intracoronal attachments. Following loss of the molars, a bilateral distal extension denture retained by attachments can be constructed.

nature. While this point is questionable, there is little doubt that a one-piece casting is more rigid and many operators would prefer to make their fixed prostheses in this way when circumstances permit.

Figure 201 shows an example of an intracoronal attachment used to join two sections of a prosthesis. Placement of the attachment requires some care if the proximal space is not to be restricted. To prevent play between the connected sections a parallel-sided unit of adequate dimensions must be selected. Where space permits, a bracing arm should be incorporated as well. Figures 202 and 203 show the principle applied to a lower prosthesis where malalignment of the teeth dictated the use of four attachments.

When the prognosis of a bridge abutment is dubious, the segment of the prosthesis carried by this abutment can be joined to the main part of the structure with intracoronal attachments. Provision should be made for a bracing arm. Should the

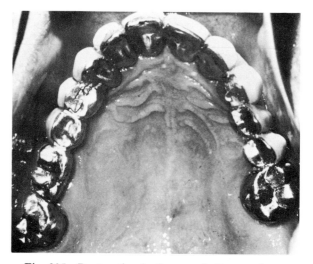

Fig. 205   Restoration in the mouth 10 years later.

abutment be lost subsequently, it can be replaced with an attachment-retained denture. When considering the possibility of a future bilateral denture, the attachments each side must not only be sturdy but they must be aligned with each other. Cantilevered pontics, at least on one side, can be used in some of these situations (Figs. 204, 205).

There are many other situations where this flexible treatment planning can be useful. Although the male section can be easily removed from the female unit, the female unit cannot be removed with the male section in place. This is because the female slot has a base and is only open at the occlusal surface. It is, therefore, vital to ensure that the prosthesis and restorations are planned so that the male part of the attachment is joined to the section of the prosthesis carried by the dubious abutment.

No matter how rigid intracoronal attachments may appear to be a small degree of play is inevitable, particularly after they have been used a while. The length of span must be considered when connecting it to another section of a prosthesis. Take for example a first molar distally displaced and connect it with a fixed prosthesis to an attachment distal in the canine. After a period of months the patient is likely to complain that the prosthesis moves slightly and on examination a minute degree of play will be found. For the sake of argument, assume the span of the prosthesis to be 30 mm. Just 1 degree of play in the attachment will allow movement of 0·5 mm of the distal section. In practice, the reverse appears to be the case with the pontics effectively cantilevered from the molar until the minute play is taken up. Incorporating a bracing arm will prevent this complication. Alternatively, the attachment can be placed distally, or bucco-lingually, in a cantilevered pontic thereby reducing the length of span of the distal section.

Intracoronal attachments therefore allow a considerable flexibility in treatment planning. Demanding upon both operator and technician they cannot be employed in a haphazard manner. Nevertheless, their popularity shows just how many are prepared to take the time and trouble to ensure they are employed in a correct manner.

THE CHANNEL SHOULDER PIN SYSTEM

If a design study were undertaken to improve the retention and stability of a conventional intracoronal attachment and lingual bracing arm, it would probably result in the development of something resembling the Channel Shoulder Pin system (CSP). This technique was originally developed by Steiger and is admirably described in his book (Steiger and Boitel, 1959). This design gives a remarkably firm bracing action and resistance to rotational displacing forces. The removable section is retained primarily by a series of parallel-sided pins, secondarily by the vertical surfaces of the unit, and is guided into place by retention grooves (Figs. 206–210). The clinical procedures place special emphasis on impression techniques, methods of location, and jaw relation records, for not only must the two sections interlock with precision, but the occlusal surfaces must be accurate. The difficulty of making occlusal adjustments to the sections of the crown covered by the removable part of the attachment should be borne in mind. Both parts of the attachment have to be produced in the laboratory and the processes are exacting. Unlike most attachment work, a rigid surveyor will not suffice for these techniques which require precise milling facilities. Examples of two popular models of milling machines combined with surveyors are illustrated (Figs. 211, 212). While the CSP system gives excellent results, it can only be recommended when both operator and technician have had experience with other types of attachment.

The multiple parallel-sided pins, together with the

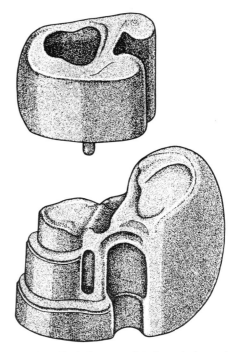

Fig. 206 Simplified diagram of C.S.P. design. The small round holes are for drainage of the pin holes. This design provides excellent retention and stability.

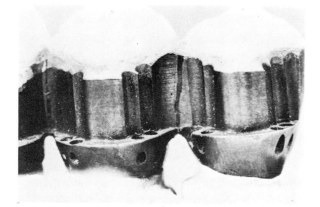

Fig. 207 Lingual view of C.S.P. type units showing drainage channels.

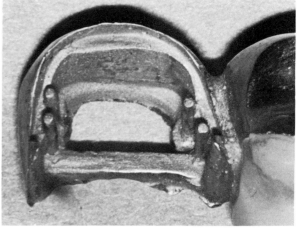

Fig. 209 The removable section, showing four parallel-sided pins and two guiding grooves.

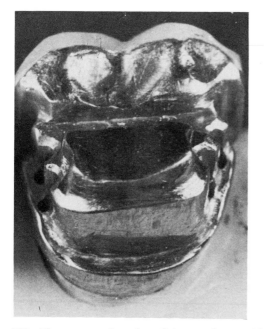

Fig. 208 The cemented section of the attachment. Note the large areas for contact in both the horizontal and vertical plane.

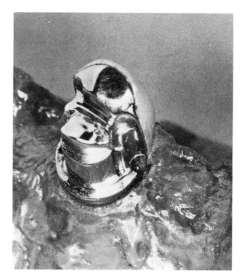

Fig. 210 Another example of the C.S.P. principle.

other frictional surfaces used in this technique, have a much greater frictional surface area than an intracoronal attachment of equivalent length. The CSP system, or modifications of it, can therefore be used, albeit with some difficulty, where lack of vertical space would preclude the use of other types of attachment. Figures 213–216 show an example of a modified CSP principle where the vertical space available for an attachment was particularly limited.

The Channel Shoulder Pin system works equally well for lower restorations and Figs. 217–220 show examples.

A major problem of maintenance is a bent pin, for the actual culprit has to be identified and straightened or removed before the restoration can be placed in the mouth. It is apparent that this retainer is not suitable for clumsy patients or those with a tendency to make their own adjustments! A broken pin is easier to repair. A small hole is drilled through the gold over the pin in question and a new one inserted through the seated denture into the hole in the crown. The pin is then connected with resin,

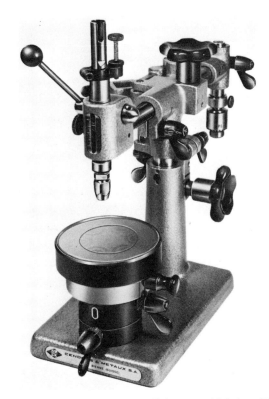

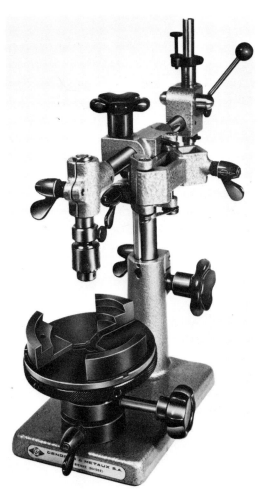

Fig. 211   The Bachmann Parallelometer (right) and Milling Instrument (above).

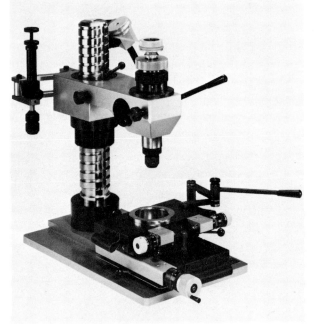

Fig. 212   The MP.2000 parallelometer.

preferably Duralay, and the denture removed from the mouth and handed to the laboratory.

Due to the problem of construction many operators have devised their own simplified versions of the CSP system. Where there is adequate crown height one can dispense with the pins, relying on the parallel surfaces, grooves and shoulders to give stability and retention. Once the principles of the CSP design and construction have been mastered, the operator is free to design his own retainer according to the needs and space available for each retainer. There is certainly no merit in complexity for complexity's sake.

A far simpler laboratory-produced attachment is shown in Fig. 221. The outer layer slides over the inner section and is supported by a shoulder running around the gingival portion of the inner layer. Parallel retention grooves add to the frictional

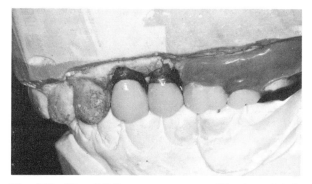

Fig. 213   The C.S.P. system or a modification of it is particularly useful where lack of vertical space precludes the use of other attachments.

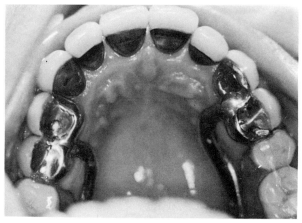

Fig. 216   The restoration in the mouth.

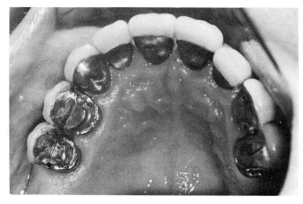

Fig. 214   Occlusal view of the restoration.

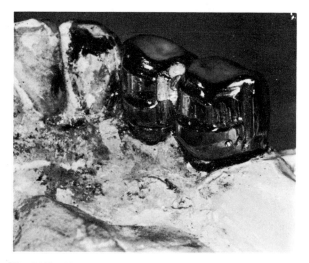

Fig. 217   Channel Shoulder Pin on two lower premolars. Note the vents to allow the removal of debris from the retention holes. The guiding groove is clearly visible.

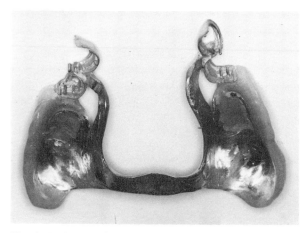

Fig. 215   Impression surface of the denture to show the retention pins within the attachments. The modification of the C.S.P. technique was dictated by lack of space and the position of the opposing cusps.

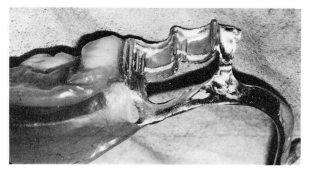

Fig. 218   The removable section of the prosthesis, showing the long, slightly tapered, guide and the shorter parallel-sided retaining pins.

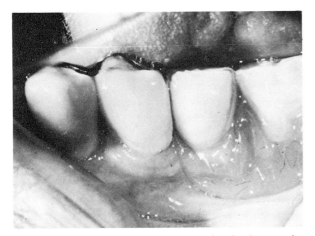

Fig. 219   Mirror view of the restoration in the mouth.

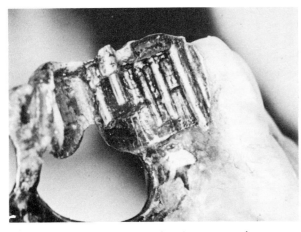

Fig. 220   C.S.P. unit after 9 years service.

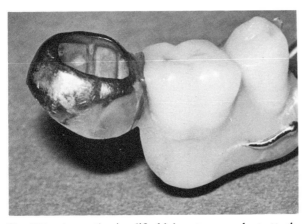

Fig. 221   A greatly simplified laboratory-product attachment which works well, provided there is sufficient vertical space available.

surface and, although the efficiency of the device cannot match that of the CSP type of assembly, it is considerably easier to produce.

THE SEMI-PRECISION REST

A semi-precision rest can be considered as an intracoronal attachment with tapered sides. Like a precision attachment it provides occlusal support, but the bracing action may be less and it cannot be relied upon by itself to produce adequate retention.

When an abutment tooth is to be crowned, guide planes can be incorporated on the proximal surface. Furthermore, the rest seat can be deepened and contoured to the operator's requirements (Fig. 222). As the rest seat is deepened, the ability to transmit lateral forces is increased until the bracing action may be considerable. In these circumstances it is

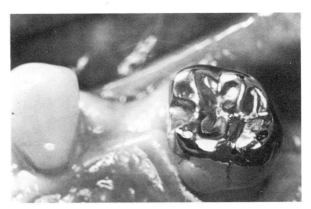

Fig. 222   A simple occlusal rest seat. Note the prepared guide plane.

possible to dispense with a bracing arm and to construct a unit consisting of a rest and a retaining arm (Figs. 223, 224).

While the components resemble those of an intracoronal attachment and bracing arm, in principle their roles are reversed. Unlike the precision attachment, it is the arm that provides the retention and the semi-precision rest the bracing action. In practice, of course, the functions are by no means separated. There are operators who prefer to make comparatively rigid bracing arms with semi-precision rests. The results are perfectly satisfactory although adjustments are difficult and the restoration unnecessarily complex. Semi-precision retainers are comparatively neat and simple to employ. They are usually more economical than their precision counterparts yet allow the construction of an effective, good-looking restoration without buccal arms to mar the appearance (Figs. 225–227).

Semi-precision rests may be carved in wax with the aid of a surveyor and then produced in the laboratory. Alternatively, preformed resin patterns may be purchased that are incorporated in the waxed up crown and subsequently burnt out with the wax (Fig. 228). The male section of the unit is normally cast as part of the framework of the removable prosthesis. A lingual arm is essential (Figs. 229, 230). These attachments can also be placed bucco-lingually in a pontic in a similar manner to other intracoronal attachments (Fig. 231).

The design and positioning of the occlusal rest influence the functions it will serve. Blatterfein (1969) has suggested that the design be considered from four aspects, proximal form, occlusal form, gingival floor form, and proximal surface placement.

The depth and taper of the rest seats are important considerations of the proximal form (Fig. 232). If some measure of retention together with bracing action is required, the rest seat depth should not be less than 3 mm and the convergence of the lateral walls should not exceed 5°. Increasing the angle of convergence of the walls facilitates insertion and removal of the prosthesis, but decreases the bracing and retentive action of the unit. These properties are rapidly reduced as the rest seat depth increases.

The occlusal outline is basically rectangular (Fig. 233). For strength and ease of manufacture, a neck width of not appreciably less than 3 mm is recommended, unless a prefabricated unit is employed. A rectangular shape does not resist displacement of the prosthesis away from the abutment tooth (Fig. 234). When semi-precision rests are placed either side of a bounded space this problem is of no significance. Where distal extension prostheses are concerned it does mean that a rigid component of the framework must resist this movement. Relying on a flexible lingual retainer to resist distal displacement would be foolhardy.

A preformed pattern with inclined walls has apparent advantages where distal extension prostheses are concerned. Circular or dovetail forms may be used.

Inclined and chanelled floors provide additional resistance to displacement. However, it must be appreciated that they complicate construction and cleaning (Fig. 235).

Retention is provided by the lingual arm, usually engaging a dimple on the lingual surface of the

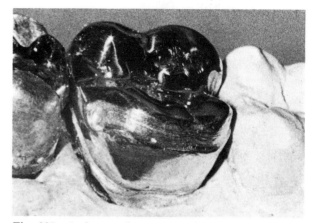

Fig. 223 A deepened rest seat with a lingual retaining arm. The depression at the mesial section of the arm is clearly visible.

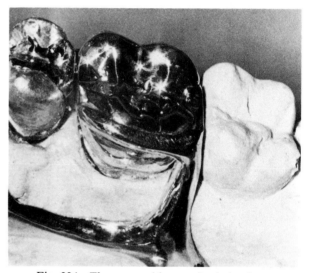

Fig. 224 The removable prosthesis in place.

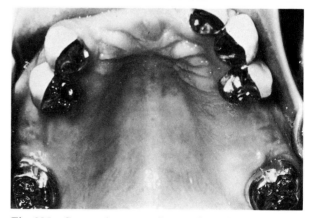

Fig. 225 Crowns incorporating semi-precision retainers.

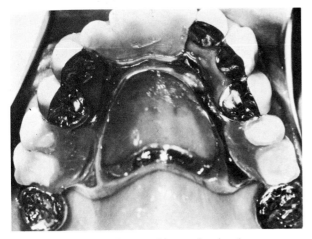

Fig. 226   Removable section in place.

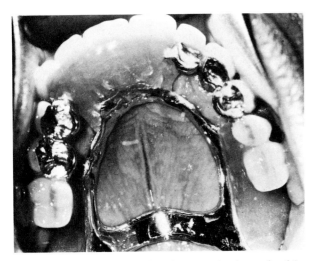

Fig. 227   Another example of a prosthesis retained by semi-precision attachments. Note absence of buccal retainers.

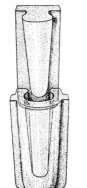

Fig. 228   The Stern resin pattern for a semi-precision attachment.

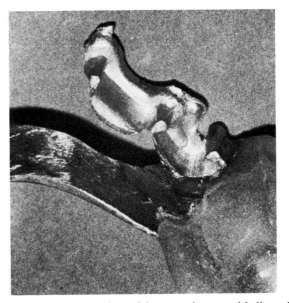

Fig. 229   Stern semi-precision attachment with lingual bracing arm.

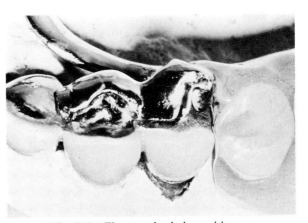

Fig. 230   The prosthesis in position.

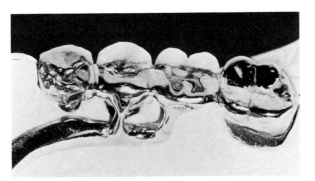

Fig. 231   Stern semi-precision retainer placed bucco-lingually in a pontic with associated bracing components.

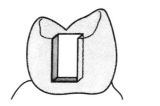 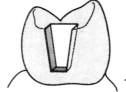

Fig. 232 Depth and taper of the rest seats influence the retention and bracing action obtained. Convergence of more than 5° significantly reduces the retention obtainable from the lateral walls of the box.

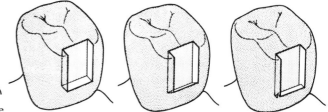

Fig. 235 A flat gingival floor is normally recommended. Inclined or channelled floors may improve the resistance to displacement but are difficult to produce and clean.

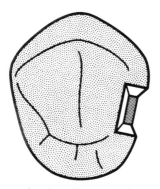

Fig. 233 The occlusal outline is basically rectangular. For strength and ease of manufacture a neck width of not less than 3 mm is recommended.

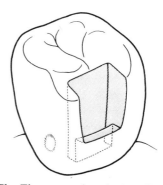

Fig. 236 The Thompson dowel. A well tried laboratory produced unit that enjoys popularity after more than four decades of use.

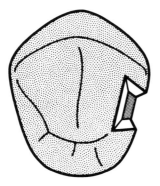

Fig. 234 Dovetail designs resist movement of the denture away from the tooth. They are desirable features of the preformed patterns, but complicate the construction of laboratory-produced units.

crown. The free end of the arm must therefore be flexible, although the arm will be rigid near its origin. The arm then contributes to the stability of the prosthesis and helps prevent wear of the rest.

The Thompson dowel semi-precision intracoronal retainer is an excellent example of a unit that enjoys popularity after more than four decades of use

(Fig. 236). Koper (1973) and McLeod (1977) have analysed the unit in some detail. Apart from support and bracing, a small degree of hinge potential is provided. Movement in the opposite direction is prevented by components acting as indirect retainers such as the distal wall of the gingival well below the shelf and the occlusal part of the axial wall above the shelf. Retention is provided by a minor connector engaging a dimple on the lingual aspect of the crown. Koper, Knowles and McLeod, have pointed out that Thompson was not entirely correct in assuming that the axis of hinge movement was the mid-well area of the dowel. It is more likely to be in line with the inner shelf line of the retaining abutment. However, there is another point that should be considered. The design of this unit goes back to the days when considerable hinge movement was felt desirable. For this reason, the retaining dimple was placed in line with the dowel, or rest seat. Had this not been done, the retaining arm would have jumped out of its dimple each time load was applied to the denture base.

Placing the dimple in line with the rest seat introduces a complication. How do you obtain a flexible arm that runs into the dimple adjacent to the rest seat? The normal solution was to employ a split lingual connector. This type of connector, particularly in lower restorations, has proved awkward to produce, difficult to clean, and prone to fracture.

Nowadays a well-made denture should have only the slightest tendency to move under load, and so there appears little drawback to placing the dimple away from the rest. The dimple can then be engaged by a simple flexible arm originating from the rest. Construction and subsequent maintenance is greatly simplified but does depend upon the production of a correctly made denture base.

Becker and others (1978) point out that the precursor to the Thompson dowel semi-precision attachment system was designed by Clark in 1938. Clark had a lingual retentive arm engaging a mesial lingual undercut, but Thompson later modified Clark's attachment system by placing the retention undercut directly on the fulcrum line. One drawback to the Thompson dowel concept is simply the cost of constructing a partial denture framework in gold. This can be overcome by using a chrome-cobalt major connector to which the gold alloy dowel rests are soldered. Primary retention is obtained by using stainless steel ball clasps to engage the retention dimples. The entire framework can, in fact, be cast in chrome-cobalt. Another limitation to the Thompson dowel system is the difficulty of hand carving the dowel rest seats.

Becker and others have now produced a standard dowel rest die from a handcarved rest seat. By using this die in a surveyor a standard dowel rest can be waxed up and cast. Left and right sided standard dyes are employed to conform to the design of the dowel rest as suggested by Koper. When the dowel rests are properly aligned, the lingual wall of the rest seats on the right and left abutments will be parallel. An optional lingual bracing arm is occasionally added. This in no way interferes with the 0.8 mm ball clasp retention device that is itself directly secured to the denture base. Adequate tooth substance must be removed for the dowels to be correctly positioned within the crown contours. Unlike many intracoronal attachments the Thompson dowel does not provide a positive lock. In order to overcome problems that would arise when an altered cast impression technique is employed an incisal hook is usually added to the framework. This incisal hook is particularly useful for orientating the removable partial denture framework on the master cast and for processing acrylic resin. It is subsequently removed following denture construction. Rebasing problems, however, are another matter and these should be considered along with extracoronal attachments which have similar problems.

There is, of course, no limit to the design and shape of retainers that can be produced in the laboratory to suit individual problems. Their versatility must be one of the greatest assets.

Prefabricated retentive devices such as the Tach-E-Z and C and L system (Figs. 237, 238) are available. A neat laboratory-produced system can also be employed (Fig. 239) but lacks the stability afforded by the lingual arm. As a result it may need frequent adjustment to maintain retention.

Semi-precision rests are simpler and more economical to employ than precision attachments. They require the preparation of few abutment teeth and allow the operator to design the unit for a particular situation. A partial or full coverage restoration is normally required in conjunction with a shoulder preparation. The full width of the shoulder should be carried through the proximal surfaces and carried onto both lingual and buccal surfaces. The semi-precision rest is neat, effective, and versatile. It should be considered for use where neither the clasp nor the attachment retainer is entirely suitable.

CLINICAL PROCEDURES

The key to success lies in careful treatment planning. For this, all the diagnostic aids possible must be available, including full-mouth radiographs and mounted diagnostic casts. In difficult situations, the diagnostic casts may be duplicated and the duplicate set used for practise of the preparations. It takes little time and can be a valuable aid in showing up difficulties ahead. The plaster preparations may also be used as a basis upon which the temporary crowns can be made.

Recommended abutment preparations are basically full crowns modified to accommodate the female part of the attachment. This modification may take the shape of a wide shoulder carried through the proximal surface and on to the lingual surface of the tooth. Alternatively, a box may be cut in the crown preparation to accommodate the attachment. The shoulder provides the technician with greater latitude for positioning the attachment but results in more tooth substance removal (Fig. 240). Either way one must be sure that adequate space has been made for the attachment if one is to avoid demoralising and time consuming repreparation when the work has reached an advanced state. One simple method is to take the female attachment, join it to a short piece of wire with compound or plasticine, and measure

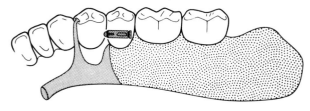

Fig. 237   The Tach-E-Z Unit. A commercially-produced spring-loaded plunger used in conjunction with a mesially placed semi-precision rest.

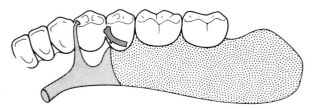

Fig. 238   The C and L unit. This commercially-produced spring clip provides additional retention to a mesially placed occlusal rest.

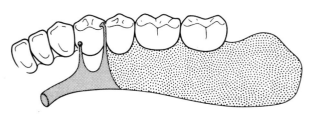

Fig. 239   A laboratory-produced retaining system employing a distally placed semi-precision rest and a lingual retaining arm engaging a dimple in the crown.

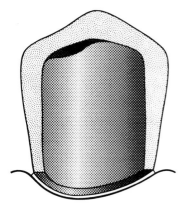

Fig. 240   A shoulder preparation results in considerable removal of tooth substance, but provides the technician with greater latitude for alignment of the attachments.

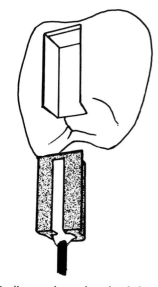

Fig. 241   Until experience is gained the attachment can be measured against the box preparation. It is easier to judge the depth of the box by cutting it before the crown is prepared.

it against the space that has been prepared for it. Up to 0·5 mm clearance is required for the surrounding gold (Fig. 241). When a lingual or palatal bracing arm is to be incorporated within the abutment crown, more tooth substance must be removed from these surfaces, otherwise the final crown will be bulky.

For those brought up on reversible hydrocolloids there is no other impression material. Certainly, the combination of stone dies and reversible hydrocolloid gives an accuracy that cannot be surpassed. Where attachments with bracing arms are to be employed, many technicians prefer a plated cast. Polyethers have grown in popularity for use where tissue undercuts are small. The high stiffness of polyether materials coupled with their medium tear energy makes them difficult to remove from the mouth. The spacing of trays should be slightly greater than those employed for silicones or polysulphides. Craig (1977) has pointed out that this stiffness also dictates care when removing gypsum products from the impression. The accuracy of polyether is among the highest of all elastomeric impression materials but its dimensional accuracy is only good if the impression is kept dry. Silver plated polyether impressions are more accurate than other materials (0·005% compared with +0·056% for polysulphide rubber) a useful property to bear in mind when plated casts are required.

Mercaptan rubbers are easier to remove from the mouth and can be silver plated. Polyether and mercaptan rubbers required a closely adapted rigid acrylic resin tray. Flexing of poorly made trays under load is one of the most common causes of subsequent problems with castings.

With all elastomeric materials problems appear to resolve around providing healthy gingival tissues, correct placement of margins, and adequate retraction.

Frowned upon by many as out of date, the copper ring technique is capable of producing excellent results. It is still used by at least one of the world's authorities on fixed prosthodontics. Having obtained individual impressions of each preparation the problem is then one of location. Metal transfer copings are recommended although Duralay resin copings can be used with care (Fig. 242). Copings must have windows to ensure correct seating and adjacent copings connected in the mouth with resin. Plaster is still the most reliable overall locating impression, it is rigid and tends to absorb the slight moisture occasionally overlooked on copings.

Having made facebow and jaw relationship recordings the master cast can be mounted on the articulator and the metal framework tested for accuracy. Intracoronal attachments are precise testers of impression accuracy. In fixed restorations errors of location show up in two ways. The prosthesis may not slide into place or it may do so by disturbing the seating of one of the crowns. Either way the fault must be found, the casting sectioned with a disc and a plaster or polyether locating impression made. Where the error is due to an inaccurate die, the casting of the preparation concerned must be removed, the remainder of the metalwork placed in the mouth, and an overall impression of the preparation made. The metalwork is removed with the impression. Polysulphides and mercaptan rubbers are best for this method.

When a removable partial denture is retained by intracoronal attachments the impression procedure is modified. The initial impression procedure is identical to that of a fixed prosthesis, but the female attachments are subsequently aligned and included in the casting. Having checked the accuracy of the abutment castings, the denture framework can be made. There is one frequent problem, however, in sectioning the cast to produce the dies, the region corresponding to the denture bearing area is often damaged, and a new impression is required. To accomplish this, construct a rigid acrylic resin tray, spaced over the castings but closely adapted over the denture bearing area. Place the castings in the

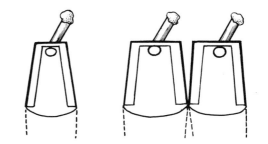

Fig. 242 Cast metal transfer copings should have small holes cut near the incisal edges to ensure correct seating. Copings on adjacent teeth should be checked to ensure they do not interfere with each other's seating.

mouth, ensure they are dry, and make an overall impression with which the castings are removed. Polyether impressions are excellent for this step. The cast can then be rearticulated and the denture framework made.

For distal extension prostheses the altered cast technique is preferred. Make the denture framework with closely adapted acrylic resin bases over the edentulous ridges. Place the abutment crowns in the mouth, check that the framework fits, and make a displacement impression using fluid wax* or zinc oxide paste. Remove denture together with abutment crowns to preserve intact details of the distal gingivae. The master cast is now sectioned to remove the areas corresponding with the edentulous ridge. This allows the crowns and connected denture to be placed on the remains of the cast. Stone can now be poured into the impression surface of the denture base to reconstitute the cast. Intracoronal attachments are particularly useful in this manner because of their precise location and lack of movement potential.

Large restorations are best inserted with a temporary non-setting cement for a period of several days. This period of trial insertion allows the restoration to be removed and polished after any subsequent corrections to the occlusal surfaces have been made. It also allows inspection of the plaque control of proximal spaces and these spaces can be modified if necessary. This trial period might also allow for slight tooth movements to compensate for any minute migrations that might have occurred while the prosthesis was being constructed.

The precise location necessary for intracoronal attachments can be disturbed by the layer of cement between crown and preparation; it would be disastrous to spoil the whole restoration at this late stage by such an error. To prevent this mishap, no crown

* Korecta Wax, Kerr Mfg. Co., Michigan.

or group of crowns should be cemented unless all the other components are placed into the mouth before the cement has hardened. Following removal of excess cement, patients with removable prostheses can be sent away for twenty-four hours with instructions not to remove their dentures.

At the next visit, the occlusion and articulation are checked. The adaptation of the denture base to the mucosa is checked with disclosing paste. If an error has occurred in this respect the denture will need to be rebased immediately.

With the aid of a large mirror the patient is shown how to remove the prosthesis and to re-insert it. A demonstration model or diagram is useful to explain the term 'path of insertion'. Above all, the danger of applying force to the prosthesis must be stressed. With a bilateral prosthesis considerable leverage can be exerted if only one side is moved.

Cleaning instructions should reinforce not only plaque control, but also denture hygiene. The female units may be cleaned with an 'interspace' toothbrush that is also useful for cleaning around the male attachment.

Once the patient can manipulate his prosthesis he may be seen one week later, and subsequently in one month for the final post-insertion checks and post-treatment radiographs. Regular six-monthly examinations should then suffice.

ADJUSTMENT OF RETENTION

Clumsy adjustment of intracoronal attachments is the one clinical procedure that is most likely to result in breakage. It must be carried out very carefully according to the detailed instructions given by manufacturers and in small stages.

With a precise path of insertion and large contact areas, only the smallest adjustments are required to produce a surprising difference in retention. Attachments such as the Stern G/L with auxiliary retentive features require special adjustment instruments. For most of the European attachments, spring replacements or retaining clip adjustments may be necessary. A screwdriver of the correct size should be available. With the correct instrument adjustment takes only a few moments, without it the attempt may not only fail but damage the attachment as well.

Intracoronal attachments with small slots, like the Stern G/A and McCollum units, can be adjusted with an annealed razor blade. The razor blade is simply inserted into the slot thereby opening it very slightly.

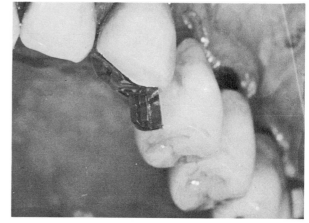

Fig. 243   The smallest of the Crismani units. The retention is entirely frictional and can be adjusted by very carefully opening out the male section by means of a fine jeweller's screwdriver.

Other types of attachment such as the Chayes and smallest Crismani can be adjusted with a small jeweller's screwdriver (Fig. 243).

Over a period of years there seems to be a tendency for the female sections of the attachments to open slightly; this type of wear or distortion occurs more rapidly with patients who tend to use excessive force when inserting their prosthesis. A lingual bracing arm reduces this type of wear and also lessens the effect of such wear as it occurs. Oversize male attachments, available for some of the Stern range of units, are useful for repairing this type of damage.

REMAKING A REMOVABLE PROSTHESIS

Remaking a removable prosthesis retained by intracoronal attachments presents one particular problem – that of reproducing the slots of the female section of the attachments.

Bartlett (1966) has described a method of using mercaptan rubber base. The material is carefully syringed into the bases of the attachment slots and then around the adjacent restorations. More viscous material is then inserted in a special tray, and the impression subsequently silverplated.

Before the silver-plated impression is poured in artificial stone, the depressions corresponding with the abutment teeth are filled with acrylic resin and joined by pieces of wire. Male attachments are then selected and tried in place in the mouth and a score mark made corresponding with the maximum depth

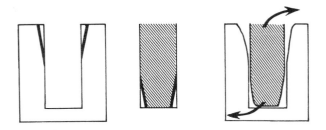

Fig. 245   The pattern of wear is usually more pronounced at the gingival portion of the male section and the occlusal third of the female section. This wear may result not only in loss of retention, but also in loss of bracing action.

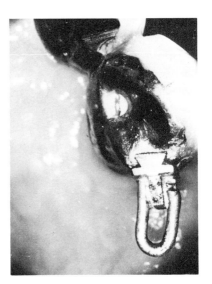

Fig. 244   Tagging soldered to the male section of the intracoronal attachment to facilitate its withdrawal in the impression.

to which they seat. The attachments are then inserted on the silver-plated cast to ensure that they seat in a similar manner.

A simpler method is to place the male attachments in the mouth to engage the corresponding female slots. Additional tagging is soldered to these male units (Fig. 244) enabling them to be removed in an overall impression. Where possible, the tagging of the male units should be joined by wire and united to it with self-polymerising acrylic resin. If this procedure can be carried out before the overall impression is made, the localisation within the impression should be precise. Plaster gives the most satisfactory localisation but its use requires judicious preliminary waxing out of proximal spaces and other undercut areas. If mercaptan rubber base is employed, the tagging and connecting elements must be scrupulously dried. Before the impression is cast, matching female units with additional tagging are inserted over the male sections of the attachments. In this way the new master cast incorporates the actual female sections of the attachments.

TECHNICAL CONSIDERATIONS

Most manufacturers provide detailed technical advice on the use of their attachments. The operator should be familiar with some of the factors involved as several technical aspects influence the design of the restoration.

An intracoronal attachment provides a removable prosthesis with direct retention, resistance to dislodgement along the path of insertion, and also first-class resistance to horizontal and rotational displacing forces. The direct retention is provided by the entire frictional surface area together with a mechanical retentive device, if this is incorporated. The lateral aspects of the attachment play an important part in its resistance to horizontal and rotational displacing forces. These lateral aspects are usually small and in many attachments they cannot be adjusted once worn. An attachment with a spring-loaded tensioning device may have its retention increased by substituting a spring with greater tension. However, this does not directly affect its ability to resist horizontal and rotational displacing forces, so that while the prosthesis might stay in place, it might still feel slack to the patient. This example may overstate the case because increasing the retention of an attachment is not without effect on its bracing action, but it does show the importance of designing the prosthesis to protect the lateral surfaces of the attachments. The pattern of wear is seldom even and is usually more noticeable at the gingival portion of the male unit and the occlusal third of the female slot (Fig. 245). Where patients have been clumsy, the female slot may in fact be distorted.

Distortion of the female section may also be seen in a mesio-distal direction but is usually limited to the area adjacent to the occlusal surface (Fig. 246).

Most attachment wear occurs when a prosthesis is being inserted and removed. Wear of attachments can and does take place while they are in position but it appears that the amount of wear that takes place is comparatively small. Attachments serving the functions of connectors between two fixed prostheses wear far less than those anchoring a removable prosthesis to its abutments.

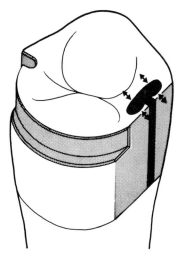

Fig. 246   The occlusal section of the slot is most prone to distortion.

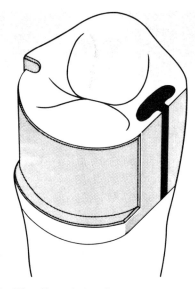

Fig. 247   The lingual bracing arm should be of the greatest possible vertical extent with an additional groove to aid retention. The groove contributes to a more rigid arm.

A patient may insert and remove the prosthesis several times a day so that the attachments may wear over a period of years. Few patients can consistently slide their prosthesis in and out of place without a few false starts. Each time they make a mistake the appliance will jam and must go back to its original position before a fresh attempt is made. It takes little imagination to visualise the effect upon the attachments.

Lingual bracing arms are most effective methods of providing additional guide planes. They help the patient find the correct path of insertion, protect the lateral surfaces of the attachment when mistakes occur, and aid the patient insert and remove the prosthesis. The vertical wall should be of the greatest possible extent and aligned with the attachment (Fig. 247). Where lingual space is restricted the step can be made near the occlusal surface and a skirt of gold carried down the lingual surface of the tooth (Fig. 248). Where space permits, two steps can be made in the lingual surface to strengthen the arm. If possible the lingual arm should be carried around the tooth above the next proximal space (Fig. 249). Making a groove for the free end of the bar will strengthen this component and aid retention. It will also resist any tendency to distort the attachment in a mesiodistal direction.

Wear of an attachment in the mouth is usually caused by inadequate heat treatment and by its resistance to horizontal and rotational displacing forces. While these forces may cause the attachments to wear, the effect they may have on the supporting structures of the teeth and denture-

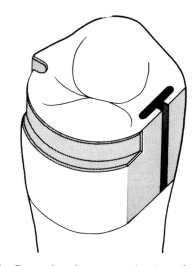

Fig. 248   Step placed near occlusal surface reduces bucco-lingual space requirements.

bearing areas are more serious. This is one reason why careful planning is so important, for only in this way can the prosthesis be designed and constructed so that it carries out its functions while being subjected to the minimum of displacing forces. Loads falling on the prosthesis can be reduced by attention to jaw relationship records and by keeping the occlusal table as narrow as possible, for this decreases the force required to penetrate a bolus

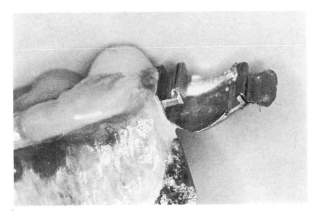

Fig. 249 Extended lingual bracing arm.

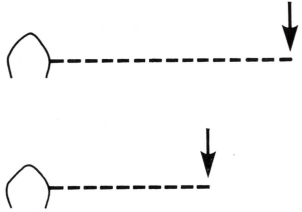

Fig. 251 Where possible, a distal extension prosthesis should have a short artificial occlusal table, for it reduces the leverages exerted by vertical and horizontal loads.

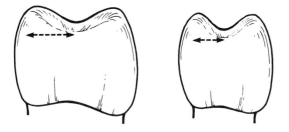

Fig. 250 The force require to penetrate a bolus of food is reduced if the occlusal table is kept narrow. The torques resulting from masticatory and non-masticatory contacts are also lessened.

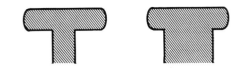

Fig. 252 A wide neck decreases the frictional area available for the attachment.

of food. It also reduces the torques resulting from masticatory and non-masticatory contacts (Fig. 250). A short occlusal table reduces the leverages of vertical and horizontal loads applied to the attachments of distal extension prostheses (Fig. 251).

Nearly all vertical and horizontal loads applied to the base will be transmitted to the abutment tooth through the neck of the male attachment. The severest loads are likely to be applied when the patient inserts and removes the prosthesis, especially before he has learnt to find the path of insertion. While an attachment of adequate neck width must be chosen, the illustration shows that a wide neck considerably decreases the amount of frictional area available for retention (Fig. 252). In making the compromise, the functions served by the attachment must be borne in mind. For example, an attachment retaining a distal extension prosthesis is likely to be subjected to far greater loads than one joining two sections of a fixed prosthesis.

Aligning the female sections of the attachments

within their respective crowns finally determines the path of insertion of the denture. It is a critical stage carried out in the laboratory on the mounting base of an absolutely rigid surveyor. The path of insertion is chosen at the treatment planning stage and should be clearly marked on both side and back of the diagnostic cast to show the degree of antero-posterior and lateral tilt required. In selecting the path of insertion, the contours of the edentulous areas must be considered (Fig. 253). If this is not carried out, the denture base extension will be jeopardised. Small alterations to this path may be necessary to make up for minor discrepancies between the alignment of the preparations and their planned alignment.

Most manufacturers provide a small surveying rod, modified to fit the female attachment at one end and the surveyor arm at the other, so that with the aid of this mounting jig, the attachment can be carried into place (Fig. 254).

If each attachment is carefully positioned in its waxed-up crown in this manner, all the attachments will be mutually parallel provided that no movement of the mounting table has occurred. Of course, the cast must be solidly clamped to the surveyor table, while the table itself must lock rigidly in place.

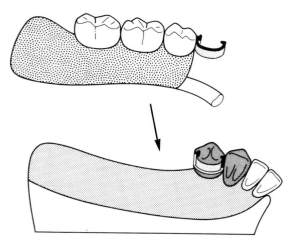

Fig. 253   The contours of the denture base area must be considered when deciding upon the path of insertion.

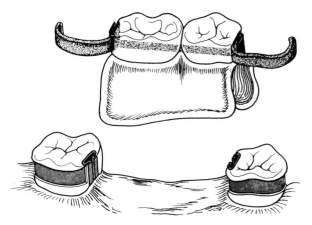

Fig. 255   The male attachments either end of a unilateral prosthesis may be soldered to a metal structure running the length of the restoration.

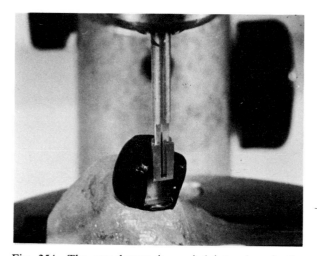

Fig. 254   The attachment is carried into place in the waxed-up crown by means of a special surveying rod fitting at one end of the attachment and the surveyor arm at the other end.

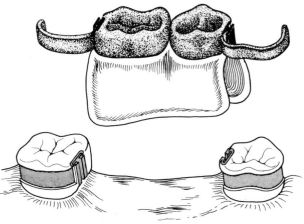

Fig. 256   The attachments can be soldered to gold occlusal surfaces.

This is the stage at which the step should be cut in the lingual surface of the waxed-up crown to accommodate the bracing arm.

The female part of the attachment can be soldered to the cast crown, or the crown can be cast around the attachment. The first method is usually the more popular. The female part of the attachment is slid out of the waxed-up crown leaving behind a rectangular space. The crown is then cast and the final localisation of the attachment is carried out on the surveyor when the attachment is carefully inserted into its rectangular box. The attachment is then held in place with Duralay* or inlay wax, so that it can be invested and soldered. This technique gives the technician greater control of the final localisation and removes any possibility of inaccuracies due to the attachment moving during the casting process. Accidental flow of gold into the attachment is also prevented. In fact, this technique has to be used for most of the normal yellow gold alloys.

Attachments made of highly-platinised alloys, such as those used with bonded porcelain/gold, usually require a different technique. In this case the crown is cast around the attachment, taking care to ensure that the internal surface of the attachment is filled with investment or a suitably shaped carbon

* Reliant Dental Mfg. Co.

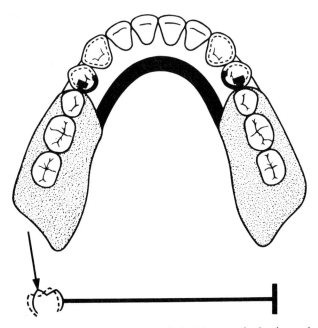

Fig. 257 A bilateral prosthesis is able to resist horizontal loads between the teeth and mucosa of both sides, while rotational loads applied to one side are resisted by the retainers of the opposite side acting with considerable mechanical advantage.

rod. This removes the need to use a special solder with its potential difficulties in bonding.

Carbon rods are provided by some manufacturers to hold the attachment in the investment and prevent the flow of gold within the attachment.

When constructing a unilateral prosthesis the male attachments on either end of the saddle may be joined by a gold bar running the length of the saddle (Fig. 255).

A more satisfactory and neater method is to join the attachments to the metal of a gold occlusal surface (Fig. 256). By connecting the male attachments the following advantages are gained:

1. The retention of the attachments to the acrylic resin is improved. There is then little danger of the patient tearing the denture base away from the male attachments.

2. Processing changes of the acrylic resin will have minimal effect on the location of the attachments.

3. Accidental breakages of the acrylic resin of the base are unlikely to affect the all-important location of the attachments.

Where bilateral prostheses are concerned, the major connector provides valuable cross-arch bracing. As a result of this bracing action, horizontal loads are resisted by an increased surface, and rotational loads applied to one side of the jaw are resisted by the retainers of the opposite side, acting with a considerable mechanical advantage (Fig. 257).

The major connector can only serve these functions if it is sufficiently rigid, while the attachments should be joined to the major connector. Small joining bars within the denture base may be necessary for this purpose. The connector must be able to resist forces applied when the patient inserts and removes the prosthesis.

Incorrect heat treatment of attachments is one of the most common causes of failure. The required procedures differ according to the gold alloys employed, but manufacturers invariably give precise recommendations. Salt baths or other instruments for careful control of these procedures should have a place in any laboratory concerned with attachment work. There can be little excuse for lack of attention to these details which, if ignored, can result in speedy failure of complex and costly restorations. The heat treatment techniques therefore merit a great deal of care.

REFERENCES AND FURTHER READING

ABRAMS, L. and FEBER, M. (1962) Periodontal considerations for removable prostheses. *Alpha Omega Fraternity* (Sept.)

BARTLETT, A. A. (1966) Duplication of precision attachment partial dentures. *J. prosth. Dent.*, *16*, 1111

BLATTERFEIN, L. (1969) The use of the semi-precision rest in removable partial dentures. *J. prosth. Dent.*, *22*, 307

BECKER, C. M., CAMPBELL, H. C. and WILLIAMS, D. L. (1978) The Thompson dowel-rest system modified for chrome–cobalt removable partial denture frameworks. *J. prosthet. Dent.*, *39:4*, 384

BRECKER, S. C. (1966) *Clinical Procedures in Occlusal Rehabilitation.* Saunders, Philadelphia and London

BRODBELT, R. H. W. (1972) A simple paralleling template for precision attachments. *J. prosth. Dent.*, *27*, 285

BROWN, D. (1973) Factors affecting the dimensional stability of elastic impression materials. *J. Dent.*, *1*, 265

CALDARONE, C. V. (1957) Attachments for partial dentures without clasps. *J. prosth. Dent.*, *7*, 206

CARR, C. M. (1898) Anchored adjustable dentures. *Dent. Cosmos*, *40*, 2119

CHAYES, H. (1910) Empiricism of bridgework. *Dent. Items Interest*, *32*, 745

CHAYES, H. (1915) Principles, functions and construction of saddles in bridgework. *Dent. Items Interest*, *37*, 831

CHAYES, H. (1917) System of movable, removable

bridgework in conformity with the principle that 'teeth move in function'. *Dent. Rev.*, *31*, 87

CRAIG, R. G. (1977) Status report on polyether impression materials. *J.A.D.A.*, *95*, 126

EICH, F. A. (1962) The role of partial dentures in the destruction of the natural dentition. *Dent. Clin. N. Amer.*, 717

EVANS, G. (1888) *A practical Treatise on Artificial Crown and Bridge Work*. The S.S. White Metal Mfg. Co., Philadelphia

EVANS, G. E. (1905) *A Practical Treatise on Artificial Crown, Bridge and Porcelain Work*, pp. 304–314. S. S. White Dental Mfg. Co., Philadelphia

GILMORE, S. F. (1913) A method of retention. *Council of Allied Dental Soc.*, *8*, 118

GOLDMAN, H. M. and BURKET, L. W. (1959) *Treatment Planning in the Practice of Dentistry.* C. V. Mosby, St Louis, Mo.

GOSLEE, H. J. (1912) Removable bridgework. *Dent. Items Interest*, *34*, 731

GROSSER, D. (1953) The dynamics of internal precision attachments. *J. prosth. Dent.*, *3*, 393

HARRIS, F. N. (1955) The precision dowel rest attachment. *J. prosth. Dent.*, *5*, 43–48

HOLLENBACK, E. A. and OAKS, S. (1950) Role of precision attachments in partial denture prosthesis. *J. Amer. dent. Ass.*, *41*, 173

KNOWLES, L. E. (1963) A dowel attachment removable partial denture. *J. prosth. Dent.*, *13*, 679–687

KOPER, A. (1973) An intracoronal semiprecision retainer for removable partial dentures: the Thompson dowel. *J. prosth. Dent.*, *30*, 759–768

McCOLLUM, B. B. and STUART, C. E. (1955) *A Research Report, Basic Course in Postgraduate Gnathology*, pp. 45–46. Scientific Press, South Pasadena

McCRACKEN, W. L. (1964) *Partial Denture Construction*, 2nd edn., p. 167. C. V. Mosby, St Louis, Mo.

McLEOD, N. S. (1977) A theoretical analysis of the mechanics of the Thompson dowel semi-precision intracoronal retainer. *J. prosth. Dent.*. *27:1*, 19–27

MILLER, C. J. (1963) Intra-coronal attachments for removable partial dentures. *Dent. Clin. N. Amer.*, 779

MORISON, M. L. (1962) Internal precision attachment retainers for partial dentures. *J. Amer. dent. Ass.*, *64*, 209

NEUROHR, F. G. (1939) *Partial Dentures.* Lea and Febiger, Philadelphia

PARR, M. (1888) Removable Bridges in Evans, G., *A Practical Treatise on Artificial Crown and Bridge Work.* The S. S. White Metal Mfg. Co., Philadelphia

PEESO, F. A. (1894) Metal cap for the anchorage of a bridge. *Busy Dentist*, *1*, 36

PEESO, F. A. (1916) *Crown and Bridgework for Students and Practitioners.* Lea and Febiger, Philadelphia

PREISKEL, H. W. (1966) The use of internal attachments. *Brit. dent. J.*, *121*, 564

SCHUYLER, C. H. (1953) An analysis of the use and relative value of precision attachment and the clasp in partial denture planning. *J. prosth. Dent.*, *3*, 711

SHERER, J. W. (1949) Sherer spring lock attachment. *Dent. Digest*, *55*, 163

SINGER, F. and SCHÖN, F. (1966) *Partial Dentures.* Kimpton, London

STEIGER, A. and BOITEL, R. (1959) *Precision Work for Partial Dentures.* Stebo, Zurich

TERREL, W. H. (1951) Specialised frictional attachments and their role in partial denture construction. *J. prosth. Dent.*, *3*, 339

THOMPSON, M. J. (1949) Reversible hydrocolloid impression material: its treatment and use in operative prosthetic dentistry. *J. Am. Dent. Assoc.*, *39*, 708–720

THOMPSON, M. J. (1957) Solution for specific problems in replacing missing teeth with partial denture. *Ill. Dent. J.*, *26*, 251–253

CHAPTER 7

Extracoronal Attachments

The term extracoronal attachment can be applied to those units having part or all of their mechanism outside the contour of a tooth. These increasingly popular attachments have their main application with distal extension prostheses; however, they may be used to retain restorations for bounded spaces. For descriptive purposes, three groups of extracoronal attachment can be considered.

1. Projection units

This large group project from abutment crowns and requires no box preparation, but the projections complicate plaque control. Projection units can be subdivided into two groups.

    (a) Rigid projection units.

    (b) Projection units allowing play between the two sections.

2. Connecting units

These units provide a joint between two sections of a removable prosthesis; they do not anchor a prosthesis to a tooth. The joint commonly allows movement between the two sections of the denture. The Axial Rotation and Rotation joints designed by Steiger and Boitel are good examples.

3. Combined units

Combined units consist of two attachments; a hinge type of connecting element outside the tooth joined directly to an intracoronal attachment. The male sections of combined attachments may be interchangeable with those of an equivalent intracoronal attachment. No projection remains when the denture is removed but box preparations are required. By their very nature these units tend to be complex and cumbersome.

PROJECTION UNITS

The design of most units is a compromise between conflicting requirements. The problems are best understood by considering a hypothetical parallel sided block soldered to the distal aspect of an abutment crown for the retention of a distal extension prosthesis. A closely fitting female unit engages this rectangular projection.

The height of the projection governs the length of the path of insertion, the retention available, and its ability to resist rotational loads around a sagittal axis. Apart from retention, the height of the unit is an important feature of wear resistance (Fig. 258).

The lateral surface area counteracts side to side and 'fish-tail' movements of the denture base. This surface area is a function of height and length. The width of the attachment affects its strength and also provides bulk for the incorporation of retaining devices (Fig. 259). The shape of the unit will need to be modified to prevent sliding or undesirable tilting movements (Fig. 260).

While bulky extracoronal units may look impressive on specially constructed demonstration models, the restrictions of the mouth must be considered.

Vertical space is a precious commodity and the cry is often heard for shorter and still shorter attachments. Careful design may overcome some of the drawbacks of short attachments. Incorporation of bracing arms may compensate for the reduced lateral surface area while meticulous construction of the attached denture base will reduce the forces applied. Metal occlusal and lingual surfaces around the attachment will reduce the overall space requirements.

The mechanical advantages of a long attachment have been mentioned but when applied to the mouth the drawbacks may be intolerable. First of all the problems of plaque control increase with the length of unit. Secondly, a greater length requires more

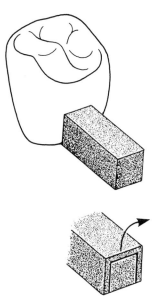

Fig. 258   Hypothetical rectangular unit. The height of the projection governs the length of the path of insertion, the retention available, and its ability to resist rotational loads around a sagittal axis.

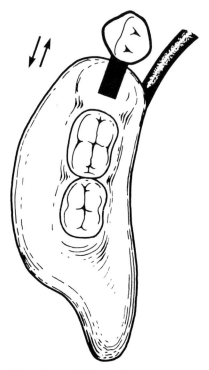

Fig. 260   The shape of the unit must prevent posterior displacement and undesirable rotations.

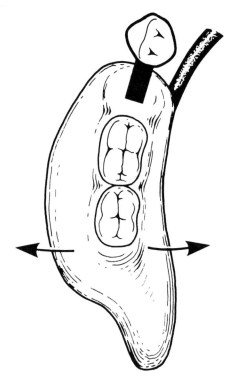

Fig. 259   Lateral surface area counteracts side to side movements of the denture base. The width affects the strength and provides bulk for the provision of retaining devices.

space within the prosthesis for the attachment. If the attachment is not aligned with the long axis of the edentulous ridge, as is frequently the case to simplify plaque control, the longer attachment may produce an unacceptable lingual bulge in the prosthesis.

The additional lateral surface contact area provided by a bracing arm is a useful way of overcoming the effects of reducing the length of the attachment. The width of the attachment is limited by two considerations, the bucco-lingual space available, and difficulties of plaque control. Rounding the base of the attachment may be helpful in this respect (Fig. 261). If some of the difficulties of designing projection units are understood the way is clear to appreciate the correct application of projection units.

Rigid extracoronal attachments tend to be somewhat more bulky than those allowing a degree of play. If the lateral surfaces of these units are sufficiently large and parallel sided, they may be used in conjunction with intracoronal attachments, useful for certain types of unilateral distal extension prostheses. Other applications include the restoration of bounded spaces and of bilateral distal extension gaps.

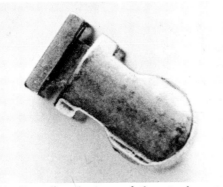

Fig. 261   Rounding the base of the attachment will be helpful to plaque control.

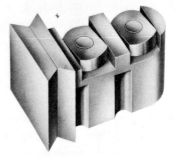

Fig. 264   The attachment assembled.

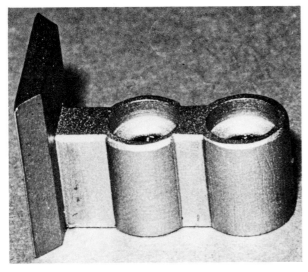

Fig. 262   The female section of the Stabilex attachment.

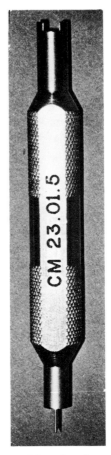

Fig. 265   Screwdriver for changing the pins.

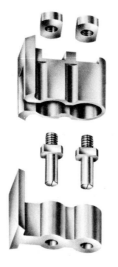

Fig. 263   The Stabilex attachment, to show removable male pins.

If one takes for example the Stabilex unit, the mechanical efficiency of the attachment is self evident (Figs. 262–265). It provides a rigid connection between male and female sections, with additional retention provided by pins. The retention of the pins is adjustable but the extra pin may be unscrewed and replaced if necessary. A special screwdriver is made for the purpose. While this robust attachment provides extremely effective retention, it is bulky. Plaque control is difficult, while the attachment requires more than 4 mm of vertical space. Perhaps the greatest drawback is its length that complicates the construction of the prosthesis, plaque control, and restricts application to situations in which there is generous space available.

The Conex attachment (Fig. 266) shares a common ancestry with the Stabilex, but is far smaller mesio-distally. A series of refinements has reduced the bulk of the unit, facilitated plaque control, and improved retention. Its applications and popularity have thereby grown. The parallel sides provide a precise path of insertion that resist rotational forces. The central retaining pin may be unscrewed and replaced. Two types of pin may be employed (Fig. 267), providing frictional retention or a mechanical lock. The retention can be so effective that a special separation device is produced to help part the two sections (Fig. 268). The

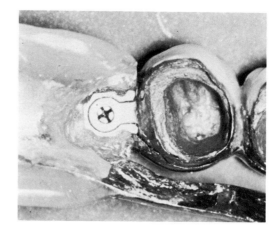

Fig. 267a   Lateral rotational forces are resisted by metal to metal contact. A bracing arm is, nevertheless, advisable.

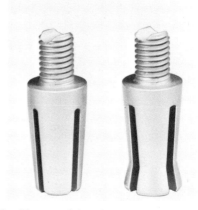

Fig. 267b   Two models of retaining pin are available producing frictional retention (left) or an additional mechanical lock (right).

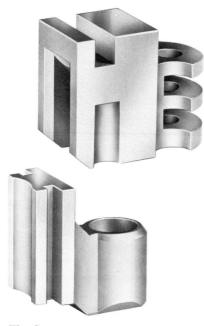

Fig. 266   The Conex attachment. A series of refinements have reduced its bulk, facilitated plaque control, and improved retention.

retention of the central pin may be adjusted by inserting a special instrument the opposite end of which may be used to unscrew the pin (Figs. 269–271). The manufacturers do not recommend soldering to the removable section of the attachment. Instead, special additional tagging is produced for soldering purposes. This additional tagging is screwed to the back of the attachment (Figs. 272, 273).

A modified Conex attachment is now produced that enables the operator to screw the removable section of the prosthesis in place (Fig. 274). This may have application for certain tooth supported prostheses provided that adequate plaque control is

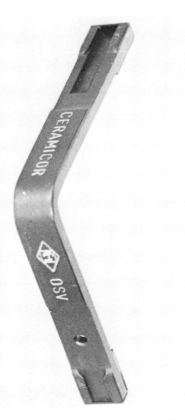

Fig. 268   Separation device to allow the dental surgeon and technician to part the two sections of the attachment in the laboratory.

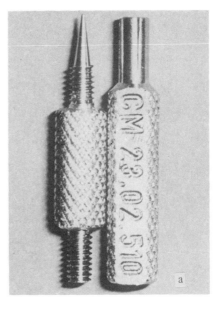

possible. The retention of the special pin (Fig. 275) is adjusted with the longer screw. This longer screw is also used to hold the pin in place. In exceptional circumstances, the attachment can be converted to a removable unit by cutting off the screw extension (Fig. 276).

Most Conex applications will be for the retention of removable prostheses, especially distal extension dentures. Where unilateral distal extension spaces are to be restored the parallel sides of the Conex allow it to be used in conjunction with intracoronal attachments on the contralateral side (Fig. 277).

The manufacturers feel that bracing arms are unnecessary due to the generous lateral surface area of the attachment. They may well be correct, but where buccolingual space permits the arm helps with seating and removing the restoration (Fig. 278, 279). When employed correctly, Conex attachments provide excellent results and plaque control presents few problems (Fig. 280). Other uses of these attachments include the retention of small restorations for bounded spaces (Fig. 281). Conex

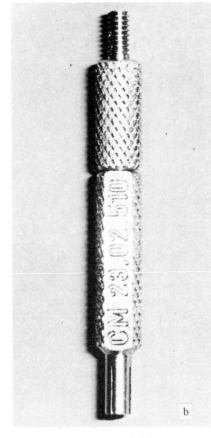

Fig. 269   Conex adjusting tool (a) dismantled, (b) assembled. The pointed end spreads the retaining pin and increases the retention.

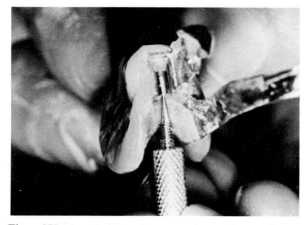

Fig. 270 Increasing the retention of a Conex attachment.

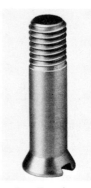

Fig. 273   Tagging screw.

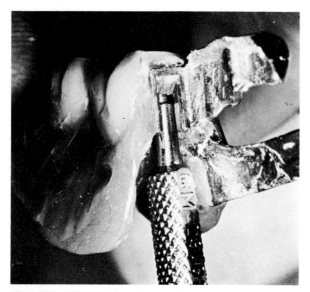

Fig. 271   Unscrewing the retaining pin of a Conex attachment.

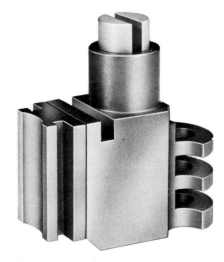

Fig. 274   Modified Conex allowing the construction of a screw-retained fixed prosthesis.

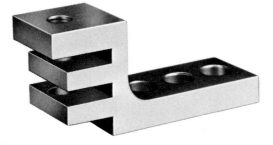

Fig. 272   Additional tagging for the removable Conex unit.

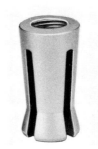

Fig. 275   Special pin for retaining the 'fixed' Conex.

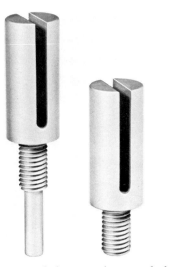

Fig. 276 The extended screw is passed through the occlusal surface of the attachment to adjust the retention of the pin and to secure it in place. In exceptional circumstances, removal of the screw extension can be employed to convert the attachment to a removable unit.

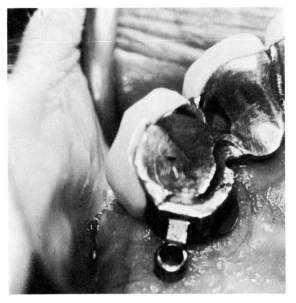

Fig. 278 Abutment crowns with recess for bracing arm.

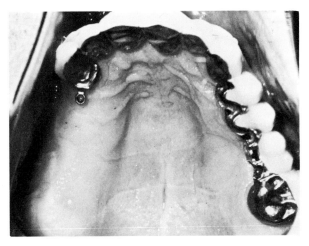

Fig. 277 The parallel sides of the Conex attachment permit it to be used in conjunction with intracoronal attachments.

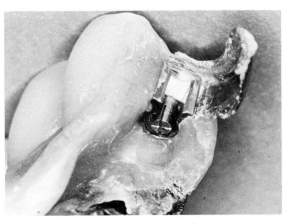

Fig. 279 Bracing arm on denture.

attachments may be used in conjunction with intracoronal attachments and telescopic crowns, provided they have parallel sides.

The Scott attachment is a laboratory-produced extracoronal system that may be rigid or allow movement, depending on the inclusion of an axial-rotational joint. There are few restrictions to its use provided that abutments of adequate strength are present and sufficient vertical and bucco-lingual space exists for the attachment. The design allows the projecting unit (the connector) to be placed away from the gingival margin with considerable advantages to oral hygiene practice (Fig. 282). This section of the prosthesis may be purchased as a plastic blank that may be cut to size on the master cast (Fig. 283). Retention is provided by the frictional grip of the removable telescopic crown on the tapered connector. This arrangement compensates

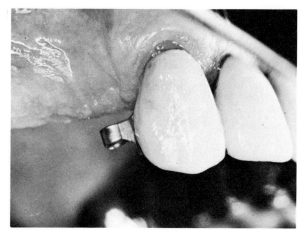

Fig. 280   Eighteen month post insertion result. Given sufficient vertical space, adequate plaque control is straightforward.

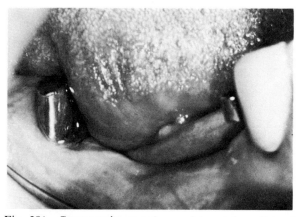

Fig. 281   Conex units may be used to retain unilateral restorations for bounded spaces. They may be employed in conjunction with intracoronal attachments or parallel sided telescopic crowns.

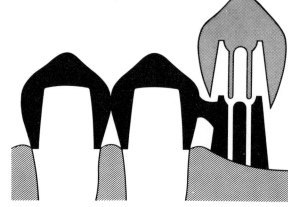

Fig. 282   The Scott attachment. The projecting unit may be placed away from the gingival margins with considerable advantages to plaque control.

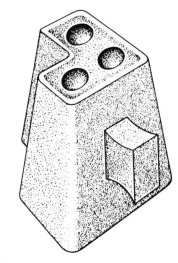

Fig. 283   Diagram of the projecting unit of the Scott attachment. This unit may be obtained as a plastic blank and cut to size on the master cast.

for wear, as the outer section simply slides further down over its counterpart. Supplemental retention is provided by parallel-sided iridio-platinum pins supplied with the attachment and these are incorporated when the pattern of the removable section (telescopic crown) is constructed in wax. Scott (1968) feels the attachment with play has applications where distal extension prostheses are concerned. Apart from the retention of distal extension prostheses, this versatile unit may be used to retain removable anterior prostheses (Figs. 284–289). Its design allows close adaptation to the underlying mucosa.

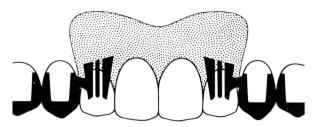

Fig. 284   The Scott attachment used to retain a removable anterior restoration. Its design allows close adaptation to the underlying mucosa.

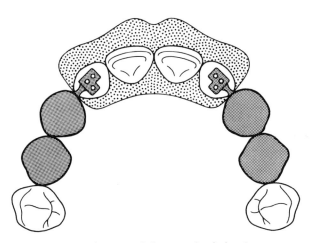

Fig. 285   Diagram of the prosthesis in place.

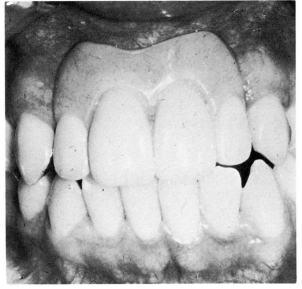

Fig. 288   The restoration assembled.

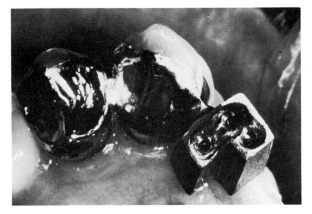

Fig. 286   Occlusal view of Scott attachment in the mouth.

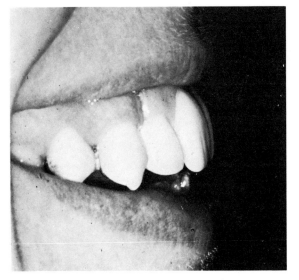

Fig. 289   Lateral view of restoration.

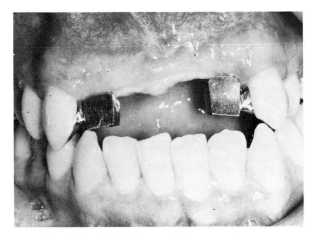

Fig. 287   Labial view of Scott attachment.

Extracoronal projection units with play between the components have become extremely popular. While it is only possible to describe a small number, the principles involved apply to the entire group.

Any movement occurring between two sections of the attachment may well decrease loads applied to the abutment crowns. Instead of being applied to the periodontal tissues, additional load will be placed on the edentulous ridge, a structure prone to resorption. Furthermore, many units, such as hinges, allow a degree of movement without significant limitation so that a vicious circle may be initiated. Increased denture base movement contributes to further resorption and yet more base movement. This problem becomes worse when the movements allowed are in more than one plane. Why are these types of attachment so popular? The answer lies in the compact size and versatility of many of them. However, possible drawbacks must be appreciated.

Consider a hypothetical attachment allowing vertical play. The denture base is entirely mucosal supported until load is transmitted through the attachment. Now suppose this hypothetical sliding attachment is spring controlled (Fig. 290). A replacement spring slightly too long would result in the entire denture base being lifted out of contact with the mucosa (Fig. 291). On the other hand a spring that had become permanently deformed would transmit little load to the abutment teeth. The partial denture, now without its occlusal support, would then be likely to damage the mesial section of the edentulous ridge. Unfortunately the minute size of attachment springs and the forces applied often result in speedy permanent deformation (Fig. 292). Since this type of mishap can occur with all types of spring-controlled attachments, it is essential that springs be changed regularly, usually at six-monthly intervals. Attachment manufacturers carefully control the spring lengths; nevertheless it is most important to ensure that the ends of the springs have not been damaged, and that the springs are pushed completely home.

Now examine hinge movement. While the distal abutment gingivae may be spared occlusal load, plaque control will be complicated by the projection. In theory load distribution will be uneven, with more load applied to the distal section of the edentulous ridge than mesially. For a well-made denture with negligible base movement this point may be of academic interest. However, many hinges wear with time and then allow a degree of lateral play and rock that is far from satisfactory.

The alignment of hinges has been the subject of controversy for some time. The views of the two rival camps deserve further thought and may be expressed as follows:

1. The hinges should be aligned with the sagittal plane to prevent jamming of the hinges during rotation.

2. The hinges should be aligned with the midline

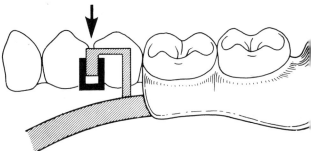

Fig. 290 A hypothetical attachment allowing movement simply in a vertical direction. Even load distribution to the mucosa occurs only when it is of even displaceability, while denture base movement relative to the papilla behind the distal abutment tooth may cause damage.

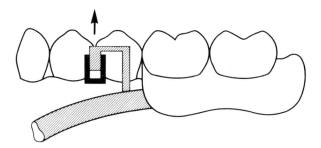

Fig. 291 A replacement spring, slightly too long would have a tendency to lift the base away from the mucosa.

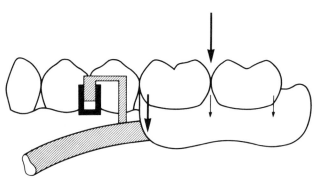

Fig. 292 If a spring loses its resiliency and becomes deformed, damaging loads can be applied to the gingivae and to the mucosa distal to the abutments. Springs should be changed at six-monthly intervals, preferably sooner.

of the ridges so that no buccal or lingual movement of the base accompanies rotation.

There is little doubt that hinges aligned with the sagittal plane will not jam and will provide

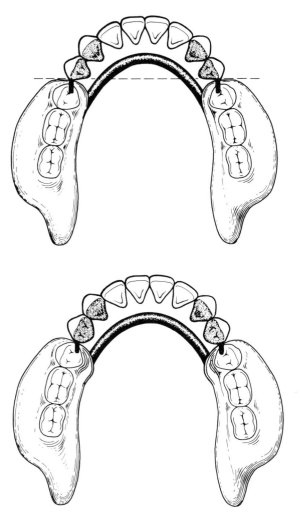

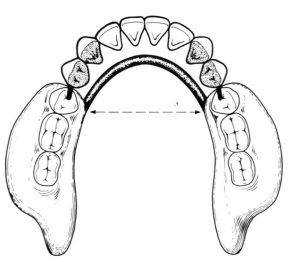

Fig. 294   Only a minute flexion of the major connector of the denture base is necessary to permit distal base movement of 0·3 mm.

Fig. 293   Hinges aligned with the sagittal plane provide unrestricted movement. However, a lingual bulge may be produced in the denture and the justification for such an arrangement is questionable.

unrestricted movement. But what price is paid for sagittally aligned hinges and is this sacrifice worthwhile? First of all, a lingual bulge is produced in the denture; the longer the hinge the bigger the bulge (Fig. 293). Secondly, the bases either side may not be of equal length. In that case a cantilevered pontic would be necessary to align the attachments. To join an extracoronal attachment to a cantilevered pontic is to produce a cantilevered extension of nearly two units, to which a distal extension prosthesis is attached. This arrangement is not only unnecessary, but contributes to a most unfavourable prognosis of the distal abutment.

The argument for sagittally aligned hinges is based on the presumption of an entirely rigid major connector. However, Heckneby's work has shown that neither the denture base resin nor a lower major connector can be considered rigid under load, particularly as the total base movement should not exceed 0·3 mm (Fig. 294). Occasionally, tales are told of patients who chew simultaneously on both sides. Such freaks, if they exist, have yet to be found. While many of the pleas for sagittally aligned hinges do not stand careful scrutiny, this does not mean that hinge type attachments can be twisted at any angle to each other (Fig. 295). Provided the denture has been well made divergencies of up to twenty degrees should produce little problem. Once this figure is exceeded vertical loads and tilting forces may be applied to parts of the attachment unable to resist these forces. A loose denture and damaged attachment might ensue.

Aligning the attachment with the edentulous ridge reduces the bucco-lingual space required (Fig. 296). In the days of large denture base movements, this arrangement ensured there was no lingual component to the rotation of the denture. The only practical problem today is that the entire base of the attachment may be in contact with the mucosa and this may complicate plaque control.

Twisting the attachments to an alignment slightly lingual to the ridges is a sensible compromise (Fig. 297). It introduces few mechanical problems and

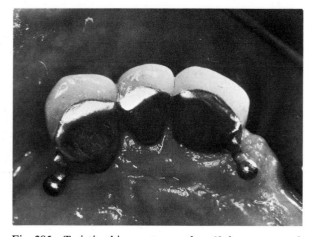

Fig. 295   Twisting hinges at more than 60 degrees to each other changes load distribution to their surfaces and can result in damage to the attachment and a poorly retained prosthesis.

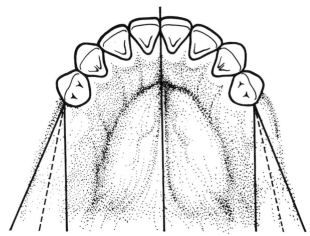

Fig. 297   Bisecting the angle between the edentulous ridge and the sagittal plane is usually a sensible compromise. Plaque control is simplified without the problem of lingual space involvement.

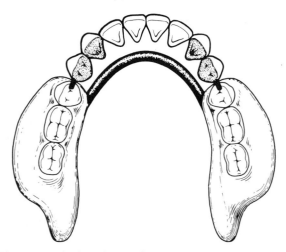

Fig. 296   Aligning hinges with edentulous ridges reduces buccolingual space requirements but often complicates plaque control.

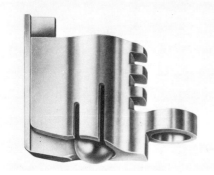

Fig. 298   The Dalbo extracoronal attachment.

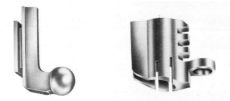

Fig. 299   Male section for use with bonded porcelain to gold techniques. The female section is made in a yellow gold alloy.

simplifies plaque control as the distal section of the attachment will overlie the distal slope of the mucosa.

The Dalbo extracoronal attachments are excellent examples of units allowing play between the two sections. Manufacture has been refined over quarter of a century during which time the attachments have shown themselves to be versatile and robust. The male unit is soldered to the surface of the abutment crowns forming a projection to which the female element, buried within the denture, can be joined. The male portion of the Dalbo design projects as an L-shaped bar with a ball joint on the lower extremity. The female section fits over the bar and engages the sides of the ball connection of the male (Figs. 298–300). This lock between the socket and the ball provides the direct retention of the unit, which is adjustable by gently bending the finger

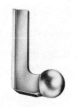

Fig. 300 Male section for use with conventional yellow golds.

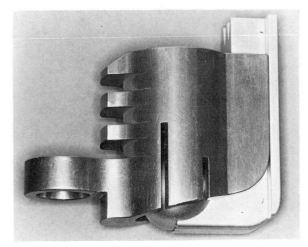

Fig. 301 Contact between lateral facing surfaces provides excellent resistance to lateral forces. Contact between the vertical surfaces prevents the distal denture base rotating away from the mucosa.

springs around the open end of the socket. Dalbo units are available in two sizes, with a matrix height of 5 mm or 6 mm. Each of these attachment heights is available in two configurations with the base of the L-shaped male unit longer in one than the other. The increased lateral surface area of the longer unit provides additional resistance to rotational and lateral displacing forces at the expense of additional bulk. These two configurations are sometimes known as bilateral and unilateral. However it would be an unwise operator who attached a unilateral distal extension prosthesis without a major connector to even the largest of these units – or to any other for that matter.

Dalbo units provide excellent resistance to both distal and lateral displacing forces. Furthermore, they incorporate a most effective tilt-preventing device that maintains the denture base in contact with the mucosa (Fig. 301). This is one of their important advantages over a clasp retainer requiring auxiliary indirect retention. Tilt-prevention is achieved by contact of the two parts of the attachment (Fig. 302), so that if a satisfactory impression technique has been used, the denture is both well-retained and stable. It is, of course, necessary to provide adequate and splinted abutments.

The design of the conventional Dalbo attachment allows some vertical play, for loads in this direction are transmitted through a coil spring to the ball connector of the male attachment (Fig. 303). The different sizes of Dalbo have dissimilar springs and containers for spares should be clearly marked (Fig. 304). An important check is to ensure that a polished facet on top of the ball is visible to show that loads are being applied to it; otherwise the prosthesis is mucosal borne. Springs introduce maintenance problems and complicate jaw relation recording and rebasing procedures. A solid spacer may be used to replace the spring (Fig. 305). A new addition to the range is the miniaturised female section without the spring chamber (Figs. 306–309). The complications of the spring are removed, and the vertical space required for the attachment

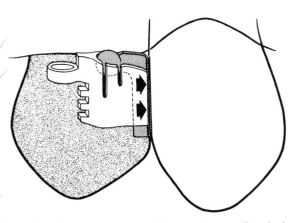

Fig. 302 Provided the remaining teeth are splinted, the tilt-preventing properties of the Dalbo and similar attachments can be employed to provide a well-retained and stable prosthesis.

virtually halved. Small wonder this unit is becoming one of the most popular denture retainers. The male attachments employed are identical with the conventional variety so that it is possible to replace conventional Dalbo units with the miniaturised variety (Fig. 310).

The drawbacks, however, must be understood. The reduced height of the female unit decreases the lateral surface area of contact and the attachment is weaker than its conventional counterpart and less well able to resist lateral loads. It is for this reason

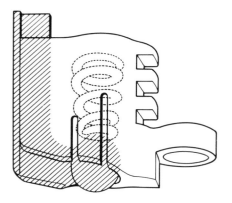

Fig. 303   Diagram of the attachment to show how vertical loads can be transmitted through a coil spring.

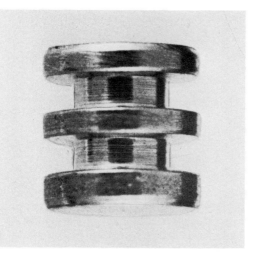

Fig. 305   A solid metal spacer may be used to replace the spring.

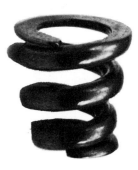

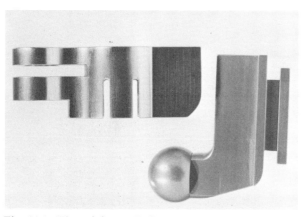

Fig. 306   The miniature Dalbo extracoronal attachment. Spring complications are removed and vertical space requirements virtually halved.

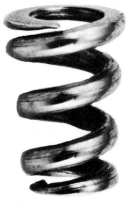

Fig. 304   Springs for the two heights of female sections. Containers for spare springs should be clearly marked.

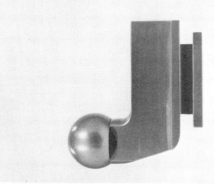

Fig. 307   The male section of the miniature Dalbo is identical to the conventional unit.

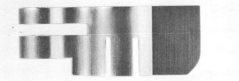

Fig. 308   The female miniature Dalbo.

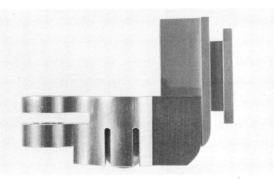

Fig. 309   The assembled unit. Note the gain in vertical space achieved by the modified female.

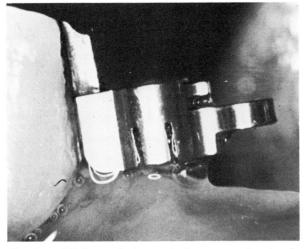

Fig. 310   Miniature Dalbo replacing conventional unit. The reduced vertical space requirement is apparent.

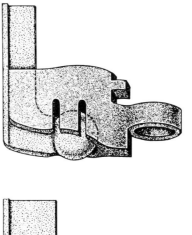

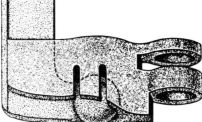

Fig. 311   The lower miniature Dalbo based on the 'unilateral' male section is normally employed. The upper diagram shows the unit based on the 'bilateral' male configuration – useful for replacement dentures.

that the manufacturers recommend the longer 'unilateral' variety of miniaturised Dalbo attachment as the increased length helps counteract the effect of the decreased height (Fig. 311). When using the 'bilateral' miniaturised Dalbo, it is apparent that exceptional care must be taken to ensure the minimum of lateral forces are applied. This is an extremely useful attachment with which to replace a conventional unit that is causing problems through lack of vertical space.

Dalbo extracoronal attachments require no buccal retainers or lingual bracing arms. The appearance of the completed restoration should be excellent while the retention and tilt preventing properties are extremely effective. Since the attachments do not interfere with the apparent contour of the abutment crown, they are particularly useful where buccolingual space is restricted (Fig. 312). Common examples are lower canine teeth that are frequently too thin to accommodate an intracoronal attachment (Figs. 313–314). Patients learn to handle Dalbo attachments remarkably quickly and require less skill in handling them than intracoronal attachments.

Like other extracoronal attachments vertical loads are transmitted away from the long axes of the abutment teeth and require the use of splinted abutments on a well constructed denture. This problem should not be accentuated by placing the attachment on the distal aspect of a cantilevered pontic.

A notable feature of this attachment is that laterally applied and tilting forces are resisted by metal to metal contact; not by acrylic resin to metal contact. This feature must contribute to the strength for which the attachment is well known.

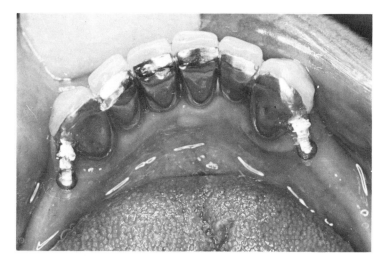

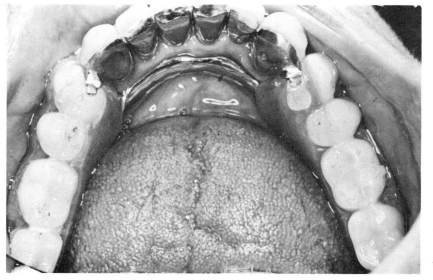

Fig. 313 Extracoronal attachments are particularly useful where lower canines are the abutments. The shape of these teeth generally precludes the use of intracoronal attachments.

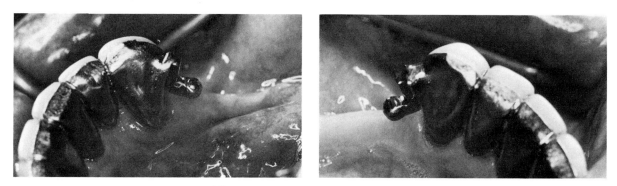

Fig. 314   Abutments 8 years later.

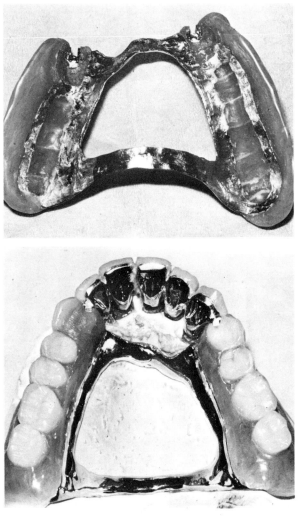

Fig. 312. An example of an upper partial denture retained by two Dalbo extracoronal attachments. A clasp-retained denture made for this situation might have been unsightly and poorly retained.

The projection across the gingivae is a complication shared with other extracoronal units. With the base of the attachment in contact with the mucosa one must avoid small, irregular spaces that are difficult to clean (Fig. 315). It is important to keep as small as possible the transition zone between the distal section of the attachment where the space is readily cleansible and the mesial section that contacts the gingivae. A slight lingual twist to the attachment increases the slope at which the mucosa falls away and reduces the transition zone (Fig. 316).

While alignment with the sagittal plane is not recommended, it is essential that the attachments align with each other in the vertical plane. This is achieved with a rigid surveyor using a paralleling mandrel supplied by the manufacturers. The path is normally selected to give an approach from the distal aspect of the abutments to facilitate positioning of the attachment.

Extracoronal attachments are extremely sensitive to poor plaque control (Fig. 317), yet there is one point that is so often overlooked – denture hygiene. If the acrylic resin of the denture is cut away from the attachment to leave a 'relief chamber', the space will fill with debris and plaque that will be difficult to remove.

Space requirements often dictate that the base of the attachment be placed in contact with the mucosa. The curved base, however, helps to simplify plaque control and covers a relatively small area – far less than an inadequately recessed intracoronal attachment. Sound periodontal tissues before prosthodontic therapy and adequate maintenance subsequently are essential for success. Patterns of wear on the occlusal surface are desirable features, provided they are not excessive. They demonstrate that the denture is partly tooth supported (Figs. 318–320).

The Dalbo units are straightforward to use but the nature of their construction makes them prone to misuse as well. While the axes of the hinges do not require alignment, divergencies of 60° are sometimes attempted. In these instances the entire load distribution to the unit is altered, and there is little to prevent tilting of the denture following distortion of the female section of the attachment (Figs. 321–324). The miniature females are more prone to this type of mishap.

Like other extracoronal units the shape of the Dalbo units make them useful for combined restorations where, for example, there is an anterior space between two small groups of teeth (Figs. 325, 326). Even a well-made partial denture will have a tendency to rock around the abutments in this situation, but a poorly constructed denture is capable of causing appreciable damage (Figs. 327, 328). A better approach is to restore the anterior space with a fixed prosthesis, thereby splinting the remaining teeth (Fig. 329). Extracoronal attachments can be employed to retain the bilateral distal extension denture (Figs. 330, 331). A similar restoration can also be constructed when only two lower canines remain (Fig. 332), provided their bone support is adequate.

This type of restoration is frequently opposed to a

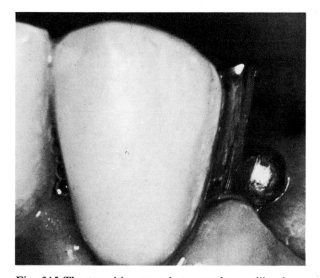

Fig. 315 The transition zone between the readily clean-sable distal section and the area of contact between the attachment and the mucosa must be kept as small as possible.

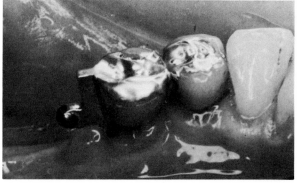

Fig. 317   Inadequate plaque control combined with continual denture movement frequently lead to this type of denture damage.

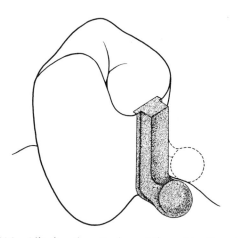

Fig. 316   Aligning the attachment lingual to the midline of the ridge increases the slope at which the mucosa falls away from the base of the unit. The size of the transition zone is reduced and plaque control simplified.

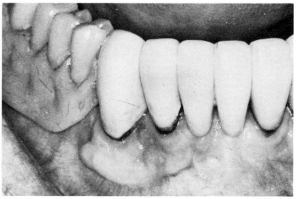

Fig. 318   Dalbo retained denture illustrating free mucosal graft three years postoperatively.

complete upper denture. It is essential that this complete denture be stable when the entire restoration has been completed; it would hardly be satisfactory to provide a complex lower prosthesis that made the upper denture unwearable. Stability in this case can be achieved only with correctly positioned teeth arranged to provide a balanced articulation. It cannot be achieved if the metal framework of the fixed prosthesis is completed before the jaw relation records are made, for this framework actually determines the position of the lower anterior teeth.

The jaw relationship records and trial insertions should be carried out as if the lower restoration were to be simply a partial denture, and the correct position of the teeth recorded in this way (Fig. 333). Their position can be recorded on the master cast by means of a plaster mask, and the metal structure then completed. When the assembled restoration is first inserted a check record is essential.

Dalbo attachments may be used to restore bounded spaces, virtually as substitutes for intra-coronal attachments. When applied in this way they lose their hinge action potential, and their vertical movement is best prevented. Their advantage of not requiring an abutment box preparation makes them useful for anterior prostheses in younger patients, and occasionally posterior ones as well, provided

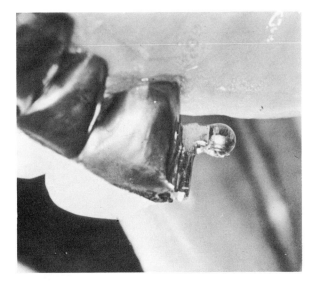

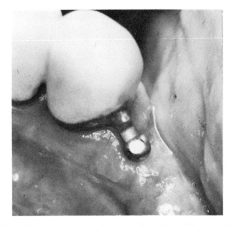

Fig. 320   Transmission of vertical occlusal forces through the miniature attachment produces slight flattening of the occlusal surface.

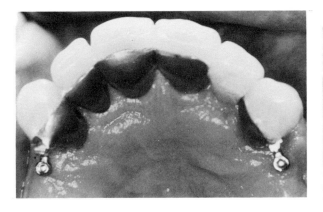

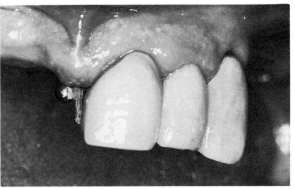

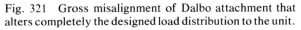

Fig. 321   Gross misalignment of Dalbo attachment that alters completely the designed load distribution to the unit.

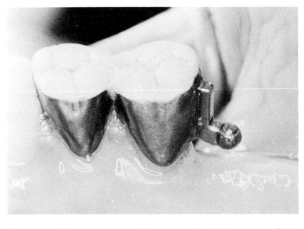

Fig. 319   Seven year results. Note the slight wear of the attachment sides and the wear of the occlusal surface by the spring. Wear patterns on the occlusal surface are desirable, if small, demonstrating transmission of vertical occlusal forces.

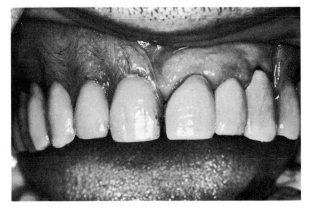

Fig. 322   A surprisingly well retained restoration.

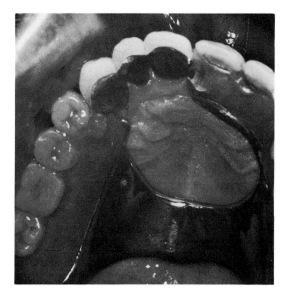

Fig. 323   However, note the palatal bulge caused by the incisor attachment.

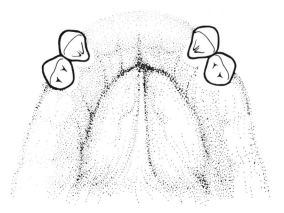

Fig. 325   Extracoronal attachments may be used in conjunction with combined restorations where there is an anterior space between two small groups of teeth.

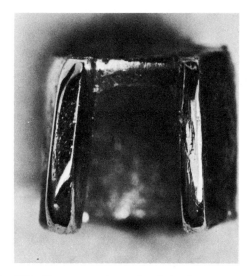

Fig. 324   Damage to the walls of the female attachment section caused by misuse. These walls were originally parallel.

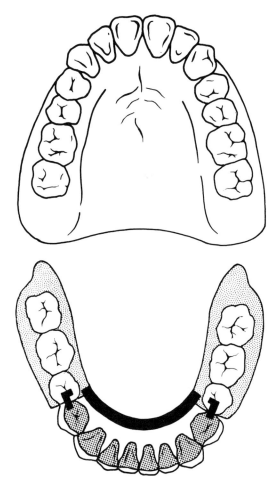

Fig. 326   The fixed anterior prosthesis splints the abutments while the attachments provide excellent retention for the removable prosthesis.

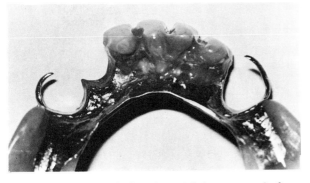

Fig. 327 A poorly designed partial denture made for a similar situation.

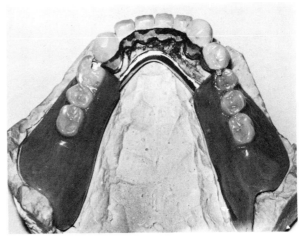

Fig. 330 The restoration on the master cast.

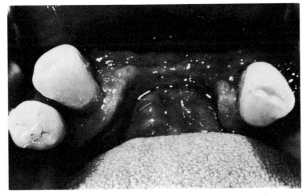

Fig. 328 The resulting damage in the mouth.

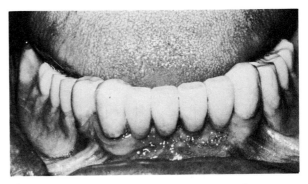

Fig. 331 The restoration in the mouth.

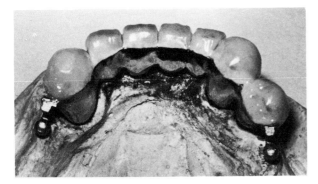

Fig. 329 The anterior space can be restored by a bridge.

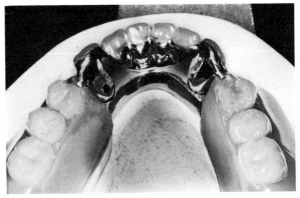

Fig. 332 An anterior space restored by a fixed prosthesis to which two extracoronal attachments are joined, acting as retainers for a removable bilateral distal extension denture.

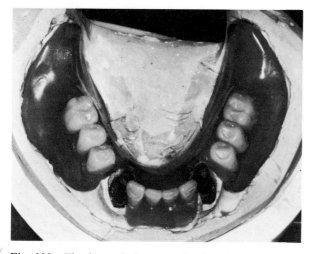

Fig. 333 The jaw relation records should be made and the positions of the teeth decided before the metal framework of the fixed prosthesis is constructed. A check record is essential when the assembled prosthesis is first inserted.

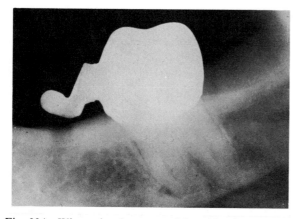

Fig. 334 Where the abutments either side of a space tilt towards each other, the attachments have to project a considerable distance from the crowns of the abutments. An impossible plaque control problem results.

there is sufficient vertical space for the attachment. The advantages and disadvantages of fixed and removable prostheses have already been discussed and apply to these extracoronal units. Extracoronal attachments like the Dalbo, should not be used where the abutment teeth on either side of the saddle tilt towards each other. An impossible plaque control problem results leading to gingival and periodontal damage (Figs. 334–336).

When used correctly, extracoronal attachments

provide a neat well-retained restoration, with many of the advantages of a partial denture. Mucosal coverage is possible, the restoration may be removed for cleaning, and it may be rebased should further alveolar resorption occur (Fig. 337).

Some attachments require individual technical procedures but the majority follow remarkably similar patterns. The abutments are surveyed to check for misalignment (Fig. 338), corrections carried out and the impression made in the material of choice. The crowns are then waxed-up (Fig. 339), and the attachments carried into place with the aid of a special mandrel (Fig. 340). Where bonded porcelain to gold techniques are employed, the attachments are left in the waxed-up crowns which are then cast (Figs. 341–343). With conventional yellow gold alloys the attachments are removed from the waxed-up crowns and subsequently soldered in place after casting.

Following construction of the major connector an important clinical task is to ensure that the location of the two sections of the attachments is identical in the mouth and on the master cast.

Retention

Thanks to its effective ball and socket connection the Dalbo attachment is remarkably wear-resistant. With the aid of a carving instrument the edges of the lamellae can be bent inwards by a minute amount. This procedure should be carried out in careful stages, one attachment at a time, and the prosthesis reinserted after each adjustment. If inadequate resin has been removed from the free edge of the female unit a small amount can be taken away with a heated discarded probe run along the outside edge of the attachment. Rotating instruments skid off the gold and remove too much resin.

Occlusal support

This vital aspect is one of the weaker points of the conventional spring-controlled attachment. Permanent deformation of the spring is insidious, is seldom noticed by patients, and results in the denture becoming entirely mucosal borne. Problems with springs is the one criticism levelled at the unit by Rantanen (1972) in his survey of attachment-retained partial dentures. Springs may not just deform, they may break or fall out. The period between spring changes varies with the loads applied but six months should be regarded as the maximum (Fig. 344). Spring damage or loss can be detected by careful examination of the articulation as it

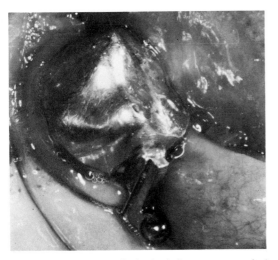

Fig. 335 Buccal view of gingival damage around abutment crown.

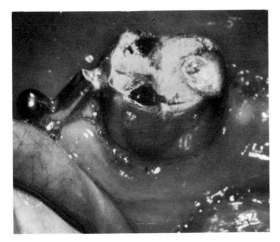

Fig. 336 Lingual view of abutment crown.

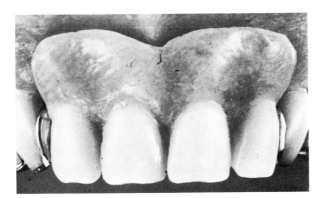

Fig. 337 An example of a removable anterior prosthesis retained by two extracoronal attachments.

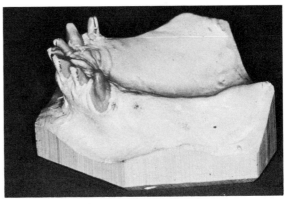

Fig. 338 Checking the alignment of the preparations.

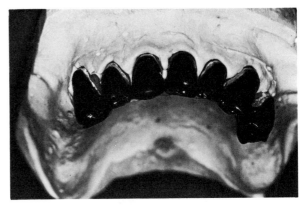

Fig. 339 The crowns waxed up

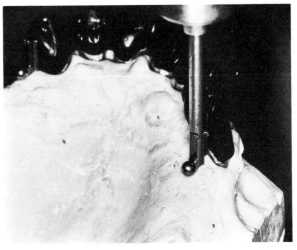

Fig. 340 Alignment of the attachments with a paralleling mandrel.

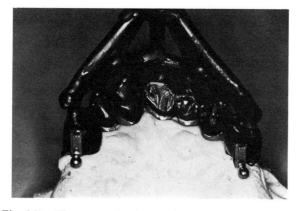

Fig. 341   The sprues in place. With conventional yellow gold technique the attachments are removed before the crowns are cast, and subsequently soldered.

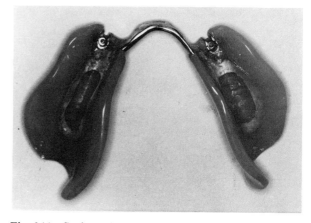

Fig. 344   Springs should be changed at no longer than six monthly intervals.

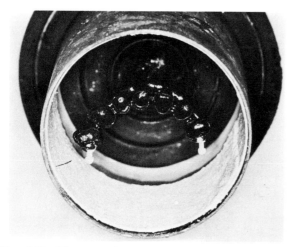

Fig. 342   The waxed-up crowns prior to investment (bonded gold to porcelain).

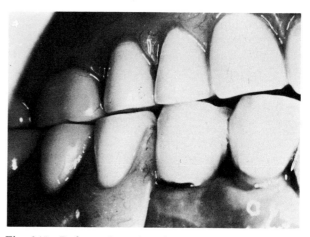

Fig. 345   Deformation of spring has lead to the mesial artificial tooth becoming out of occlusion.

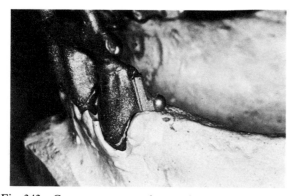

Fig. 343   Crowns cast on to the attachments (bonded gold to porcelain).

results in the mesial denture tooth coming out of occlusion (Fig. 345). Some wear of the ball is both normal and desirable showing that it is carrying load. Failure to check this important point can lead to the prosthesis losing tooth support resulting in damage to the edentulous ridge (Fig. 346).

The old spring is simply removed with a well used probe, and the chamber examined to ensure that no broken pieces or debris remain. The new spring can then be carried into place on the shank of an old bur from which the head has been removed. The wider end of the spring is inserted first. Spring containers must be carefully marked to ensure the two sizes are not confused.

In view of the complexities of springs, operators

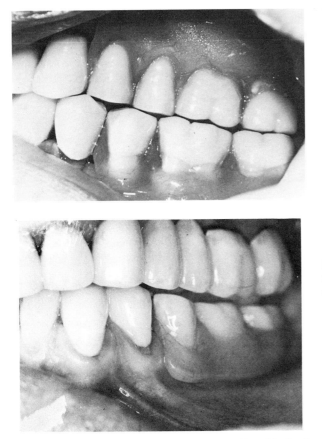

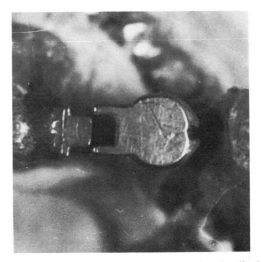

Fig. 347 Hinge movement occurring during the displacement impression procedure will defeat the entire purpose of the technique.

Fig. 346 Two examples illustrating the results of lack of maintenance.

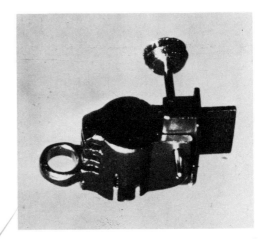

Fig. 348 The Pin-Dalbo. A modified Dalbo attachment allowing the two sections to be locked together during impression or rebasing techniques.

may prefer to substitute the metal spacer where loads dictate the use of conventional Dalbo attachments. The miniature attachments do not suffer from this problem but it is unwise to use them for long bases opposed by natural teeth. Even miniature Dalbo attachments should be inspected to ensure that a shiny spot is present that shows occlusal loads are being transmitted through the attachment.

Rebasing

Partial dentures retained by intracoronal or rigid extracoronal attachments can be treated as clasp-retained prostheses. The precise path of insertion and the absence of movement ensures the denture is correctly seated while the impression is made. Dalbo, and other similar extracoronal attachments, do not have this advantage. While vertical play can be prevented by using the metal spacer, the distal hinge movement is virtually uncontrolled. Since it

is only natural to apply load to the artificial teeth when making the impression some hinge movement will inevitably occur. With the Dalbo attachments the two flanges will be separated. If the resin is now processed with the flanges in this relationship, the denture will be free to rotate away from the mucosa until the flanges touch (Fig. 347). Apart from derangement of the occlusion, this allows the back of an upper denture to drop or a lower denture to lift. Ingenious modifications of the Dalbo such as the Pin-Dalbo (Fig. 348) and Dalbo M (Mensor 1968) have been developed to prevent such evil fortune.

Rebasing is not a five minute operation. It is an exacting and demanding technique requiring considerable time and clinical expertise.

The resin should be cut away from the occlusal and lingual aspect of the female attachment. Occasionally the buccal facing may need to be sacrificed. It will now be possible to see the precise relationship of the two sections of the attachment when the denture is seated. Furthermore, seating load can be applied directly to the attachment and not to a point distal to it. The rebase impression can now be made ensuring that the relationship between the attachment sections remains undisturbed. This relationship is even more critical with the miniature units in view of the small contact area and the relatively large leverages around them (Figs. 349, 350). Once the material has set, excess is removed from the region of the attachment and the abutment crowns and the attachment relationship is then examined with care. As an additional safeguard the denture base can be checked for movement. The denture is then removed in an overall alginate impression that records details of the entire arch. Before the impression is cast, dowels are placed in each attachment and become incorporated in the cast. These locating dowels prevent movement of the attachment during processing (Fig. 351). Most manufacturers produce such dowels for their attachments. Without them the alignment will be disturbed during processing.

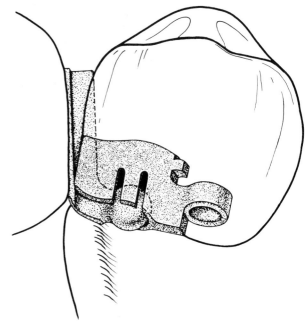

Fig. 350 The miniature attachments require considerable care as it is difficult to detect small rotations.

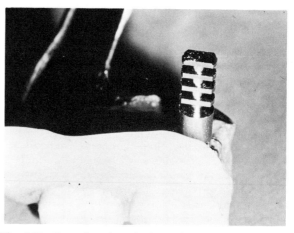

Fig. 351 Locating dowel placed in attachment. These devices maintain the location of the attachments during processing.

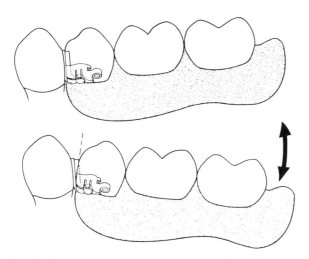

Fig. 349 Hinge movement occurring during rebasing or relocating procedures will subsequently allow the base to lift away from the mucosa until the two sections of the flange engage.

Replacing the denture in the mouth requires three important checks:

1. *Does the denture base seat correctly?* Ensure that no acrylic resin flash jams against the distal crown or attachment. No perceptible movement should occur when load is applied to the artificial teeth. The adaptation of the base can be checked with disclosing paste.

2. *Do the attachments engage?* The slight click of the socket engaging the ball should be felt. In the case of other similar attachments one should be able to feel the two sections lock together. In the absence of a satisfactory connection, examine the attachment for debris or acrylic resin that may prevent it seating. Make a small adjustment to the retention in case this has been altered during processing. If the attachments still do not engage, it is due to their having moved in the denture base during processing, usually as a result of failure to employ a rebasing jig, or locating dowel. A relocating procedure will be required and this will be described below.

3. *Check the occlusion and articulation.* This is best achieved using a check record and remount procedure. In the case of a lower restoration a centric relation record is made and the record stone or wax left on the occlusal surfaces of the denture in the mouth. The denture is removed in a full arch alginate impression. When this impression is cast it is mounted with the centric relation record against a cast of the opposing jaw that has been positioned with a facebow. Eccentric records can then be made and the occlusion and articulation perfected. Only minor corrections should be necessary unless an error in attachment location has occurred.

Relocating procedure

The aim of this difficult procedure is to correct the alignment of an attachment when all other aspects of the construction are correct. The process has to be carried out in the mouth.

First of all, the offending attachment is cut out of the denture taking care to damage neither the buccal facing nor the attachment. A lingual window is cut out of the acrylic resin to allow subsequent inspection of the relationship of the flanges (Fig. 352), and to ensure that the denture will not foul the attachment when subsequently reinserted. The denture is then inserted in the mouth, minus the attachment, to ensure it seats correctly and that the occlusion and articulation are correct.

Space under the projection of the male unit is blocked with soft wax or, better still, plaster (Fig. 353). Any self-polymerising resin that flowed into this space would lock the denture firmly in place making subsequent removal time consuming, destructive, and painful for all concerned. Only those who have suffered this misfortune can know the problems a small amount of acrylic resin in the wrong place can cause.

The gingivae and surrounding mucosa are

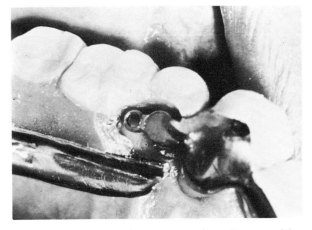

Fig. 352 Female section cut away from denture with a lingual window prepared to allow inspection of the two sections of the attachment.

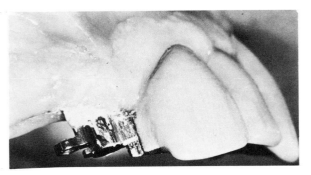

Fig. 353 Space under the attachment is blocked out with wax, or preferably plaster.

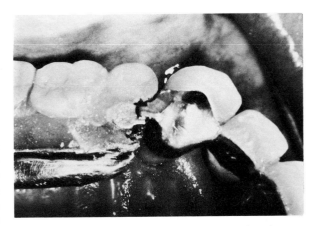

Fig. 354 Relocating the attachment to the denture with self-polymerising acrylic resin.

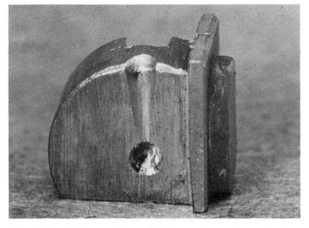

Fig. 355 Lingual view of P.R. male section showing dimple for retaining plunger and retraction slot. Note the large lateral facing surface.

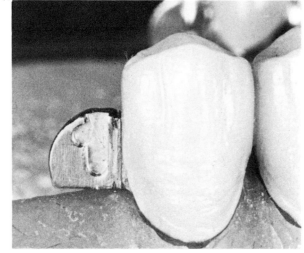

Fig. 357 Buccal view of the receptacles for locating projections.

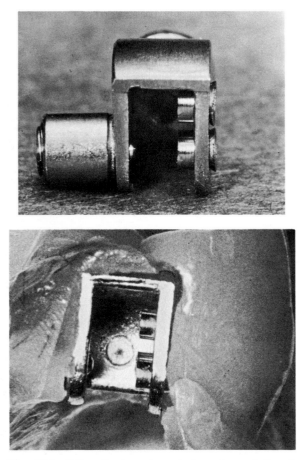

Fig. 356 P.R. attachment, anterior view of female section. Retaining plunger is on the left and the two locating projections on the right.

protected with vaseline and the attachment positioned on its counterpart. Check to ensure sufficient resin was removed to allow the denture to seat into its correct position without applying load to or tilting the attachment. The most common problem is slight load to the retention ring of the attachment causing tilting. Further resin will need to be removed in this instance and it is at times like this we appreciate the bulk occupied by different attachments. The location of miniature Dalbos is particularly critical. Suppose the top of the flange failed to touch by 0·2 mm. The number of degrees the base was free to rotate would be about double compared with a similar error on the conventional Dalbo unit.

With the denture firmly seated and the attachment correctly located, lock the two together with the aid of a small amount of self-polymerising resin inserted through the lingual window (Fig. 354). When the resin has completely covered the denture, ensure that adequate retention has been obtained, and that the location is correct. The remaining defect in the denture resin can then be repaired in stages, thereby minimising the effects of acrylic resin contraction.

Finally, remove excess resin from the free edges of the socket using a heated blunt probe.

The proper use of rebasing dowels will virtually eliminate the need to relocate attachments after rebasing. Accidents apart, the relocating procedure will be required when attachments need to be replaced and is frequently employed when a second denture is to be made after the abutment crowns have been cemented.

The PR extracoronal attachment must be one of the most robust constructed (Figs. 355–357). It features very large lateral surfaces. Retention is provided by a spring-loaded plunger, mounted lingually, engaging a dimple in the male section. A retraction slot is prepared to guide the plunger into place. The two small projections on the buccal side of the female unit govern the movement potential. The lower projection limits the vertical travel and the upper one restricts hinge movement. From the mechanical point of view the attachment has obvious advantages, particularly as a range of useful ancillary devices is available.

Plaque control and size restrictions are the limiting factors. The smaller of the two attachments is 4·5 mm tall, 5 mm long, and 5·4 mm wide. The larger unit measures 5·5 mm×6 mm×5·9 mm. Where space permits these units have obvious merit. Left and right sided units are made, and elements compatible with yellow gold or bonded porcelain to gold are available.

The Ceka attachment system has gained steadily in popularity and scope. It is among the most versatile of all attachments. When used as an extracoronal retainer, the male retaining pin is attached to the denture and engages the centre of a ring that is joined to the abutment tooth. The retaining pin is conical in shape, while the female section is tapered from top to bottom (Fig. 358).

Two configurations of retaining pin are provided, one allowing vertical play of 0·3 mm together with associated hinge movement, the other permits no vertical travel (Fig. 359). The circular shape of the attachment will not prevent rotation around a vertical axis. For this reason lateral bracing arms are essential. The arms will help with the seating of the prosthesis, and prevention of movement of unwanted hinge movement (Fig. 360). Guide planes should be used in conjunction with lateral bracing arms. The attachment should be considered as a direct retainer.

The diameter and shape of the female ring is now standard throughout the Ceka range. The following group represent differences in the retaining element. It should be understood that if a properly constructed bracing arm with occlusal rest seat is constructed, the difference between 'rigid' and 'resilient' retaining pins become solely of academic interest.

The 600 series are resilient and must be used in conjunction with the correct spacers (Fig. 361). The 700 series are comparatively rigid. The retaining pin may be unscrewed from its base allowing replacement to be made without difficulty. It is also possible to change from a resilient configuration to a rigid configuration and vice versa. The base of the

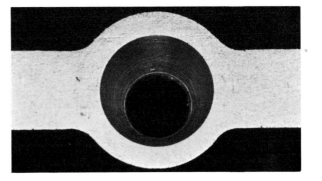

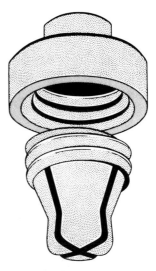

Fig. 358 The Ceka attachment system consists of a standard sized tapered female ring (top), engaged by a conical shaped retaining pin. The retaining pin (bottom) may be unscrewed and replaced.

retaining pin may be soldered to the framework of the partial denture (S-type) (Fig. 362) or buried in the acrylic resin (KS type) (Fig. 363). A choice of yellow gold or stainless steel is provided for the KS rings. An alternative arrangement, the 300 series, allows the base to be bolted to a minor connector of the partial denture (Fig. 364).

Where vertical space is restricted the Mini retaining element is useful. The retaining pin forms its own base thereby allowing a significant reduction in vertical space (Fig. 365). The Mini configuration reduces the height of the units to 2·45 mm for the rigid and 2·75 mm for the resilient attachment.

The female sections are produced as part of a bar that is sectioned close to the attachment. Palladium gold and yellow gold versions are available. Alternatively, a high heat modification, the Irax is

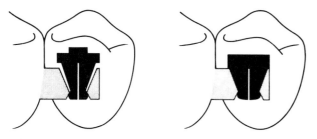

Fig. 359   Two types of retaining pin are available for the Ceka attachment. One allows some vertical play and rotational movement; the other provides a comparatively rigid union.

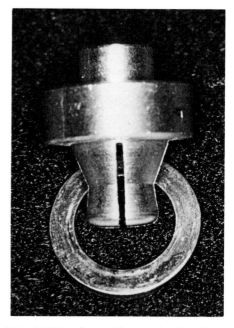

Fig. 361   '600' series resilient male pin with spacer.

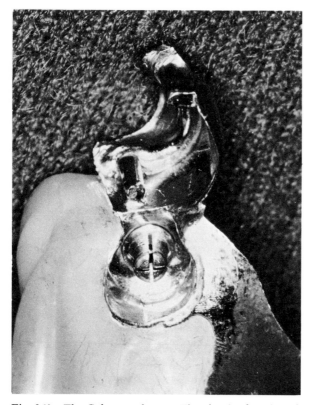

Fig. 360   The Ceka attachment. The circular female unit is joined to the abutment tooth and the conical-shaped male section is attached to the removable prosthesis. Note the bracing arm and occlusal rest seat.

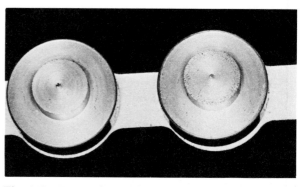

Fig. 362   Bases of retention pins designed for soldering to denture connector (S-type).

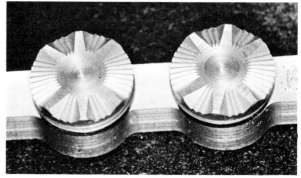

Fig. 363   Retention pins with bases for incorporation in acrylic resin of denture base (KS-Type).

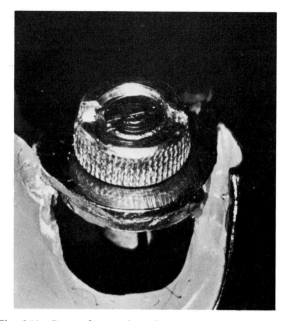

Fig. 364 Base of retention pin bolted to denture connector ('300' series).

manufactured for use with porcelain bonded to gold techniques (Fig. 366).

A recent addition to the range is a plastic pattern that can be invested and burnt out thereby allowing the attachment and crown to be cast as one. The pattern includes a liner of platinized alloy that becomes incorporated within the casting, thereby ensuring precision of fit and adequate wear resistance. This type is known as the OL series (Fig. 367). A small notch in the pattern allows a plastic bar, straight or bent, to be made up and cast, thereby incorporating the attachment in a bar connector. The latest pattern of the OL series includes a preformed distal guide plane. A new, non precious alloy has

now been produced for use with the Ceka OL series.

The vertical space requirement for the conventional Ceka range is at least 5 mm and the Mini retaining pin requires about 4 mm of vertical space. These measurements can be reduced slightly by employing a cast metal occlusal surface. The diameter of the ring is 4 mm. Additional bucco-lingual space is required for the facing, and for an adequate thickness of material for strength. Breakages are usually, and unfairly, blamed on the attachments. The common cause is failure to appreciate the space requirements.

Where buccal space is limited the attachment can be positioned slightly lingual to its normal position and a lingual metal surface employed to reduce the bulk of the prosthesis. If bucco-lingual space is restricted it is not the best attachment for the situation.

When used to retain distal extension prostheses the applications are similar to other extracoronal units, apart from the need for bracing arms and some additional occlusal support (Fig. 368). The attachments need to be aligned in the vertical plane and this is achieved with a special mandrel (Fig. 369). The connecting strut should be as short as possible, to reduce leverages applied to the abutments, and the ring placed close to the mucosa. The positioning of the ring should take into account ease of plaque control without which the prognosis of the restoration must be hopeless.

The distal surface of the abutment crown should incorporate a guide plane against which the mesial section of the denture will fit. This adaptation will help prevent the distal section of the denture base lifting away from the mucosa. The bracing arm will provide additional guide plane activity.

Additional resistance to rotational forces is provided by carrying the metal framework around the

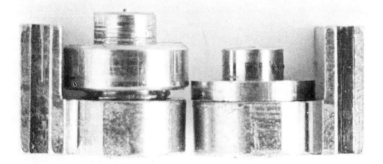

Fig. 365 Miniature and conventional retaining pins in place. The retaining pin of the miniature unit cannot be unscrewed.

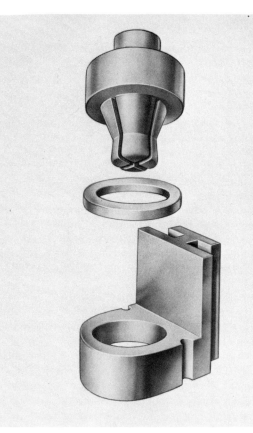

Fig. 366 The Irax Ceka unit for use with bonded porcelain to gold techniques. It includes a ready made guide plane.

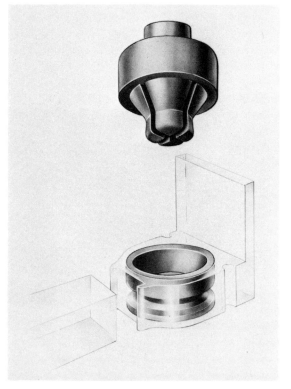

Fig. 367a The OL series features a plastic pattern with a liner of platinized alloy. The liner becomes incorporated within the casting ensuring precision of fit.

ring. The metal surface simplifies cleansing apart from adding to the strength of the restoration. Ingenious technical adjuncts are provided to allow the framework to be waxed up around a special former and subsequently finished and polished with matched instruments (Fig. 370). These instruments are included in one of the most comprehensive kits produced for an attachment (Fig. 371). It includes adjusting tools, locating dowels, soldering dowels, finishing instruments, riveting tools, and specially modified pliers for holding the attachments. Small wonder that this system is so popular in the laboratory.

The Ceka attachment is versatile, robust, and relatively simple to employ.

If the clinician is to obtain the best results from these attachments he must be familiar with some of the technical aspects.

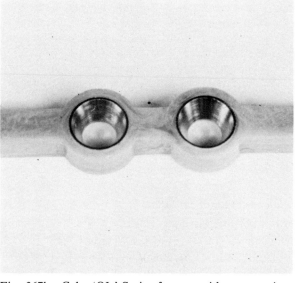

Fig. 367b Ceka 'OL' Series for use with non-precious or gold alloys.

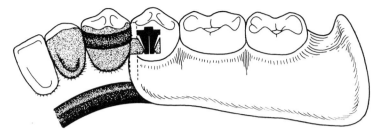

Fig. 368   The bracing arm, an essential feature of the design, provides stabilization and additional occlusal support. It is particularly useful for rebasing and relocating procedures.

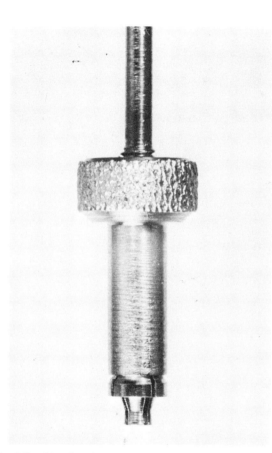

Fig. 369   Mandrel for alignment of attachment. Twisting the knurled knob releases the tension and allows it to be withdrawn without disturbing the ring in the waxed abutment.

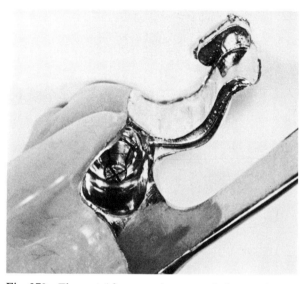

Fig. 370   The metal framework surrounds the attachment simplifying plaque control and contributing to the strength of the restoration.

ments of this nature should be carried out extremely carefully and in stages.

When loosening the retention of the attachment care must be taken not to cross the leaves of the retaining pin. A special instrument is provided to slacken retention, H9 in the Ceka kit. If this is not available long nosed pliers may be carefully employed (Figs. 375, 376).

When inserting a prosthesis for the first time the retention of the pins should be slackened as much as possible.

Adjustments for retention

The special adjustment tool for the Ceka attachment incorporates a wedge shaped blade (Fig. 372). The other end of the instrument incorporates a device for unscrewing retaining pins. This blade should be carefully inserted between the leaves of the male pin without levering them apart (Figs. 373, 374). Adjust-

Rebasing

The principles involved in rebasing dentures with Ceka attachments are similar to those described before. Resilient Ceka attachments require the spacer to be inserted over the male section before the impression is made. The denture should be seated by load applied to the bracing arm and

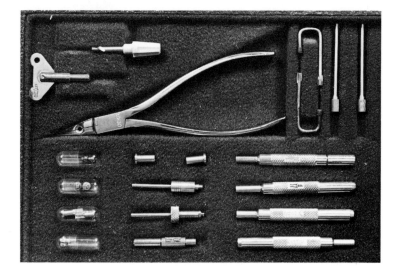

Fig. 371 Possibly the most comprehensive ancillary kit available for any attachment. This Ceka assembly includes devices for adjustments, alignment, riveting, soldering, together with locating dowels for rebasing.

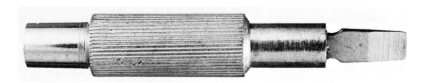

Fig. 372 Wedge shaped blade for increasing the retention of the Ceka pins. The opposite end is used for replacing retention pins.

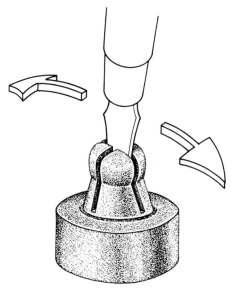

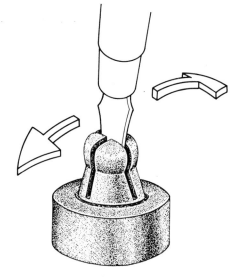

Fig. 373 Retention is increased by inserting the wedge and sliding it from side to side.

Fig. 374 The leaves of the retention pin should never be levered apart.

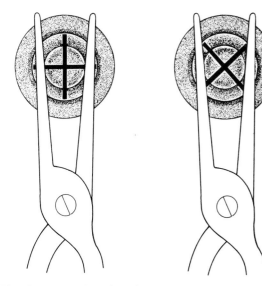

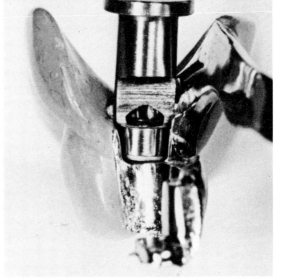

Fig. 375 Retention should be slackened with the special tool. Long nosed pliers may be used carefully in this manner.

Fig. 376 Incorrect use of pliers to slacken retention resulting in crossing the leaves of the retention pin.

Fig. 377 Ceka locating dowel in place. Its use is essential during rebasing procedures.

occlusal rest. If these structures are correctly seated, the denture has been seated in its proper position in the mouth. A locating dowel is available to prevent attachment movement during curing of the resin (Fig. 377).

Relocation

The objectives of this difficult procedure have been described already. If the Ceka attachment fails to engage, the male pin can be unscrewed with the special instrument. A shim of platinum foil is placed in the screw base and the male pin replaced and tightened. This process may be repeated. If the attachment engages, the riveting tool is then employed to prevent accidental loosening of the male pin. This artificial lengthening of the male pin may not solve the problem, in which case a relocating procedure similar to that described previously will be required.

The shape of the Ceka female dictates particularly careful blocking out of the space under and around the attachment, and one must not forget to insert the spacer when resilient attachments are employed. Bracing arms and associated occlusal rests ensure correct seating of the denture during the process and contribute to the accuracy with which the process can be undertaken.

CONNECTING UNITS

These units connect two parts of a removable prosthesis, allowing a certain limited amount of play. They have an apparently similar function to a long and flexible major connector but act in a more precise and predictable manner.

The Steiger joints are good examples of this type of unit. They work well and illustrate clearly the principle involved. The Steiger joints were developed between the Wars for joining a denture to its retainers, usually removable sections of crowns. Steiger recommended his excellent CSP system for the removable crowns, although a simpler telescopic system will usually suffice. The joints may be also used for joining a denture base to the major connector of a clasp-retained denture.

The female section of the attachment consists of a vertical sleeve soldered to the removable crowns or the clasp-retained section of the denture. The male unit is a flattened rod, attached to the denture saddle, and fits within the sleeve. The two parts of the attachment are held together by a small screw passing through the female sleeve and into the male section.

Two basic types of joints are manufactured:

(a) The axial rotation joint (Fig. 378)

This connector allows a limited vertical movement, as a small window is cut out of the female section around the screw. The male section is therefore free to travel up and down within the narrow confine of the window. Rotation and lateral movements can be provided by dismantling the attachment and very slightly trimming the male unit. This joint can be incorporated within the Scott attachment.

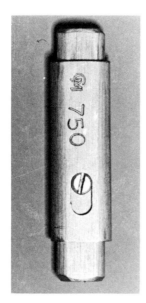

Fig. 378   The Axial Rotation Joint. The small window around the screw determines the vertical travel allowed by the joint.

(b) The rotation joint (Fig. 379)

This attachment is similar to the Axial Rotation Joint but there is no window around the screw (Fig. 380). Vertical movements cannot therefore take place.

Steiger originally envisaged the Axial Rotation Joints as connectors for distal extension dentures. He felt that the screw should be at the top of the window when the teeth were apart (Fig. 381), and should move downwards as load was applied to the artificial teeth. Since the most favourable distribution of load to the edentulous ridge occurs with a combination of vertical and rotational movements, it was suggested that a small amount of metal be removed from the mesio-gingival and disto-occlusal sections of the male unit. The amount of relief required was extremely small. For example, Steiger calculated that it was only necessary to remove 0·07 mm of metal to allow the average distal extension

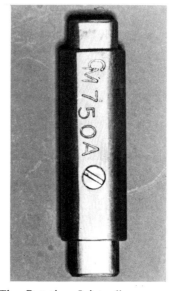

Fig. 379   The Rotation Joint allows no vertical play between the two sections of the attachment.

denture to rotate by 2 mm. When this approach was used, the adjustments were carried out by trial and error. The prosthesis was left in place for several days and then removed and taken to pieces. The shiny spots on the mesio-gingival and disto-occlusal portions were shaved with a hand instrument, and the procedure repeated a week later. In this way, it was felt the degree of movement within the attachment could be adjusted to meet individual requirements. The mesio-occlusal and disto-gingival portions of the male unit were never adjusted, for they prevented the distal portion of the denture saddle lifting away from the mucosa (Fig. 382).

The Rotation Joint was designed for the unilateral distal extension prosthesis, for this type of denture is usually tooth- and mucosal-supported on one side and entirely tooth-supported on the opposite side. Since vertical movement could be damaging to the teeth on the tooth-supported side, Steiger designed the Rotation Joint to allow only slight rotational and lateral movements in order to minimise torques transmitted from the distal extension base on the opposite side (Fig. 383). A typical unilateral distal extension design would, therefore, incorporate an Axial Rotation Joint connecting the distal extension base to the retainers and major connector, while the retainers on the opposite, tooth-supported, side would be connected through a Rotation Joint.

The Steiger joints are models of careful design, and are one of the few attachments in which the amount and direction of the movement allowance

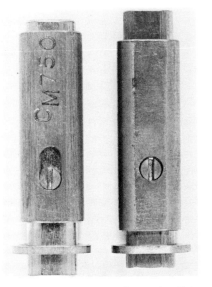

Fig. 380   The Axial Rotation and Rotation Joints side by side illustrating the soldering rings.

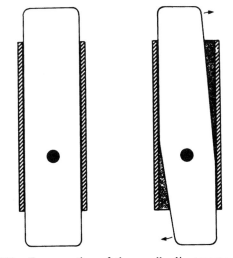

Fig. 382   Exaggeration of the small adjustments necessary to allow slight rotation within the Axial Rotation Joint. The metal is shaved only from the mesio-gingival and disto-occlusal sections of the male unit. The other surfaces prevent the denture base moving away from the mucosa and should not be touched.

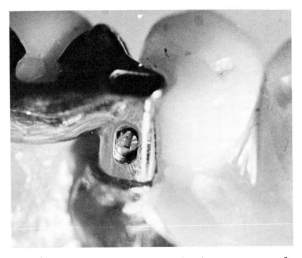

Fig. 381   The Axial Rotation Joint is a connector for bilateral distal extension dentures. Steiger felt that the screw should be at the top window with the teeth apart and should move downwards as load is applied to the artificial teeth.

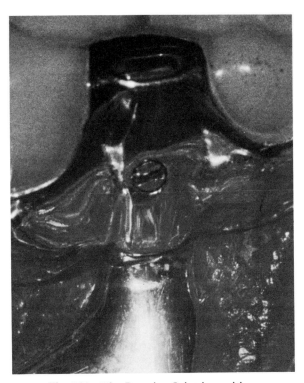

Fig. 383   The Rotation Joint in position.

can be determined precisely by the operator. If appreciable wear takes place, both parts of the attachment can be removed from the mouth and a replacement soldered on. Many of Steiger's original prostheses have stood the test of twenty or thirty years use. As denture designs and impression techniques improved, it was found that even the slight movement allowance provided by Steiger's original designs gave too much vertical play and led to damage of the distal papilla of the distal abutment tooth. Boitel now finds that better results are obtained by using the Rotation Joint for bilateral distal extension base prostheses as well. The window around the screw can be very slightly widened to allow a minute amount of vertical play. Dismantling and shaving the male attachment is unnecessary for the slight wear taking place between the two units provides the requisite amount of freedom.* It is difficult to calculate the degree and direction of movement that will be allowed by a long flexible major connector. The Steiger joints are small and the movement they allow and the direction in which this movement occurs can be determined with precision. However, it can be seen that a well designed and constructed denture requires little, if any, movement around the natural teeth.

COMBINED ATTACHMENTS

These units consist of a hinge connector joined to an intracoronal attachment. The hinge unit is buried within the denture so that when it is in position, the attachment closely resembles a rigid intracoronal attachment. Combined attachments usually fit identical female slots to the intracoronal attachments produced by the same manufacturer, so that after tooth loss it may be possible to make a denture substituting a combined attachment for an intracoronal attachment.

Crismani combined units are illustrated as being typical of this group. Two types of Crismani are available, one allowing a purely hinge motion (Fig. 384), the other allowing lateral play in conjunction with the hinge motion (Fig. 385). Movements of both types are spring controlled. Lateral play is allowed so that a divergence of the abutments will not prevent the hinge action. Access to the spring is available by dismantling the attachment by means of a small screw in the base (Fig. 386).

Combined attachments are commonly misused to retain unilateral distal extension prostheses. Follow-

Boitel, R., personal communiations.

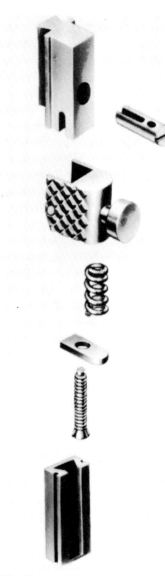

Fig. 384   The Crismani combined unit dismantled. This attachment allows only a spring-controlled hinge movement.

ing loss of a molar tooth, it is tempting to convert a unilateral posterior 'removable bridge' into a unilateral distal extension denture, merely by substituting a combined attachment for the mesial intracoronal unit. In most cases, however, such a prosthesis nearly always requires support from the other side of the arch.

When the restoration is small, for example, where a second molar is replaced with an artificial tooth narrower bucco-lingually and mesio-distally.

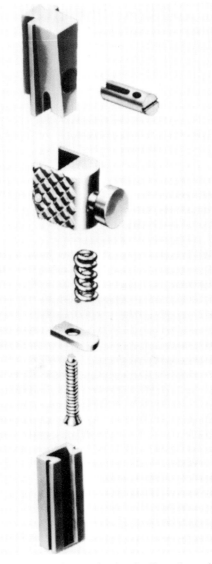

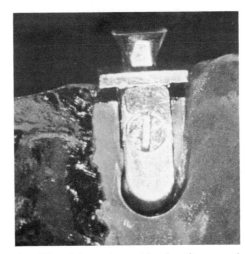

Fig. 386 The Crismani combined units may be dismantled by means of a screw in the impression surface.

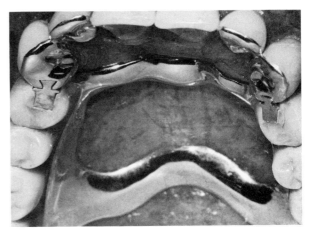

Fig. 385 This Crismani combined unit allows lateral play together with a spring-controlled hinge movement.

Fig. 387 Bilateral distal extension denture retained by Crismani combined units.

bilateral support may be considered unnecessary. Provided the abutments are sufficiently rigid, such as a firm second premolar and first molar, a cantilevered fixed prosthesis can be considered. The prognosis of this type of restoration is more favourable when it is opposed by artificial teeth. Whatever the restoration, a 'stress-breaking' attachment should never be used as an excuse for anchoring an unstable denture to a natural tooth.

Combined attachments may be used to retain distal extension prostheses where the strength of the abutment is questionable (Fig. 387). They are more bulky than intracoronal units, and may interfere with the occlusal surface of the first tooth on the denture. Acrylic-resin artificial teeth are nearly always required. Lingual bracing arms are recommended where space allows, and the retention of all these units is adjustable in the same manner as the intracoronal attachments.

CLINICAL PROCEDURES

The importance of sound periodontal tissues has been stressed throughout this text. Occasionally mucogingival surgery, together with orthodontic therapy, may be necessary to reposition abutments, ensure peridontal health, and to obtain adequate space (Figs. 388–390) for the retainers.

Impression techniques

As a distal extension base derives important support from the mucosa, this aspect will be considered in some detail. Since the mucosa is displaceable, the denture base will tend to sink under occlusal load until an equilibrium is reached between the displacing forces and a combination of mucosal resistance and support from the teeth. The mucosa of the denture-bearing area is seldom of even displaceability or thickness, and there can be substantial base movements where the mucosa is poorly supported. The potential base movement can be reduced by using an impression technique that adapts the impression surface of the denture to the shape the mucosa will assume under occlusal load. The base would then have less distance to travel before mucosal resistance developed. On the other hand, it would be undesirable to have the mucosa subjected to continuous, heavy load from the denture base. The compromise suggested by Applegate (1955) was to record mucosal displacement just below the level that produced surface ischaemia or blanching of the mucosa, with the teeth out of contact.

If it were possible to obtain with one impression details of all the teeth of one jaw, the abutment preparations, and a displacement impression of the denture-bearing area, subsequent procedures would be considerably simplified. Improved elastomeric impression materials have made this possible (Fig. 391) and produce excellent impressions of the abutment preparations and their surrounding structures in their correct relationship to one another. Since the viscosity of the materials varies, the amount of mucosal displacement obtained cannot be determined, and a subsequent impression of the denture-bearing area may be advisable. Another problem rests with the impression tray, for it is usually necessary to employ an acrylic resin tray in order to obtain close adaptation to the teeth and denture-bearing areas.

Acrylic resin trays of this type are prone to flex under load because of their size and because some operators weaken them by retention holes for the impression material. The tray may be strengthened by a rib running around it. With the knowledge now available about the visco-elastic properties of mucosa, it is possible to obtain an impression of the entire arch to include abutment preparations and denture bearing area. This is difficult to achieve and can only be useful on a master impression if the patient has previously worn a denture. When it is possible to obtain such a master impression it simplifies all subsequent stages.

In many instances this one step impression will not be possible and an altered cast technique indicated. When at least six, and preferably more, teeth remain in a dental arch with a reasonably prominent curvature, the displacement impression can be made before the metal framework is constructed.

The abutment preparations are completed, and impressions of them made in the material of choice.

An acrylic resin tray is constructed on the cast of this impression. The tray consists of a rigid U-shaped strut of acrylic resin fitting over the occlusal surfaces of the teeth. The tray handle is attached to the mid-point of the strut, and the two distal ends of the strut support close-fitting trays covering the mucosa of the denture-bearing area (Fig. 392). This type of tray requires precise location onto the teeth, so that at three widely spaced points occlusal stops are provided between the strut and the teeth. In view of the precise location required, this procedure can be used only where there are widely spaced contacts. It could not be used where there are remaining six anterior teeth in a square arch, for they would be virtually in line.

At the next visit, the temporary crowns are removed, and the tray checked in the mouth. The extension of the trays should resemble that of a complete denture, and some relief around the mylohyoid muscle will be required. It is essential that the three occlusal stops make proper contact.

Applegate and co-workers developed a series of impression waxes of known viscosity at mouth temperature.* The hardest of these waxes (No. 1) was designed for use in extending the borders of the denture base, and the softest (No. 4) for use in recording details of the impression surface. The mucosal displacement is obtained when an excess of wax is expelled around the borders of the tray or denture base, rather than by direct pressure applied by the dentist. The amount of mucosal displacement depends upon the the viscosity of the wax. Since this has been predetermined, the mucosal displacement is controlled.

---

* Korecta Wax, Kerr Mfg. Co. Inc., Detroit, Michigan.

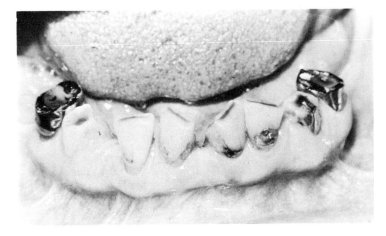

Fig. 388   Malpositioned abutments and inadequate clinical crown height.

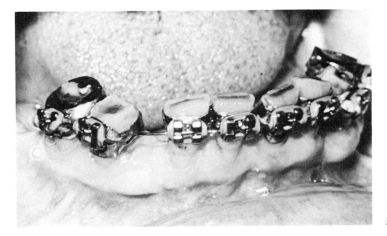

Fig. 389   Preliminary mucogingival surgery followed by orthodontic therapy.

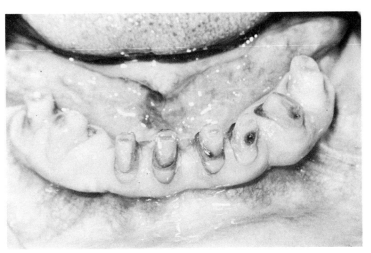

Fig. 390   Outlined preparations.

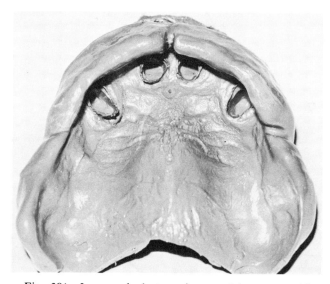

Fig. 391   Improved elastomeric materials can provide details of all the teeth of one jaw, the abutment preparations, and a displacement impression of the denture-bearing areas.

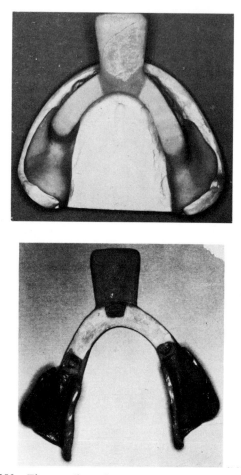

Fig. 392   The acrylic resin tray for making an impression of the denture-bearing mucosa.

The impression wax is best manipulated by softening it in a container surrounded by hot water at approximately 200 °F (Fig. 393). Most commercially available thermostatically-controlled water baths can be readily adapted, and it is seldom that more than the two types of wax will be required, although intermediate grades are available. The impression wax can be applied with a small paintbrush; a brush with medium stiff bristles 1 cm (3/8″) long is suggested by Applegate. A separate brush should be used for each wax, as it is important that the waxes should not be contaminated.

A thin layer of wax is painted on the impression surface of the tray which is then inserted in the mouth. The tray is seated by applying finger pressure over the occlusal stops, never over the denture base area. The bulk of the wax will cause displacement of the mucosa and excess wax will be squeezed out around the periphery of the base. When the area is large, it is helpful to dip the impression tray in hot water just before seating it. While it is true that dipping the tray in water may leach out some of the constituents of the impression wax, the results appear to be satisfactory and it does overcome the problem of having some parts of the impression warmer than the others when the impression wax first contacts the mucosa. When correctly supported the impression wax (No. 4) appears glossy. The impression surface should be chilled and dried thoroughly with compressed air before an addition

is made, and every care taken to ensure that the occlusal stops of the tray are in contact. The length of time required for the wax to flow varies with the size of the saddle, but at least four minutes is usually required.

If the impression has been overbuilt, it may show up by a very high gloss on the impression surface and by the occlusal stops which may not seat home. In these circumstances it is best to scrape out the wax and start again. When a satisfactory impression has been obtained, the impression tray with its recording of the denture-bearing area cannot now be replaced on the cast. Instead, the edentulous ridges are cut off the cast, and the impression tray is reorientated back on the cast by means of the occlusal stops (Fig. 394). The master cast obtained in this manner provides an accurate representation of the residual ridge mucosa under slight load, in its

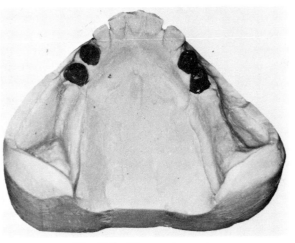

Fig. 395   The master cast.

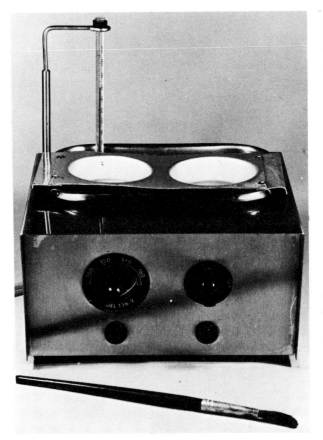

Fig. 393   A thermostatically-controlled water bath suitable for melting impression waxes.

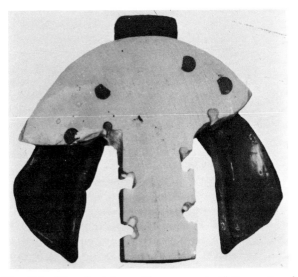

Fig. 394   The edentulous ridges are cut off the cast and the impression tray localised by means of its occlusal stops. Note the keyways placed in the residual cast.

correct relationship to the abutment preparations and to the remainder of the dental arch (Fig. 395).

Unfortunately the number or arrangement of the natural teeth frequently fail to provide widely spaced occlusal stops. Another impression procedure is then required.

Rigid extracoronal attachments can be treated like intracoronal units. An impression of the abutment crowns is made with an elastomeric material. Copper tube impressions of individual teeth, transfer copings and a subsequent locating impression may seem dated to some, but are accurate and useful for dealing with awkward problems (Figs. 396, 397). However it is made, the impression of the abutment crowns must include details of the entire edentulous area. At a subsequent visit jaw relations are recorded. The abutment crowns with attachments can then be made together with the metal framework of the denture and the counterparts of the attachment.

Closely adapted acrylic resin bases covering the edentulous areas are then constructed on the master cast and joined to the major connector. The precise path of insertion provided by the attachments ensures that the location is unquestionable. The abutment crowns can now be placed in the mouth uncemented and the denture slid into place and the bases checked for extension (Fig. 398). The impression in fluid wax can now be produced, but virtually indistinguishable results can be obtained with one of the more viscous zinc oxide eugenol pastes.* One practical tip is to remove the abutment crowns attached to the denture as this ensures that the area of the distal gingivae is recorded intact

* Kelly's Paste, Chicago.

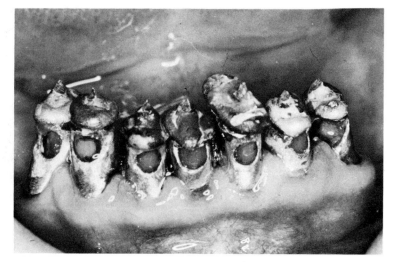

Fig. 396 Metal transfer copings in position. A dated technique but accurate nevertheless.

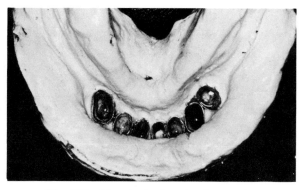

Fig. 397 The plaster locating impression.

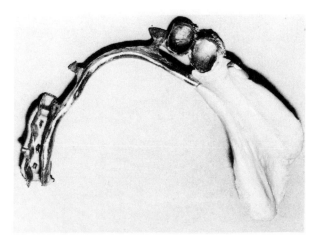

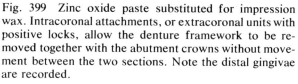

Fig. 399 Zinc oxide paste substituted for impression wax. Intracoronal attachments, or extracoronal units with positive locks, allow the denture framework to be removed together with the abutment crowns without movement between the two sections. Note the distal gingivae are recorded.

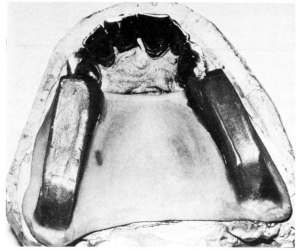

Fig. 398 Upper prosthesis showing close-fitting tray joined to the crowns by means of the attachments.

(Fig. 399). The master cast is now sectioned, removing the area corresponding to the denture base. This allows the assembled prosthesis to be slid into place on the remains of the cast and stone subsequently poured into the impression areas to reconstitute the master cast.

The advantages of rigid attachments with precise paths of insertion and withdrawal become apparent when techniques of this nature are described. But how does one deal with extracoronal attachments with hinge and vertical play? Obviously the one step

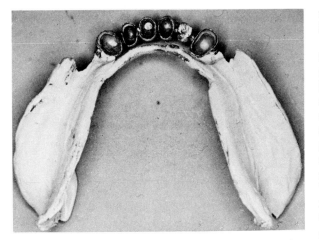

Fig. 400 Dalbo-retained denture base. Movement between base and retainers could occur during removal and there is inadequate reproduction of the intervening structures. An overall elastomeric impression is required to unite the two sections of the prosthesis in their correct relationship, to record the surrounding structures, and to facilitate removal of the impression.

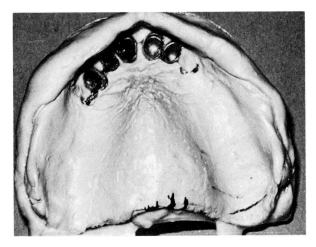

Fig. 401 An overall alginate impression has been employed to remove the two sections of the prosthesis in their correct relationship.

impression is the most convenient when possible otherwise an approach similar to the following is required.

The impression of the abutment crown preparations and entire arch is made according to the preferred technique as described for rigid attachments. Jaw relationships are recorded, the master cast mounted on an adjustable articulator and the metalwork for crowns and denture framework made including the attachments (Fig. 400).

Once the resin bases have been made the prosthesis may be tried in the mouth. Apart from the movement potential within the attachments a problem is the small handling area available for the operator. The resin should not obscure vision of the attachment in any way and seating load must be applied directly over the attachment. One can then proceed with the impression provided the location of the attachments is correct. If not, the attachments may be cut from the resin and relocated in the bases. The displacement is then made using fluid wax or zinc oxide eugenol. Excess material is cleaned from the attachments to ensure they are correctly seated and that no tilting has occurred. If all is well, alginate impression is loaded in a stock tray and inserted over teeth, crowns and base. Both sections of the restoration are removed in this overall impression in their correct relationship to one another (Fig. 401). Apart from removing denture and crown, the alginate records details of the surrounding tissues. The dies of the preparations are inserted into their respective crowns and a new master cast produced. Subsequent jaw relations will be necessary to mount this new master cast and for this reason some operators attempt to combine this stage with the impression procedure. This combined result is somewhat easier to achieve with upper impressions than with lower impressions. However, fast setting artificial stone can be placed on the occlusal surface of the resin tray before the overall impression is made.

A trial insertion of the posterior teeth is made at the next visit and eccentric records remade. Both denture and crowns can then be completed.

Inserting the prosthesis

The adaptation of the abutment crowns and that of the denture are rechecked. The attachment positions and their engagement are examined as well. Before the crowns are cemented, further attention should be paid to the jaw relation records. Many of these prostheses oppose complete upper dentures, and it is essential that the jaw relation records be checked with great care if the stability of the upper dentures is not to be impaired. When natural teeth are in opposition, it is equally important to check the jaw relations, in this instance to ensure that undue loads are not placed upon the dentures.

Since mucosal displaceability makes the use of articulating paper unreliable, a check record procedure is carried out. A centric relation record is

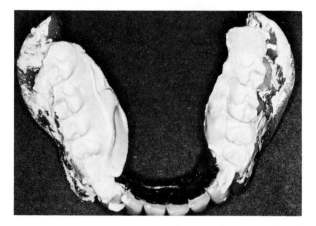

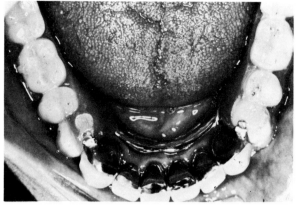

Fig. 402 The check record made when the restoration is inserted in the mouth but before cementation of the crowns.

Fig. 404 The completed restoration in the mouth.

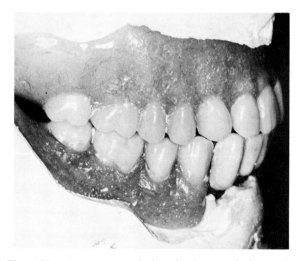

Fig. 403 By means of the check record the entire restoration is remounted on the articulator. Small errors of jaw relationship can then be corrected with the denture bases mounted on unyielding cases.

made in plaster or fast-setting artificial stone with the teeth just apart (Fig. 402). The entire prosthesis is now remounted on the articulator (Fig. 403), and corrections can be speedily made with the bases mounted on unyielding plaster.

When the crowns have been cemented, the patient must be shown how to insert and remove the prosthesis (Fig. 404). Time should be set aside to demonstrate how the entire prosthesis should be cleaned, while the importance of maintenance needs to be stressed.

Care taken in the construction of the restoration will be rewarded by a long interval before rebasing is required. However, the potential for movement and periodontal breakdown that may be caused by a lapse of plaque control must never be forgotten. Neither must the hazards of springs and other such devices be overlooked however tempting they may be to use.

Extracoronal attachments have many valuable applications. They are robust, versatile, and gaining ever-increasing popularity. Regular inspection and maintenance is essential if they are to provide satisfactory long-term service.

REFERENCES AND FURTHER READING

APPLEGATE, O. C. (1955) The partial denture base. *J. prosth. Dent.*, *5*, 636

GOODMAN, J. J. and GOODMAN, H. W. (1963) Balance of force in precision free-end restorations. *J. prosth. Dent.*, *13*, 302

HECKNEBY, M. (1969) Distribution of load with the lower free-end partial denture. *Acta odont. scand.*, *27* (Suppl. 52), 140

KABCENELL, J. L. (1970) The resilient partial denture. *N.Y. St. dent. J.*, *36*, 492

LUBESPÈRE, A. and ROTENBERG, A. (1976) *Attachements et Prothèses Combinées.* Julien Prélat, Paris

MARSHALL, W. S. (1938) Precision attachments and their advantages in respect to underlying tissue. *J. Amer. dent. Ass.*, *25*, 1250

MENSOR, M. C. (1968) The rationale of resilient hinge-action stressbreakers. *J. prosth. Dent.*, *20*, 204

NALLY, J. N. (1961) The use of prefabricated precision attachments. *Int. dent. J.*, *11*, 192

PREISKEL, H. W. (1969) Precision attachments for free-end saddle prostheses. *Brit. dent. J.*, *127*, 462

PREISKEL, H. W. (1971) Impression techniques for attachment-retained distal extension removable partial dentures. *J. prosth. Dent.*, *25*, 620

RANTANEN, T., MÄKILA, E. and YLI-URPO, A. (1972) Investigations of the therapeutic success with dentures retained by precision attachments. II. Partial dentures. *Suom. hammaslaak. toim.*, *68*, 73

RUSHFORD, C. B. (1974) A technique for precision removable partial denture construction. *J. prosth. Dent.*, *31:4*, 377–383

SCHILLI, G. (1959) *Ein Beitrag zur Versorgung einseitiger Freindlücken mit Hilfe des Dalbo-Gelenkes*. Dissertation, University of Freibürg im Breisgau, W. Germany

SCOTT, J. and BATES, J. F. (1972) The relining of partial dentures involving precision attachments. *J. prosth. Dent.*, *28*, 325

SCOTT, W. R. (1968) A removable telescopic external attachment with an axial-rotation joint. *J. prosth. Dent.*, *20*, 216

STEIGER, A. A. (1951) Abutment preparation for removable crown and bridgework with a new system of attachment. *Dent. Mag. (Lond.)*, *68*, 183

STEIGER, A. A. and BOITEL, R. H. (1959) *Precision Work for Partial Dentures*. Stebo, Zürich

TABET, G. (1961) Classifications cinématiques des attachements rupteurs des forces. Indication à prothèse décollétée. *Rev. franc. Odonto-stomat.*, *8*, 6

WATT, D. M. (1972) Dimple-hinge attachments for partial dentures. *Dent. Practit.*, *22*, 12

CHAPTER 8

Neuromuscular Control of Overdentures

A. G. Hannam

Mastication may be considered as a patterned motor act in which both central and peripheral feedback play a major role. There has been a considerable expansion of research in the area, especially over the last decade or two, and this research has been the subject of several recent reviews (Kawamura 1974; Sessle and Hannam 1976; Anderson and Matthews 1976; Dubner et al. 1978).

The masticatory pattern is cyclical and apparently influenced by a rhythmical 'pattern generator' in the brainstem. The latter can be activated, or altered, by corticofugal signals, or by peripheral inputs from areas such as the teeth, the joint capsules, and the muscles. Sensory afferent input from intra- and peri-oral sites may therefore be viewed as a means for providing information that can be used for a variety of purposes. It may have a modulating influence on the pattern generator; it is clearly important in permitting conscious perception via the thalamo-cortical route, and if the stimulus is severe enough, it may also be responsible for evoking protective, reflex behaviour in the muscles of the jaws and face.

The peripheral feedback of information concerning jaw displacement, interocclusal force, and position of the food bolus is essential not only during the learning process when complex patterns of motor activity are encoded by the central nervous system, but also during function in the mature animal, when regulation and adjustment of elements of the chewing cycle are constantly necessary. The variable form of the chewing stroke (Gibbs et al. 1971; Ahlgren 1976; Hannam et al. 1977), the irregular nature of interocclusal forces (Graf 1975) and the changing position of the food bolus during natural mastication in man (Wictorin 1972) all testify to the flexibility demanded of the neural control system.

No anatomically separate receptor group is solely responsible for signalling information about a given parameter of the chewing cycle, although one particular group may have a dominant influence. Thus, even though mechanoreceptors in the temporomandibular joint capsules have long been held to be partly responsible for signalling the position and, presumably, speed of movement of the mandible in space (Thilander 1961; Storey 1976), receptors in other locations, like the tongue, lips and masticatory musculature probably participate as well in the overall feedback of information concerning jaw separation. Similarly, while mechanoreceptors in the periodontal tissues may provide an important source of information about the nature of occlusal forces (Anderson et al. 1970; Hannam 1976a) it is also probable that other mechanoreceptors in tendon, fascia and periosteum signal information to the central nervous system. The multiple sources of sensory input available during function may account for the remarkably adaptive behaviour of patients with severe occlusal handicaps. They may also account, in part, for the lack of really dramatic alterations in sensorimotor performance when controlled experiments are carried out on subjects with known deficiencies.

Considering the differences between subjects with complete dentures and overdentures, it seems reasonable to assume that there are fairly clear-cut distinctions between the neural feedback available in each case. Yet research involving direct behavioural comparisons between complete and overdenture patients is sparse.

Overdentures may impart a mechanical stability which itself enables an improved neuromuscular performance by the subject. In addition, the retention of denervated tooth roots, and the consequent preservation of some of the periodontal innervation may result in an enhanced perception of occlusal forces, thereby improving the subject's ability to grade them. It is also possible that the preservation of a portion of the periodontal innervation contributes towards a perceptive sense that can be used by the overdenture patient to discriminate changes in the size or texture of small objects held between the teeth, or to assist him in the detection of light tooth contacts. These possibilities are discussed below.

The stability offered by an overdenture might be expected to provide a more resistant platform for the generation of force by the masticatory musculature than the base supplied by a complete denture. It is already known that subjects with an intact, natural dentition are able to produce about 5 or 6 times the interocclusal force, measured in the molar area, than can be produced by subjects wearing complete dentures (Wennström 1971b); and that in comparison with the latter group, the retention of enough mandibular teeth to support, in part, a lower Kennedy Class 1 partial denture increases the maximum attainable level of force in the same region (Wennström et al. 1972). There are, of course, various factors which can account for these differences, but in the absence of more direct evidence, it can be reasonably assumed that a stable occlusal foundation is more conducive to the development of high interocclusal forces than an unstable one. Furthermore, it has been shown that denture instability in complete denture wearers has a profound influence upon their perception of the hardness of interocclusal objects (Langer and Michman 1968). The suggestion that an unstable denture base will impair a subject's ability to grade normal, and especially strong, interocclusal forces (Wennström 1971b) seems reasonable.

The sensory discriminability for small particles held between the teeth of both dentate subjects and edentulous subjects wearing complete dentures may change according to the function being performed. This seems to be less acute during natural chewing than under more artificial laboratory conditions (Öwall and Møller 1974), and implies that alterations in peripheral and central nervous activity can affect perceptual thresholds. Even though direct evidence does not exist, it is likely that the sensory experience attending function with an unstable denture results in a lessened discriminatory sense for fine particles. Afferent signals produced in response to a moving denture base probably impair the effects of signals contributing to discrimination rather than enhance them.

Denture instability, however, does not necessarily affect all discriminatory senses in the oral environment. It has been shown, for example, that a subject's ability to estimate the degree of jaw separation is not drastically altered in the presence of unstable dentures (Siirilä and Laine 1972). Furthermore, considerable functional adaptation of the neuromuscular apparatus may occur over the life of

the prosthesis. Öwall (1974) has demonstrated that discriminability for small particles held between the teeth of complete dentures improves with the age of the dentures. Findings such as these may partly account for the remarkable neuromuscular control shown by some patients with highly unstable prostheses.

When considering the role of the periodontal innervation during mastication with overdentures, it seems obvious that the preservation of some periodontal sensory input would provide a decided neurophysiological bonus to the overdenture-patient (Loiselle et al. 1972; Kay and Abes 1976). It is, however, not so easy to demonstrate this.

Studies carried out on experimental animals have shown unequivocally that the tooth supporting tissues are well innervated. These studies have focused upon mechanoreceptors that have been assumed to lie within the periodontal ligament, and which have probably included adjacent sites like the gingiva and alveolar periosteum (Hannam 1976a). The morphological and physiological characteristics of the mechanoreceptors are now reasonably understood and both have been the subject of recent reviews (Anderson et al. 1970; Griffin and Malor 1974; Hannam 1976a; Byers and Holland 1977). These receptors are capable of responding to forces as low as 1–2 gm applied to the teeth, and to tooth displacements of the order of a few microns. Individually, the receptors are directionally sensitive, and are able to discriminate between small increments in the magnitude of applied force, especially in the lighter ranges (Hannam and Farnsworth 1977). This discriminability is illustrated in Fig. 405. The receptors are also sensitive to the rate of change of force (Pfaffman 1939; Hannam 1969). Taken together, these observations explain why low sensory thresholds to applied force can be demonstrated in man. Thresholds of the order of 1·5 gm are normal for anterior teeth, and seem to be unaltered by denervation of the tooth pulp (Linden 1975). They are lower in anterior than in posterior teeth (Anderson et al. 1970).

The primary role of the periodontal mechanoreceptor population would appear to arise from its proven ability to signal information about interocclusal pressures to more central destinations. The receptors function primarily as sensors for a system controlling the generation of masticatory force, and experimental evidence supports this assumption. Pressure on the teeth has long been known to cause reflex inhibition of jaw closing motoneurones in man and other experimental animals, simultaneously activating the jaw opening muscles in some species

(Goldberg 1976a, b; Matthews 1976) and causing contralateral jaw movements in others (Lund et al. 1971). It is possible that these receptors may be part of a positive feedback system operating at a cortical level, and they are probably important in the generation of jaw closing forces during normal mastication in the dentate subject (Sessle 1976).

In one of the few studies of force discrimination in man, Bonaguro et al. (1969) have shown that sensory discriminability for externally applied stimuli on single anterior teeth seems to be optimal between 50 and 500 g, although some discrimination is still possible outside this range. When dentate subjects are asked to grade the amount of interocclusal force they produce by voluntary contraction of the jaw closing muscles, a situation in which neural elements other than the periodontal innervation must also be included, they can reproduce between 6 and 8 levels with some accuracy over ranges of 8 kg at the incisors (Hannam 1976b) or 30 kg in the first molar region (Wennström 1971a).

The precise contribution of a small number of retained, denervated tooth roots to the feedback system responsible for the grading of interocclusal forces cannot be specified. However, experiments conducted so far would imply that, given adequate stimulation, their afferent innervation is capable of signalling information that is potentially useful for the perception and control of such forces over a very wide range. Unfortunately, there are as yet no studies which answer the vital question whether a subject wearing overdentures regulates these forces with more precision than one with complete dentures.

Maximum comfortable levels of bite force, measured in the molar zone of complete denture wearers, are about 1/5 those of subjects with their natural teeth (Wennström 1971a). If the large difference in operating ranges is ignored, complete denture wearers seem to be able to grade interocclusal forces as well as dentate subjects, at least when their ability to produce different categories is measured (Wennström 1971a, b).

The value of retaining some periodontal innervation is well illustrated, however, in the experiments of Pacer and Bowman (1975), where the sensory discrimination of applied force was compared in groups of patients with complete dentures and overdentures. Despite their rather surprising, and as yet unexplained, demonstration that discriminatory thresholds in the range 100–500 g were slightly lower in complete denture wearers than in subjects wearing overdentures, it is clear from this work that at higher force levels the overdenture patients were better able to discriminate between different levels of stimulation (Fig. 406). The authors suggested that at low force levels the overdenture base made either light or no contact with the abutment teeth so as to lessen the periodontal contribution. At high levels of applied force, there was firm contact between the base and the retained teeth and they reasoned that such contact would ensure a neural input from the periodontium and so permit better sensory discrimination.

As expected, it has been shown that sensory input from the periodontium does not play a major role in the estimation of large degrees of jaw separation (Christensen and Morimoto 1977), a function unsuited to the periodontal innervation on intuitive

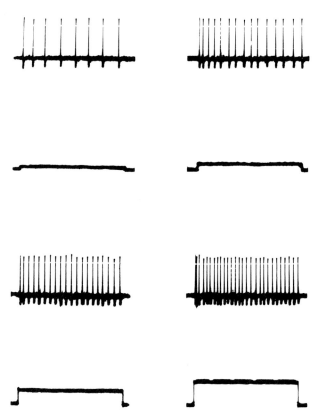

Fig. 405   Response of a single periodontal mechanosensitive neurone to forces applied to the lower canine tooth in a cat. Strain gauge records of 4 increasing amplitudes of force are shown, each applied for 500 msec. In every case, trains of nerve impulses evoked by the stimulus are shown above the strain gauge record. Changes in force amplitude are reflected by changes in the frequency of discharge of the neurone, thus providing the basis for sensory discrimination. Calibration bar represents 50 gm.

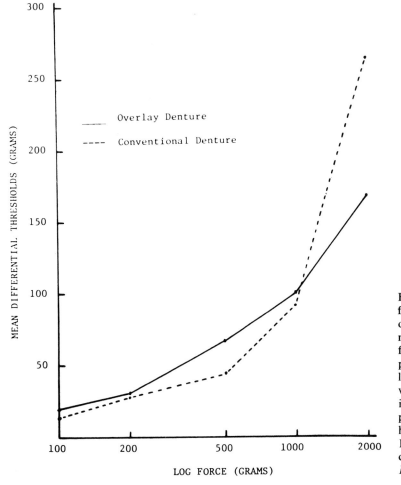

Fig. 406 Mean differential thresholds to forces applied to lower dentures from an occlusal direction, plotted against the logarithm of the applied force. Data are shown for groups of subjects wearing both complete and overlay dentures. At higher levels of force, discriminability in patients wearing conventional complete dentures is less than that in the overdenture patients, as their mean differential threshold is greater. (From Pacer, Fred J., and Bowman, Douglas C., 1975. Occlusal force discrimination by denture patients, *J. Prosth. Dent.*, *33*, 602.)

grounds alone. Other receptors, possibly those in the musculature, seem to be responsible for this perceptual sense (Siirila and Laine 1972; Christensen and Levin 1976). Moreover, there is direct evidence which demonstrates that local anaesthesia of the abutment teeth in subjects wearing overdentures does not affect thickness estimation in the 2–3 mm range (Christensen and Levin 1976).

Discriminability in assessing the thickness of very small objects held between the teeth can be affected, albeit mildly, by altering the milieu of the periodontal innervation, either by means of local anaesthesia (Siirilä and Laine 1963) or by previously loading the teeth with prostheses (Slabbert and Christensen 1978). Presumably tactile occlusal sense is influenced by input from the periodontium, if only in the perception of small particles. Complete denture wearers, for example, are approximately 6

times less efficient than dentate subjects at detecting the thickness of very small objects between the teeth (Siirilä and Laine 1969). How this tactile sense functions is not fully understood. The periodontal input may simply provide a highly sensitive mechanism for indicating the presence or absence of events in time. Alternatively, it may furnish specific information about small intrusions of the teeth and their directional changes when tiny objects are held interocclusally. The uncertainty surrounding the nature of the inputs associated in perception at this level is well illustrated by the observation that the tactile thresholds can also be influenced by masking the audible sounds of light tooth contact both in dentate subjects and in patients wearing complete dentures (Laine and Siirilä 1977).

To summarize, it seems reasonable to conclude that the retention of part of the natural dentition affords the overdenture patient a gain in neuro-muscular performance. Higher occlusal forces may be produced during mastication, and the enhanced ability of the overdenture patient to sense the amplitudes of such high forces probably enables him to grade these forces with more precision. Finally, it is likely that the overdenture patient has a better tactile sense for fine particles than his edentulous counterpart, providing the overdenture remains in contact with its abutment teeth.

REFERENCES AND FURTHER READING

AHLGREN, J. (1976) Masticatory movements in man. In *Mastication* by Anderson and Matthews. John Wright, Bristol

ANDERSON, D. J. and MATTHEWS, B. (1976) *Mastication*. John Wright, Bristol

ANDERSON, D. J., HANNAM, A. G. and MATTHEWS, B. (1970) Sensory mechanisms in mammalian teeth and their supporting structures. *Physiol. Rev.*, *50*, 171–195

BONAGURO, J. G., DUSZA, G. R. and BOWMAN, D. C. (1969) Ability of human subjects to discriminate forces applied to certain teeth. *J. dent. Res.*, *48*, 236–241

BYERS, M. R. and HOLLAND, G. R. (1977) Trigeminal nerve endings in gingiva, junctional epithelium and periodontal ligament of rat molars as demonstrated by autoradiography. *Anat. Rec.*, *181*, 509–524

CHRISTENSEN, L. V. and LEVIN, A. C. (1976) Periodontal discriminatory ability in human subjects with natural dentitions, overlay dentures and complete dentures. *J. dent. Ass. S. Afr.*, *31*, 339–342

CHRISTENSEN, J. and MORIMOTO, T. (1977) Dimension discrimination at two different degrees of mouth opening and the effect of anaesthesia applied to the periodontal ligaments. *J. Oral Rehab. 4*, 157–164

DUBNER, R., SESSLE, B. J. and STOREY, A. T. (1978) *The Neural Basis of Oral and Facial Function*. Plenum, New York

GIBBS, C. H., MESSERMAN, T., RESWICK, J. B. and DERDA, H. J. (1971) Functional movements of the mandible. *J. prosth. Dent.*, *26*, 604–620

GOLDBERG, L. J. (1976a) Motoneurone mechanisms: reflex controls. In *Mastication and Swallowing: Biological and Clinical Correlates*, by Sessle, B. J. and Hannam, A. G. Univ. Toronto Press

GOLDBERG, L. J. (1976b) Changes in the excitability of elevator and depressor motoneurones produces by stimulation of intra-oral nerves. In *Mastication*, by Anderson and Matthews. John Wright, Bristol

GRAF, H. (1975) Occlusal forces during function. In *Occlusion: Research in Form and Function*, by Rowe, N. H. Univ. Michigan School of Dentistry

GRIFFIN, C. J. and MALOR, R. (1974) An analysis of mandibular movement. In *Front. Oral Physiol. vol. 1*, by Kawamura, Y. Karger, Basel

HANNAM, A. G. (1969) The response of periodontal mechanoreceptors in the dog to controlled loading of the teeth. *Archs. oral Biol.*, *14*, 781–791

HANNAM, A. G. (1976a) Periodontal Mechanoreceptors. In *Mastication* by Anderson and Matthews. John Wright, Bristol

HANNAM, A. G. (1976b) The regulation of the jaw bite force in man. *Archs. oral Biol.*, *21*, 641–644

HANNAM, A. G. and FARNSWORTH, T. J. (1977) Information transmission in trigeminal mechanosensitive afferents from teeth in the cat. *Archs. oral Biol.*, *22*, 181–186

HANNAM, A. G., DE COU, R. E., SCOTT, J. D. and WOOD, W. W. (1977) The relationship between dental occlusion, muscle activity and associated jaw movement in man. *Archs. oral Biol.*, *22*, 25–32

KAWAMURA, Y. (1974) *Physiology of Mastication*, *Front. Oral Physiol. vol. 1*. Karger, Basel

KAY, W. D. and ABES, M. S. (1976) Sensory perception in overdenture patients. *J. prosth. Dent.*, *35*, 615–619

LAINE, P. and SIIRILÄ, H. S. (1977) The effect of auditory sense on interocclusal microdiscrimination and size discrimination of persons with natural dentitions and full dentures. *Proc. Finn. dent. Soc.*, *73*, 27–31

LANGER, A. and MICHMAN, J. (1968) Occlusal perception after placement of complete dentures. *J. prosth. Dent.*, *19*, 246–251

LINDEN, R. W. A. (1975) Touch thresholds of vital and nonvital human teeth. *Exp. Neurol.*, *48*, 387–390

LOISELLE, R. J., CRUM, R. J., ROONEY, G. E. and STUEVER, C. H. (1972) The physiologic basis for the overlay denture. *J. prosth. Dent.*, *28*, 4–12

LUND, J. P., McLACHLAN, R. S. and DELLOW, P. G. (1971) A lateral jaw movement reflex. *Exp. Neurol.*, *31*, 189–199

MATTHEWS, B. (1976) Reflexes elicitable from the jaw muscles in man. In *Mastication*, by Anderson and Matthews. John Wright, Bristol

ÖWALL, B. (1974) Oral tactility during chewing. III. Denture wearers. *Odont. Revy.*, *25*, 255–272

ÖWALL, B. and MØLLER, E. (1974) Oral tactile sensibility during biting and chewing. *Odont. Revy.*, *25*, 327–346

PACER, F. J. and BOWMAN, D. C. (1975) Occlusal force discrimination by denture patients. *J. prosth. Dent.*, *33*, 602–609

PFAFFMANN, C. (1939) Afferent impulses from the teeth due to pressure and noxious stimulation. *J. Physiol. (Lond.)*, *97*, 207–219

SESSLE, B. J. (1976) How are mastication and swallowing programmed and regulated? In *Mastication and Swallowing: Biological and Clinical Correlates*, by Sessle, B. J. and Hannam, A. G. Univ. Toronto Press

SESSLE, B. J. and HANNAM, A. G. (1976) *Mastication and Swallowing: Biological and Clinical Correlates*. Univ. Toronto Press

SIIRILÄ, H. S. and LAINE, P. (1963) The tactile sensitivity of the parodontium to slight axial loadings of the teeth. *Acta odont. scand.*, *21*, 415–429

SIIRILÄ, H. S. and LAINE, P. (1969) Occlusal tactile threshold in denture wearers. *Acta odont. scand., 27,* 193–197

SIIRILÄ, H. S. and LAINE, P. (1972) Sensory thresholds in discriminating differences in thickness between the teeth, by different degrees of mouth opening. *Proc. Finn. dent. Soc., 68,* 134–139

SLABBERT, J. C. G. and CHRISTENSEN, L. V. (1978) Discrimination of interocclusal dimensions before and after insertion of partial dentures in man. *Arch. Oral Biol., Vol. 23.*

STOREY, A. (1976) Temporomandibular joint receptors. In *Mastication*, by Anderson and Matthews. John Wright, Bristol

THILANDER, B. (1961) Innervation of the temporo-mandibular joint capsule in man. *Trans. R. Sch. Dent. Stockholm, 7,* 1–67

WENNSTRÖM, A. (1971a) Psychophysical investigation of bite force, Part I. *Swed. dent. J., 64,* 807–819

WENNSTRÖM, A. (1971b) Psychophysical investigation of bite force, Part II. *Swed. dent. J., 64,* 821–827

WENNSTRÖM, A., MARKLUND, G. and ERIKSSON, P. (1972) A clinical investigation of bite force and chewing habits in patients with total maxillary denture and partial mandibular denture. *Swed. dent. J., 65,* 279–284

WICTORIN, L. (1972) Masticatory function in cases with denture, in cases with natural teeth and the importance to digestion. In *Oral Physiology*, by Emmelin, N. and Zotterman, Y. Pergamon, Oxford

CHAPTER 9

Overdentures

Shakespeare at least had definite views upon the edentulous state. It belonged to the seventh age of man '...last scene of all, that ends this strange eventful history, is second childishness and mere oblivion; sans teeth, sans eyes, sans taste, sans everything'. These unequivocal views might have been a reflection upon the limitations of the Elizabethan prosthodontic service, but even today there appears to be a strong and ever-increasing body of opinion to support the view that maintaining a few roots in an otherwise edentulous mouth must be of considerable benefit to the patient.

An overdenture is a removable prosthesis that entirely covers at least one tooth. The idea is far from new. In 1888 Evans had described a method for using roots for retaining restorations, and in 1896 Essig described a telescopic-like coping. There is also evidence to suggest that overdentures were being made in Great Britain around 1870. Peeso was also employing removable dentures supported by telescopic crowns at this time. Later on the bar type of construction such as that designed by Dr Gilmore in 1913 was beginning to evolve.

The reasons for retaining the roots were not always clear, but it is likely that denture retention and stability must have been uppermost in clinicians' minds. Gilmore was obviously looking for denture retention and stability whereas Peeso's reference in 1916 suggests that he was interested primarily in denture support. Whatever the reasons for retaining roots they were normally devitalised. This type of construction therefore lost favour when the focal sepsis scare was at its peak. However, continental Europe did not share the enthusiasm of Hunter and his disciples so that overdentures and similar constructions continued to be made.

With the advent of a more reasoned approach and improvements in endodontics, periodontics, and prosthodontics, the principle of making dentures over retained roots has been re-evaluated. For additional details on overdentures readers are strongly recommended to read *Overdentures* by Brewer, Morrow and others (1975).

TOOTH SELECTION FOR OVERDENTURES

Complete overdentures may be indicated where the plan of treatment would otherwise dictate extraction of all the teeth in an arch. This type of construction may be particularly valuable when natural teeth are in opposition.

The following points should be borne in mind when planning overdentures:

Periodontal aspects

Adequate sulcus depth, attached gingivae, and minimal mobility are essential considerations. While preliminary mucogingival surgery may help, there must be sufficient bone support. Periodontal aspects are considered in a separate chapter.

Tooth position

Canines are key teeth in arch formation, while there is also evidence to show that physical presence of their roots decreases resorption in the intercanine edentulous area. Teeth should be retained where the occlusal force on the edentulous ridge has the greatest destructive potential (Lord and Teel 1974).

Buccal prominence

Since there will be little, if any resorption around the retained roots, the denture flange will encroach on the sulcus space. This is an important consideration in choice of teeth to be retained.

Apart from excessive lip support, problems may occur with the path of insertion. An anterior tooth with a labial inclination will complicate matters if posterior contours prevent a markedly inclined path

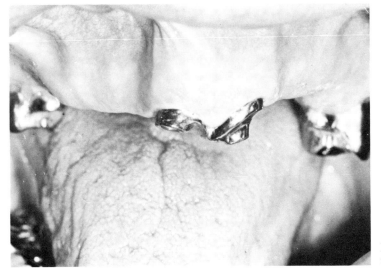

Fig. 407   Marked labial prominence around upper central incisors.

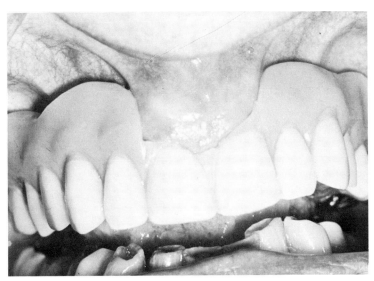

Fig. 408   Cutting away labial flange overcomes the problem of the prominence but damages border seal and weakens the denture.

of insertion. Shortened borders around roots may reduce lip support and path of insertion problems. However, they reduce the border seal and weaken the denture (Figs. 407, 408).

Endodontic factors

Richard et al. (1977) have pointed out the advantages of using hemisected molar roots for overdenture abutments. This approach is particularly useful where just one root possesses healthy attachment tissues, or where there is a furcation involvement.

The distal root is normally favoured as it is easier to root fill. A successful outcome of the treatment depends on a satisfactory root filling and a healthy periodontal environment.

It is naturally simpler and cheaper to employ as abutments teeth that already possess sound root fillings. Anterior teeth are generally easier to root fill than posterior teeth. The possibility of successfully root filling an abutment must be considered when selection is made. In addition to preserving the periodontal innervation, maintaining roots may confer the following advantages.

PSYCHOLOGICAL BENEFITS TO THE PATIENT

The stigmata and taboos of becoming edentulous have, in the past, overshadowed the practice of some forms of European continental dentistry to the extent of preserving rotting roots with purulent exudates – a state of affairs that could hardly have been further removed from the concepts of Hunter and his focal sepsis theories. Compare this with the reckless abandon with which Anglo-Saxons and their dentists have tended to discard natural dentitions. Is the English Channel so narrow?

The apparent psychological benefits will vary. For some, the emotional impact of tooth loss can be damaging, particularly when the effect on body image together with the deep emotions associated with the oral area are borne in mind. For others, the bedside glass containing dentures has been a way of life for generations. These stoical characters will often care less about the prognosis of one, two or three remaining roots than those for whom the transition from a fixed prosthesis to a so-called removable bridge has been emotionally traumatic. It is certain, however, that without active patient co-operation the prognosis of these teeth would be hopeless.

THE EFFECTS UPON THE EDENTULOUS RIDGE

In 1967 and 1969 Tallgren showed that over a seven-year period the reduction of anterior ridge height of the mandible was four times greater than that of the maxillary edentulous ridge. The mean loss mandibular ridge height was 6·6 mm whereas the maxillary loss was 1·7 mm. Tallgren's seven-year studies of alveolar bone loss around mandibular natural teeth in patients with partial dentures showed the vertical loss to be only 0·8 mm, compared with the 6·6 mm loss in those wearing complete dentures. It is apparent that this difference in rate will become more important with advancing years.

Crum and Rooney (1975), reporting a four-year study, claimed that the retention of mandibular canines for overdentures helped preserve the remaining edentulous ridge. Their figures showed there to be an average of 0·6 mm of ridge reduction in the anterior part of the mandible for patients with overdentures, whereas patients with conventional dentures lost on average 5 mm. An interesting observation was that patients with remaining canines lost less ridge height in the region between the canines than those without any natural teeth. Intelligent patients with good plaque control therefore stand to gain considerable benefits from preserving roots.

IMPROVED RETENTION AND STABILITY OF DENTURES

The degree of improvement obtained must be governed by the remaining roots.

The length of canine roots makes them particularly favourable in this respect, although virtually any soundly supported root with adequate periodontal tissues may be employed, provided an adequate zone of attached gingivae exists (Fig. 409).

The shape and size of the inner copings or root surface preparations will decide the retention and stability to be gained by the overdenture. For the purposes of discussion three categories of preparation may be considered (Fig. 410):

1. The thimble-shaped coping.
2. The domed coping or prepared root surface.
3. The use of attachments.

Preparations that may be employed depend on the vertical and bucco-lingual space available together with the loads that can be safely withstood by the roots.

1. Thimble-shaped copings

Copings such as those recommended by Miller (1958) may be placed on vital abutments.

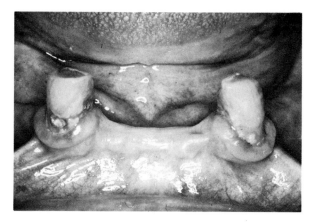

Fig. 409 Inadequate zones of attached gingivae and restricted sulcus depth worsen the prognoses of these overdenture abutments.

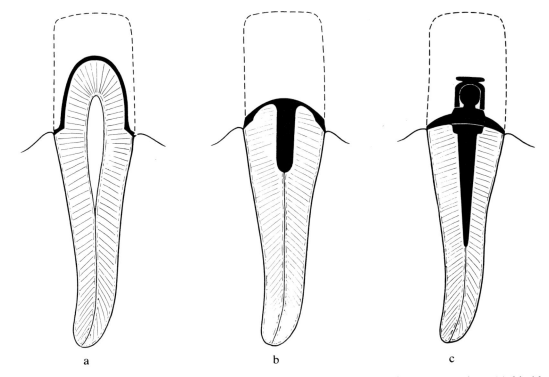

Fig. 410   Diagrams to show the vertical space requirements for the three types of root preparations: (a) thimble-shaped coping; (b) domed coping; (c) stud attachment.

Miller termed these abutment preparations 'biologic stabilizers'. He pointed out that even if a short life expectancy of the teeth was anticipated the assistance they might lend in helping the patient become accustomed to denture wearing justified the techniques. After ten years of clinical investigation he was surprised that many teeth outlived their estimated life expectancy.

Over a period of six years 46 dentures were inserted of which 34 were immediate replacement prostheses. Miller claimed evidence of lessened resorption of the ridge tissues as none of the dentures had required 'refitting'. The technique required preparations for full crowns, preferably with shoulders, and a recommendation that the normally flattened occlusal portion of the preparation be rounded or parabolic in form. By preparing the tooth in this fashion and covering it with a correctly shaped gold casting Miller suggested the loads of occlusion would only be directed along the long axes of the abutment teeth. Schweitzer (1966) Reitz, Weiner and Levin (1977) have correctly pointed out that this part of the concept, at least, might contain a measure of wishful thinking in view of the height of the preparations. The number of

remaining teeth and the path of insertion together with the question of appearance determined the extent of any labial or buccal flange, while no effort was made to provide retention from the copings.

Yalisove described an apparently similar technique in 1966 known as the crown and sleeve coping retainer, but considered it a form of partial denture retainer that could be used in conjunction with fixed prostheses. The rounded form allowed the denture to move when horizontal pressures were applied but intermittent vertical load application was possible. As Schweitzer had commented (1966), it is difficult to deny the application of horizontal loads when the inner (primary) copings occupy sufficient vertical space to allow them to be constructed over vital abutments.

Yalisove claims that devitalisation of abutment teeth is seldom necessary. The inner (primary) coping is required to protect the teeth from caries while the outer coping is essential for strength and wear resistance. According to the author over one thousand such prostheses have been made, over the last twenty years, and successful results claimed.

Nevertheless, with the patients I see, space considerations often require devitalisation of the abutment teeth so that despite the apparent simplicity and attraction of the approach, one must appreciate that the thimble coping will occupy considerable vertical and bucco-lingual space. Furthermore, the coping must be covered by an adequate thickness of denture base material and facing to withstand loads and to prevent breakage and at the same time provide a satisfactory appearance. The retention obtained for the overdenture will vary inversely with the taper of the coping. The adaptation to the coping will influence the stability obtained.

Root filling the teeth allows for greater flexibility of treatment. Mensor recommends between 3 and 8 mm of crown structure be left above the mucosa if attachments are not to be employed. In this way, a cast gold coping can be placed over the exposed surface of the tooth without requiring a post. Bearing in mind the restricted space often available, it is normally wiser to limit the height of the preparations to around 4 mm. In this case, the walls of the preparation must be virtually parallel sided, otherwise a retaining post will be required.

Copings are useful for immediate replacement dentures. When such a prosthesis is to be made, the teeth to be preserved are cut down before the extraction of the remaining teeth and insertion of the dentures. Once healing has occurred and the edentulous ridges mature, mucogingival surgery may be carried out and the teeth prepared for copings or attachments.

Making the copings before extracting the teeth has obvious short-term advantage (Fig. 411). Immediate stabilisation of the overdenture is obtained, but one is guessing at the level of the edentulous ridge. It may be necessary to remake the coping and surrounding structure at a later date. This presents little difficulty if they are not post-retained, but adds to the expense of the restoration.

Inner copings cemented to the teeth need to be made of gold. The outer copings forming part of the denture can be constructed in metal or resin. Acrylic resin copings become simply part of the denture. Schweitzer has claimed the following advantages for resin outer copings, usually cured over the final stone casts and that include accurate impressions of the inner copings:

(a) The degree of stabilisation and retention can be controlled by the operator upon insertion of the removable prosthesis. It is comparatively simple to adjust the adaptation of the outer to the inner coping.

(b) Closely spaced teeth may interfere with the placement of two layers of metal copings. However, it is often possible to use resin outer copings with the proximal resin removed. Strength requirements might be the limiting factor here.

(c) Occasional difficulties arise in seating the denture in the mouth over the inner copings. Where gold copings are used they need to be removed from the denture and a tricky relocation procedure carried out in the mouth. With resin, the entire inside surface of the crown can be removed, a small perforation drilled into the palatal or lingual surface of the denture and a new outer coping made with self-polymerizing resin in the mouth. This can be checked several times until it is finally cured. The excess resin protruding through the perforation is subsequently removed and the palatal surface repolished.

When resin outer copings are used some wear must inevitably occur and one should be prepared to re-adapt the copings periodically. Resin copings should not be used without a labial flange due to strength and retention considerations. Whatever material is selected for the outer coping space requirements cannot be assessed by guesswork and need to be planned with the benefit of mounted diagnostic casts.

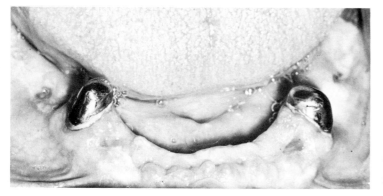

Fig. 411 Making copings before removal of the other teeth has short term advantages in stabilising immediate replacement denture. The teeth may need to be reprepared and new copings constructed when the edentulous ridge has matured.

2. Dome-shaped copings

Cutting root filled teeth down and preparing dome-shaped copings to extend only 1 or 2 mm above the ridge crest will produce a very significant improvement in the crown root ratio. Lateral loads are reduced and the space occupied is at a minimum. In this instance the roots are being used to give a measure of support against vertical loads while their contribution to retention will be negligible. The number and distribution of the roots together with the adaptation of the denture to the root preparations will determine their contribution to denture stability. This popular and effective method of preparing overdentures was developed by Lord and Teel with extremely satisfactory results. Since vertical space requirements are so small the strength of the denture is not compromised and breakages are relatively rare. In a recent survey of 250 overdentures, Reitz, Weiner and Levin (1977) found only one that had broken. Moghadam and Scandrett (1979) have described the use of magnetic retainers with overdenture copings—a technique that may hold promise.

The relatively small lateral loads applied to the roots allows this technique to be employed where neither root support nor vertical space permits the use of thimble copings or attachments. Gold copings are not always necessary. If sound tooth structure remains, and home care is adequate, caries is a relatively minor problem. Silver amalgam restorations are placed to seal the occlusal surface of the root canal and the tooth surface and restoration polished. A gold coping with short retaining post is employed only where an acceptable contour is unobtainable with the tooth surface. The absence of a coping simplifies the construction but topical application of a 2% sodium fluoride containing solution is recommended.

3. The use of attachments

Prefabricated attachments are versatile, and may provide considerable retention and stability. The third option is that of using prefabricated attachments. In terms of space required they are normally midway between the tall thimble copings and the extremely short dome-shaped preparations. The design and shape of attachments provide a significant measure of retention and stability of the overdenture. An adequate level of bone around the roots is required to say nothing of sufficient space within the overdenture to accommodate the opposite section of the attachment and still provide enough strength for the denture base.

Employing attachments adds to the expense of the restoration. Warren and Caputo (1975) felt that load distribution to the abutments might not be so favourable when applied through attachments as with tapered copings. These measurements were, however, made on dummy roots using photo elastic stress analysis.

Attachments not only require precise location between the various components but may place additional forces on their retaining posts. Nevertheless, in selected patients the benefits provided can be most worthwhile and their popularity continues to grow.

Impression techniques for use with attachments are described in the relevant chapters. Since all overdentures require support from the edentulous areas, maximum coverage is important. The buccal shelf area is a primary load bearing region for mandibular dentures, and the palate is well adapted to withstand vertical loads applied by maxillary prostheses. Border seal is no less important for overdentures as for complete dentures.

Sectional impression techniques employing transfer copings and a close fitting tray may be employed. The details are explained in the next chapter. However, elastomeric materials such as thiokol rubber give perfectly satisfactory results in a well contoured tray (Fig. 412). This allows details of the coping preparation or even of the copings themselves to be included in the master impression.

During insertion of any overdenture, attachment-retained or otherwise, there are important checks that must be made.

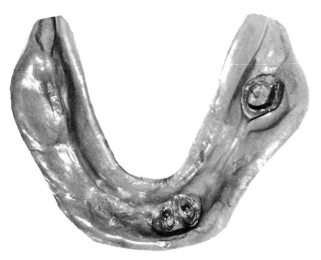

Fig. 412 Elastomeric materials are convenient for overdenture impressions involving coping construction.

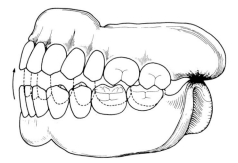

Fig. 413 The posterior premature contact may cause direct trauma, while the resultant movement of the denture bases may cause damage elsewhere.

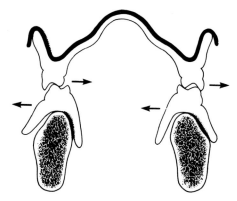

Fig. 415 Deflective contacts are difficult to see in the mouth and may cause damage to the areas heavily lined.

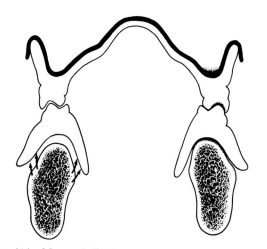

Fig. 414 Mucosal displacement may hide small discrepancies. Nevertheless, these errors of jaw relation recording are quite capable of causing damage.

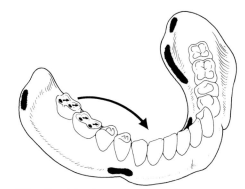

Fig. 416 Combined premature and deflective contacts may cause the dentures to rotate, resulting in complex patterns of trauma.

Base extension can be examined with the aid of disclosing paste. By painting a thin layer of material onto the impression surface of the denture base adaptation can be examined as well. Do not allow the opposing teeth to contact during this procedure as errors of jaw relation will be transferred onto the denture base. Once this step is completed the way is clear to examining the occlusion and articulation of the dentures. Limitations of vision make it extremely difficult to examine the occlusion of a complete denture in the mouth.

Premature contacts (Figs. 413, 414)

Premature contacts may cause trauma in two ways:
1. The initial contact places a heavy load in one spot, generally under the premature contact.
2. As a result of this initial contact there is a tendency for the denture bases to move, causing trauma to areas remote from the premature contact.

Deflective contacts (Fig. 415)

If accurate intercuspation does not occur as the teeth contact, deflective contacts may arise from the inclined plane action of the facets of the opposing cusps.

Combined premature and deflective contacts (Fig. 416)

The majority of jaw relation errors commonly give rise to a combination of premature and deflective contacts. It is unlikely that a premature contact would occlude with a flat plane. Flat cusped teeth do not overcome these manifestations of recording jaw relationship – they merely substitute contact of an area for several small point contacts.

POTENTIAL ERRORS IN THE CENTRIC RELATION RECORD

Even if the centric relation record appears correct at the trial insertion, there are still a number of potential sources of error before the dentures reach the patient's mouth. These sources of error may be considered as: (1) Processing changes; (2) Clinical errors.

1. Processing changes

Errors of processing technique may produce considerable occlusal changes; however, the larger errors are generally avoidable. Nevertheless, it would seem that however carefully the dentures are flasked and polished, some slight change of occlusion would result. These errors become more noticeable following removal of the dentures from the casts.

2. Clinical errors

Looking at the occlusion provides only a limited picture of what is taking place. Small movements of the denture base will hide some jaw relationship errors, while others could be masked by displacement of the mucosa underlying the denture base. The mucosa may give way under a small premature contact so that the occlusion appears correct. This excess load may cause trauma to the mucosa, yet the displacement cannot be seen by eye. Displaceable mucosa will, therefore, hide larger errors than firm mucosa. At this stage, a jaw relationship record which looks correct, can be said to be one in which the errors are sufficiently small to be hidden by displacement of the mucosa.

THE CHECK RECORD

The check record provides a method of detecting and eliminating small errors, difficult to see in the mouth. It is not a substitute for recording accurate jaw relationships at earlier stages.

The check record is best carried out when the processed dentures are first inserted in the patient's mouth. A facebow record will be required followed by an interocclusal record of centric relation made with the vertical relation increased sufficiently to prevent cuspal contact or interference. The record itself may be made of plaster, wax, or one of the occlusal indicating compounds. The interocclusal record should be kept as thin as possible, consistent with these aims. By means of this record, the dentures are remounted on the articulator (Fig. 417), the record removed, and the occlusion examined with the dentures mounted on unyielding plaster casts (Fig. 418). It is then possible to see small errors that would otherwise be masked in the mouth.

Articulating paper may be used to mark contact points, and there is no danger of smearing due to sliding contacts (Fig. 419). A wise practice is then to re-record condylar angles and check eccentric articulations.

The entire check record procedure is far from time consuming. Visits for adjustments are reduced while the patient must benefit from an occlusion and articulation adjusted with precision.

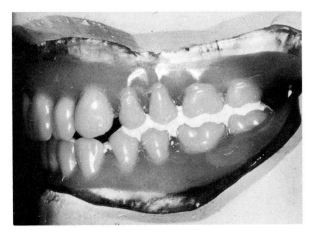

Fig. 417 The dentures are remounted on the articulator with the check record between them.

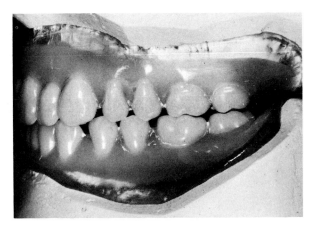

Fig. 418 The check record procedure will show up small errors otherwise difficult to detect in the mouth.

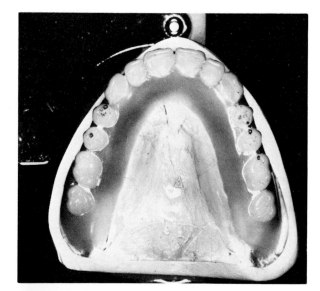

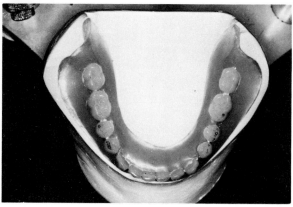

Fig. 419 With the dentures mounted on unyielding plaster casts, contact marking strips can be used as an aid to correcting the occlusion.

DUPLICATING OVERDENTURES

An increasing number of patients request spare dentures, and the following technique has provided consistently good results. The prostheses are treated as complete dentures. Where attachments are involved they are located into the spare denture according to the methods described for individual attachments.

Sticky wax sprues are added to the dentures to be copied and a wire attached, allowing the dentures to be suspended in a container (Figs. 420, 421). The container must be sufficiently large to accommodate the denture and have a floor that can be pressed upwards allowing material in the container to be removed. The container is then filled with duplicating agar (Fig. 422), although alginate material may be used as a substitute. Cooling of the agar is speeded by placing the container in a water bath with continuous flow (Fig. 423). Once hardened, the agar mould is removed from the container and split down the middle, allowing the denture to be removed (Fig. 424). The mould is now reassembled in its metal container and the void filled with tray resin (Fig. 425). This technique produces replicas of the original dentures in tray resin (Fig. 426). Undercuts are removed from the impression surfaces of the replicas which are then border moulded before zinc oxide impressions are made. A facebow record is then made of the upper replica in the mouth before the centric relation record. The next clinical visit is the trial insertion.

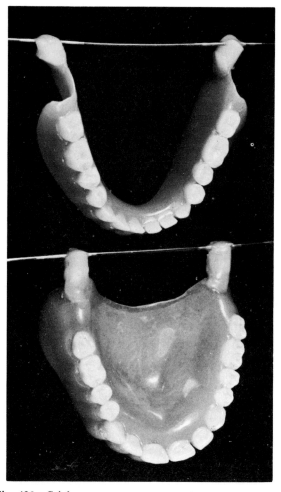

Fig. 420 Sticky wax sprues are attached to the dentures requiring duplication.

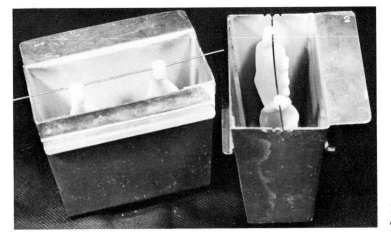

Fig. 421   Dentures suspended in a duplicating container.

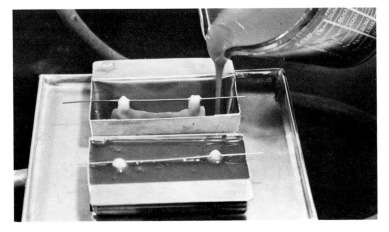

Fig. 422   Containers being filled with duplicating agar.

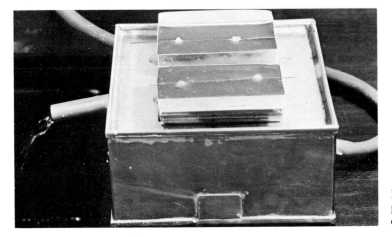

Fig. 423   Cooling of the agar speeded by placing the containers in a water bath with continuous flow.

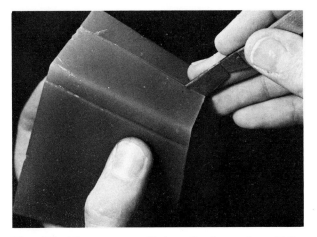

Fig. 424   The agar mould is split down the middle, allowing the denture to be removed.

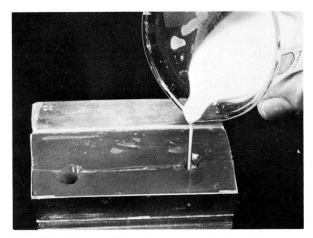

Fig. 425   The mould is then reassembled and the space filled with tray acrylic resin.

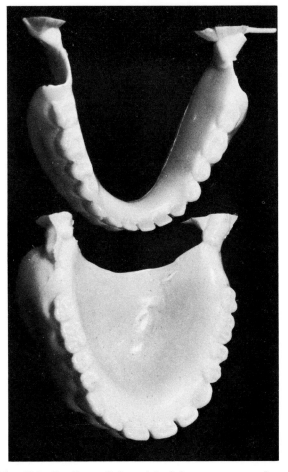

Fig. 426   Replicas of the original dentures are produced that are employed for impressions and jaw relations.

By using this technique at least two visits are saved, while the positioning of the original artificial teeth can be copied. An advantage of the technique is its flexibility as it allows improvements to be made on the originals, while preserving the basic measurements.

OVERDENTURE PROGNOSIS

It is hardly surprising that long-term surveys of overdentures are notable for their scarcity. Individual practitioners tend to favour particular techniques, while it is never easy to be absolutely objective about the results of one's own handiwork.

Surveys are invaluable but they are also difficult and time consuming to undertake. Most have been institution based and the variables of patient selection, operator technique and maintenance are seldom directly applicable to a private office. Nevertheless the warnings are clear and should be heeded before overdentures are planned.

In 1971 Rantanen and others published a survey of attachment-retained overdentures between four years and seven months old. Gingival inflammation was common and there had been loss of attached gingivae in 62% of the abutment teeth, and in 100% of abutment supporting restorations for more than three years. Cutting away the labial flange of the denture made no difference to the figures but made a significant contribution to increasing the incidence of denture fractures. Caries was found in 40% of abutment teeth.

The attachments concerned were fairly typical of those manufactured. Generally they stood up well to the loads applied. Despite instructions to the contrary the majority of subjects wore their dentures night and day thereby showing poor motivation for instruction and possible lack of interest. The authors pointed out that with the group involved the prognosis of the roots was poor and the denture was not necessarily the cause of the damage to the supporting teeth. On the contrary they felt the damage might have been worse if no prosthodontic therapy had been instituted.

A rather different picture is portrayed in the survey of Reitz, Weiner and Levin (1977). 59 overdentures involving 131 teeth were examined. Only one instance of denture breakage was recorded – far lower than most other results. A probable cause might have been the construction technique employing dome shaped copings or simple prepared root surfaces. The preparations occupy the minimum of space and weaken the denture less than any other overdenture technique. 16% of patients had caries and the application of topical fluoride-containing solutions were considered beneficial in this respect. Periodontal complications ranged from a change in tissue tone to loss of attached gingivae and pocket formation. About 30% of the patients had abutment teeth graded as failing but, even so, these teeth could be regarded as potential abutments for a few years to come.

In view of the overdentures covering the gingival margin, plaque control and denture hygiene are at a premium. The prognosis of the restoration is likely to be influenced by numerous factors including the selection of the patient treatment planning, preparation of the mouth, execution of the prosthodontic therapy and also by the maintenance therapy necessary to ensure a satisfactory result. Once this is appreciated the way is clear to providing a useful and worthwhile overdenture service from which the patient will obtain considerable benefit.

REFERENCES AND FURTHER READING

ADLER, P. (1947) Sensibility of teeth to loads applied in different directions. *J. dent. res.*, 26, 279

ANDERSON, D. J., HANNAM, A. G. and MATTHEWS, B. (1970) Sensory mechanisms in mammalian teeth and their supporting structures. *Physiol. Rev.*, 50, 171

AUGSBURGER, R. H. (1966) The Gilmore attachment. *J. prosth. Dent.*, 16, 1090–1102

BONAGURO, J. G., DUSZA, G. R. and BOWMAN, D. C. (1969) Ability of human subjects to discriminate forces applied to certain teeth. *J. dent. Res.*, 48, 236

BOTTGER, H. (1969) *Teleskopsystem in der zahnarzlichen Prosthetik*, 54s. 3. Auflage, Barth, Leipzig

BOTTGER, H. and GRUNDLER, H. (1969) *Die Praxis des Teleskop-systems* (Neuer Merkur, München 1970)

BREWER, A. A. and FENTON, A. H. (1973) The overdenture. *Dent. Clin. N. Amer.*, 17, 723–746

BREWER, A. A. & MORROW, R. M. (1975) *Overdentures*. C. V. Mosby, St Louis, Mo.

BRILL, N. (1955) Adaptation and the hybrid-prostheses. *J. prosth. Dent.*, 5, 811–824

BRODIE, A. G. & THOMPSON, J. R. (1942) Factors in the position of the mandible. *J.A.D.A.*, 29, 925

CRUM, R. J., LOISELLE, R. J. and HAYES, C. K. (1971) The stud attachment overlay denture and proprioreception. *J. Amer. dent. Ass.*, 82, 583

CRUM, R. J. and LOISELLE, R. J. (1972) Oral perception and proprioception: a review of the literature and its significance to prosthodontics. *J. prosth. Dent.*, 28, 215

EVANS, G. (1888) *A Practical Treatise on Artificial Crown and Bridge Work*. The S. S. White Dental Mfg. Co., Philadelpha

EVANS, G. (1920) *A Practical Treatise on Artificial Crown, Bridge, and Porcelain Work*, pp. 249, 8th edn. P. Blakeston's Son & Company, Philadelphia

ESSIG, C. J. (1896) *The American Textbook of Prosthetic Dentistry*, p. 439. Lea Brothers and Company, Philadelphia

GAERNY, A. (1969) *Der abnehmbare Interdentalbraum – Verschluss (I.R.V.)*. Quintessenz, Berlin

GILMORE, S. F. (1913) A method of retention. *Council of Allied Dental Societies*, 8, 118

GOSLEE, B. A. (1923) *Principles and Practice in Crown and Bridgework*, p. 6, 5th edn. Dental Items of Interest Publishing Co. Brooklyn

GUYER, S. E. (1975) Selectively retained vital roots for partial support of overdentures: a patient report. *J. prosth. Dent.*, 33, 258–263

GROSSMAN, R. C. (1964) Oral sensory threshold determination methods. *J. Dent. Res.*, 43, 833 (Suppl.)

GROSSMAN, R. C., HATTIS, B. F. and RINGEL, R. L. (1965) Oral tactile experience. *Arch. Oral Biol.*, 10, 691

HOFMANN, M. and LUDWIG, P. (1973) Die teleskopierende Totalprothees im stark reduzierten Luckengebiss. *Dtsch. Zahnarztl. Z.*, 28:2

HUNTER, W. (1906) Oral sepsis in relation to disease. *Brit. Journal Dent. Science*, 4711, 805

IGARASHI, Y. (1975) Selection of retainers in lower overlay denture in relation to the abutment tooth mobility (a laboratory study). *Bull. Tokyo med. dent. Univ.*, 22, 207–220

KABCENELL, J. L. (1971) Tooth-supported complete dentures. *J. prosth. Dent.*, 26, 251–257

KAWAMURA, Y. (1964) Recent concepts in physiology of mastication. In *Stape, P. W., Advances in Oral Biology, Vol. I*. Academic Press, New York

KAWAMURA, Y. and FIJIMOTO, J. (1958) A study of the jaw opening reflex. *Med. J. Osaka Univ.*, 9, 377

KAWAMURA, Y. and WATANABE, M. (1960) Studies

on oral sensory thresholds. *Med. J. Osaka Univ.*, *10*, 291

KORBER, K. H. (1973) *Konuskronen-Teleskope.* 3 Aufl. A. Huthig, Heidelberg

KRUGER, L. and MICHEL, F. (1962) A single neuron analysis of buccal cavity representation in the sensory trigeminal complex of the cat. *Arch. Oral. Biol.*, *7*, 491

LITVAK, H., SILVERMAN, S. I. and GARFINKEL, L. (1971) Oral Stereogenisis in dentulous and edentulous subjects. *J. prosth. Dent.*, *25*, 139

LOISELLE, R. J., CRUM, R. J., ROONEY, G. E. and STUEVER, C. H. (1972) The Physiologic Basis for the Overlay Denture. *J. prosth. Dent.*, *28*, 4–12

LORD, J. L. and TEEL, S. (1969) The overdenture. *Dent. Clin. N. Amer.*, *13*, 871–881

LORD, J. L. and TEEL, S. (1974) The overdenture: patient selection, use of copings, and follow-up evaluation. *J. prosth. Dent.*, *32*, 41–51

MacDONALD, E. T. and AUNGST, L. F. (1970) Apparent independence of oral sensory functions and articulatory proficiency. In *Second Symposium on Oral Sensation and Perception*, ed. Bosma, J. Charles C. Thomas, Springfield, Ill.

MILLER, P. A. (1958) Complete Dentures Supported by Natural Teeth. *J. prosth. Dent.*, *8*, 924–928

MOGHADAM, B. K. and SCANDRETT, F.r. (1979) Magnetic retention for overdentures. *J. prosth. Dent.*, *41*, 1, 26

MORROW, R. M., FELDMAN, E. E., RUDD, K. D. and TROVILLION, H. M. (1969) Tooth-supported complete dentures: an approach to preventive prosthodontics. *J. prosth. Dent.*, *21*, 513–522

NAIRN, R. I. (1976) The concept of occlusal vertical dimension and the importance in clinical practice, p. 58 in *Mastication*, by Anderson and Matthews. John Wright, Bristol

PEESO, F. A. (1916) *Crown and Bridge Work for Students and Practitioners.* Lea and Febiger, Philadelphia

POUND, E. (1977) Let /S/ be your guide. *J. prosth. Dent.*, *38:5*, 482–489

RANTANEN, T., MÄKILÄ, E. and YLI-URPO, A. (1971) Investigations of the therapeutic success with dentures retained by precision attachments. I. Root-anchored complete overlay dentures. *Suom. hammaslaak. Toim.*, *67*, 356

REITZ, P. V., WEINER, M. G. and LEVIN, B. (1977) An overdenture survey: preliminary report. *J. prosth. Dent.*, *37:3*, 246–258

RICHARD, G. E., SARKA, R. J., ARNOLD, R. M. and KNOWLES, K. I. (1977) Hemisected molar abutments for additional overdenture support. *J. prosth. Dent.*, *38:1*, 16–21

SCHWEITZER, J. M. (1966) Discussion of 'crown and sleeve-coping retainers for removable partial prostheses'. *J. prosth. Dent.*, *16*, 1086–1089

SCHWEITZER, J. M., SCHWEITZER, R. D. and SCHWEITZER, J. (1971) The telescoped complete denture: a research report at the clinical level. *J. prosth. Dent.*, *26*, 357–372

SHRILA, H. and LAINE, R. (1963) The tactile sensibility of the paradontium to slight axial loadings of the teeth. *Acta. odont. scand.*, *21*, 415

SWENSON, M. G. (1970) *Complete Dentures*, 6th edn. C. O. Boucher. C. V. Mosby, St Louis, Mo.

TALLGREN, A. (1967) The effect of denture wearing on facial morphology: a 7-year longitudinal study. *Acta odont. scand. 25*, 563–592

TALLGREN, A. (1969) Positional changes of complete dentures: a 7-year longitudinal study. *Acta. odont. scands.*, *27*, 539

TALLGREN, A. (1972) The continuing reduction of the residual alveolar ridges in complete denture wearers: a mixed-longitudinal study covering 25 years. *J. prosth. Dent.*, *27*, 120–132

THAYER, H. M. and CAPUTO, A. A. (1977) Effects of overdentures on remaining oral structures. *J. prosth. Dent.*, *37:4*, 374

TRYDE, G., FRYDENBERG, O. and BRILL, N. (1962) An assessment of the tactile sensibility in human teeth, *Acta. odont. scand.*, *20*, 233

WARREN, A. B. and CAPUTO, A. A. (1975) Load transfer to alveolar bone as influenced by abutment designs for tooth-supported dentures. *J. prosth. Dent.*, *33:2*, 137–148

YALISOVE, I. L. (1966) Crown and sleeve-coping retainers for removable partial prostheses. *J. prosth. Dent.*, *16*, 1069–1085

ZAMIKOFF, I. I. (1973) Overdentures: theory and technique. *J. Am. Dent. Assoc.*, *86*, 853–857

CHAPTER 10

Stud Attachments

Stud devices are among the simplest of all attachments. The male part of the unit consists of a stud-shaped projection and in the majority of attachments it is soldered to the diaphragm of a post crown: the female part fits over the male unit and is embedded within the acrylic resin of the prosthesis or soldered to a metal sub-frame. There are, however, a few systems in which the male section forms part of the denture and the female part of the root surface preparation. Few stud attachments are entirely rigid since their size makes it difficult to prevent a small amount of movement between the two components. In some attachments springs or other devices are specifically incorporated to allow a controlled degree of movement. Stud attachments have numerous applications to overdentures. Being relatively small they can provide additional stability, retention and support while the positive lock of certain units can maintain the border seal of the denture.

CLINICAL TECHNIQUES

Despite the minimal bulk of many stud attachments there are still patients for whom inadequate vertical and buccal lingual space can be found for these units (Fig. 427). Mounted diagnostic casts are important aids to check the space available before an attachment is selected (Fig. 428). Where there is inadequate vertical space, or where bone support of the roots is minimal, a short dome-shaped coping is the recommended root preparation (Fig. 429). With all overdentures the importance of sound periodontal tissues is vital to the success of the restoration. An adequate zone of attached gingivae together with reasonable sulcus depth are other important requisites for a good prognosis. The stud-retained overdenture, like all overdentures, covers the gingival margins and this potential source of irritation will be aggravated by movement of the denture base.

Meticulous plaque control and denture hygiene is essential. Failure to pay attention to these details results in irritation of the gingivae leading to rapid downgrowth of the epithelial attachment and loss of attached gingivae (Fig. 430). Irritation may lead to proliferation of the gingival tissues. It used to be felt that cutting a space in the acrylic resin of the denture base over these tissues was the answer to the problem. Cutting such a space merely provides a greater area into which the damaged gingival tissue can proliferate (Fig. 431). The denture must therefore be made inherently stable and retentive while subjected to the minimum of displacing forces. Stress breaking attachments are no substitute for a correctly designed and constructed denture. A poorly constructed complete denture will move around in the mouth; a poorly constructed denture with attachments will move around the roots, leading to damage of the gingivae, periodontal breakdown and failure of the whole restoration.

The clinical techniques described for stud attachments are applicable to other attachments as well. Following endodontic therapy the teeth are cut down to just above gingival level, thereby improving the crown root ratio. Preparation of the roots should consider the following points:

1. The margins should not be sub-gingival (Fig. 432). Where caries is present it should be removed before mucogingival surgery is carried out in order to ensure that the preparation margin does not become sub-gingival (Fig. 433).

2. Plaque control requirements dictate that the coping must not be over-contoured or bulbous in any respect. A bevel is usually required around the margin.

3. The centre of the root should be prepared to provide the greatest possible thickness of metal in the diaphragm post junction (Fig. 434). This is important for strength and for providing the largest bonding surface for precious metal posts when cast-on techniques are employed. Hollowing out the

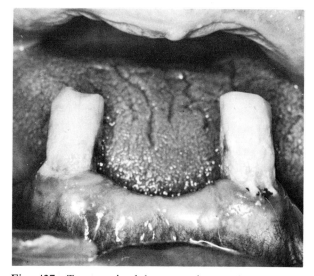

Fig. 427 Two retained lower canines and a common prosthodontic problem.

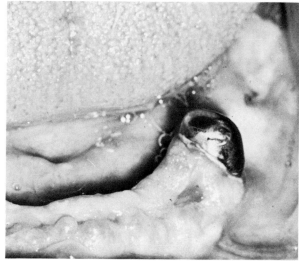

Fig. 429 Where inadequate vertical space exists for an attachment, the dome shaped coping should be considered.

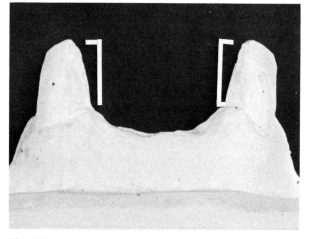

Fig. 428 The vertical space available for the overdenture is usually less than the space occupied by the canines as they are frequently over-erupted.

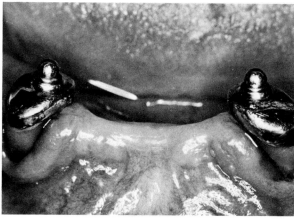

Fig. 430 Poor treatment planning can lead to rapid downgrowth of the epithelial attachment and loss of attached gingivae.

root face allows the attachment to be positioned as low as possible and minimises its encroachment upon vertical space (Fig. 435). The basic tent-shaped preparation will help prevent rotation while an anti-rotation device such as the slot should be incorporated as well. About two-thirds of the root preparation will normally face the labial aspect and one-third the lingual. In making the preparation it is helpful to visualise the eventual positioning of the attachment. Where lower canines are concerned the

attachments will normally be placed between one and two millimetres lingual to the centre of the root (Fig. 436).

4. Selection of posts. None of these methods will be of avail if the post is insufficiently retentive. Unlike the dome shaped coping considerable displacing forces may be applied to the posts when the denture is removed, particularly after initial insertion when the attachment may have been overtightened.

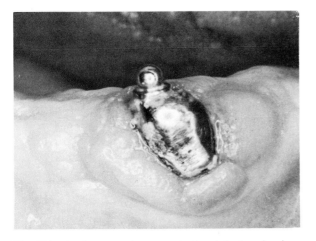

Fig. 431 Inadequate plaque control and denture hygiene, together with continued denture movement frequently lead to this type of result.

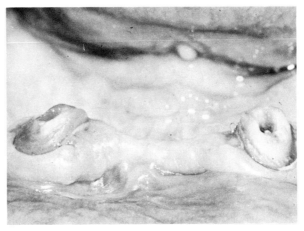

Fig. 433 It is wise to remove caries before periodontal surgery to ensure the margin does not become subgingival.

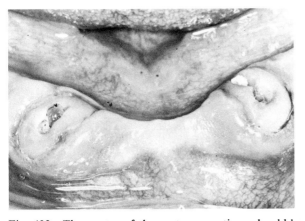

Fig. 432 The centre of the root preparations should be hollowed out to allow a greater thickness of metal at the post/diaphragm junction, and to provide more room for the attachment. The edge should not be sunk below the gingival margins.

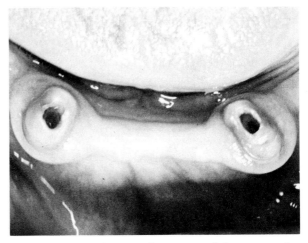

Fig. 434 Hollowing out the centre of the preparation increases the strength of the post/diaphragm junction and lowers the level of the attachment.

Laboratory produced posts

Waxing up and casting one's own post gives the operator wide choice in the preparation of the post canal. It seems by far the most common method employed yet the difficulties are seldom fully appreciated. The mechanical properties of a cast dental gold cannot be expected to match those of a wrought alloy specially produced for the purpose. There is the additional risk of debris or air contaminating the casting and contributing to a subsequent fracture.

Apart from the problems of reassessing the impression procedures, Mensor (1975) has pointed out the technical problems of matching dental investment to produce accurately fitting diaphragms and posts with the same mix. Attempting to seat an over-sized post may split the root while an undersized post reduces retention and allows shearing loads to be borne by the cement with loosening of the post ensuing. Where correctly sized posts of minimal taper are produced a cement release groove will prevent hydraulic pressure of the cement interfering with seating of the casting.

Laboratory produced posts are indicated for

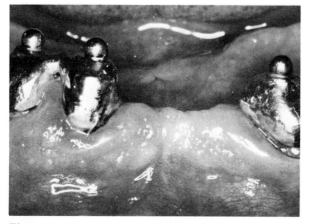

Fig. 435 Inadequate preparations lead to excessive encroachment upon vertical space and bulbous copings. Three attachments were unnecessary.

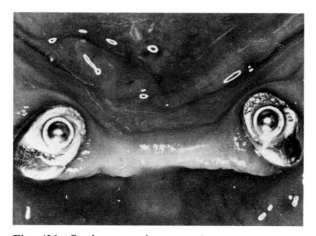

Fig. 436 On lower canines, attachments are usually placed about one to two millimetres lingual to the centre of the root.

unusually shaped or angled roots. They require to be made of generous cross section and the problem of construction should not be underestimated. Clinical and technical skills of a high order of magnitude are required.

Prefabricated metal posts

A variety of different posts are produced by several manufacturers. These wrought posts are constructed from specially formulated alloys and require less canal enlargement than an equivalent laboratory produced post.

Most precious alloy posts are supplied with matching reamers. Stainless steel posts are available for impression purposes and for temporary restorations. The Ackermann and Mooser posts are examples of tapered European posts that have been used for many years. Parallel-sided posts like the Schenker offer far more retention compared with an equivalent length of tapered post. The Schenker is an example of this design in which a step is incorporated to accommodate root taper. Mensor (1978) claims no cementation failure over a thirteen year period with the Schenker system. He recommends parallel-sided post systems be used with a cement relief groove to facilitate seating of the casting. While designed for use with engine driven reamers, any wobble occurring due to a slightly loose bearing is going to be reflected in an enlarged canal and a poorly adapted post. Mishaps of this type can be overcome by minimising reaming speeds. Specially produced chucks are available to allow latched-type reamers to be turned by hand (Fig. 437).

Prefabricated resin patterns

Rather like a compromise between the previous two methods, this system uses a matched set of burs for preparing the post space together with resin post patterns to reduce the technical problems of waxing both coping and post.

Threaded posts

Threaded posts provide additional mechanical fixation. The majority of screw-retained posts cannot be used in conjunction with stud attachments but the Kurer (1979) system is an exception.

The Kurer post-retained stud attachment is ingenious, combining the advantages of a well tried screw retained post with those of a stud attachment. The chances of accidental dislodgement of a retaining post are thereby reduced to a minimum and it can be used in comparatively short single-rooted teeth provided adequate bone support remains.

A special kit is produced incorporating a stainless steel attachment on a threaded post (Fig. 438). At the first visit, the tooth is reduced to just above gingival level taking into account that 4 mm of vertical space will be required for the attachment complex. As the female section of the modified Ancrofix attachment is somewhat wider than others care should be taken to ensure that it is not positioned too close to the labial aspect of the tooth. Furthermore it is not wise to use it where labiolingual space is restricted.

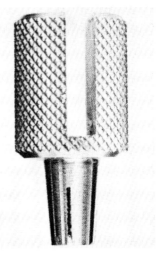

Fig. 437 The Thomas chuck. This device allows latched-type reamers to be turned by hand.

A depth reamer is used to ream the canal to the desired length and this is followed by the width reamer. The matched thread cutting instrument is used by hand, rotating forward for one or two turns and then partially reversed before repeating the procedure. Once the thread has been cut it is possible to screw the attachment directly into the tooth with the aid of a special screwdriver and the use of cement.

This technique is a rapid single visit method but most operators would prefer the root face to be covered with a cast coping. In this case a somewhat longer procedure is required.

When a coping (root diaphragm) is incorporated,

the threaded post will pass through it to be screwed into the canal (Fig. 439). To achieve this result the canal is reamed and tapped. An impression is made by placing a smooth locating dowel (called a waxing dummy by the manufacturer) in the canal (Fig. 440). This locating dowel is removed in the impression and becomes incorporated in the die. The coping is waxed up around it. A special wax facer is provided to carve the shoulder around the dowel at right angles to its long axis (Fig. 441). If this correct angle were not achieved, the shoulder of the attachment might not seat against the coping as turning the screw would alter the points of contact. Having ensured the wax is as thin as possible, the coping may be cast.

At the patient's next visit the cast coping is placed on the root face and the stud attachment on its post screwed into place with the aid of a special instrument provided in the kit. The shank of the screw may be shortened with a diamond disc. When the collar of the attachment seats on the shoulder of the coping, it is ready for cementation. The coping and attachment are cemented and screwed into place in one operation.

The next step is to incorporate the female unit in the denture. This is carried out by making an impression of the entire arch over the cemented coping and stud attachment. A special transfer unit (transfer dummy), incorporating a brass replica of the male section of the attachment, is placed in the impression before it is poured (Fig. 442). The master cast then includes a replica attachment upon which the female unit can be placed (Fig. 443), the denture waxed-up, and processed.

The advantages of this unit are self-apparent, but

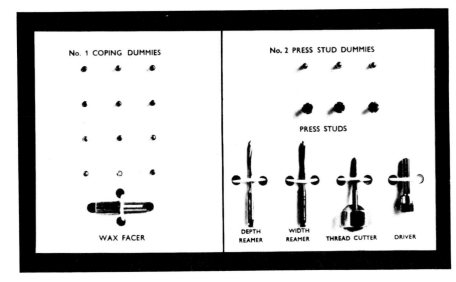

Fig. 438 Manufacturers kit for using the Kurer post retained stud attachment unit.

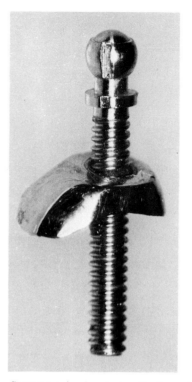

Fig. 439 Screw-retained stud attachment passing through coping. This attachment is made of stainless steel.

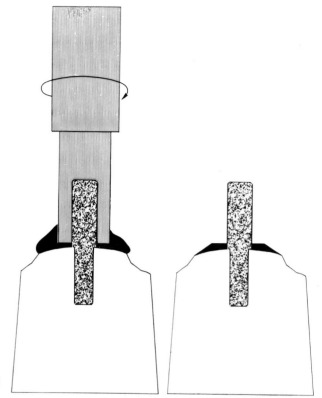

Fig. 441 Using the wax carver to ensure that the shoulder of the coping is at right angles to the long axis of the dowel.

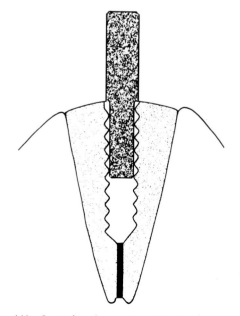

Fig. 440 Locating dowel placed in the root canal.

like all other attachments the vertical and buccal lingual space requirements must be assessed carefully beforehand. Angulation of the roots provides another complication, for the male unit cannot be aligned in the laboratory as with other stud attachments. It is true that the ball and socket design allows for some variation in this aspect and the manufacturers claim that up to 20° of divergence may be acceptable. However, wide angles of divergence are likely to increase the rate of attachment wear, despite the mechanical advantages of the stainless steel ball. This system holds considerable promise if used with discretion.

Impression techniques for stud-retained overdentures

Most complete overdentures are tooth and mucosal supported. Since the number of remaining roots is relatively small a large measure of support comes from the mucosa. Base extension principles are

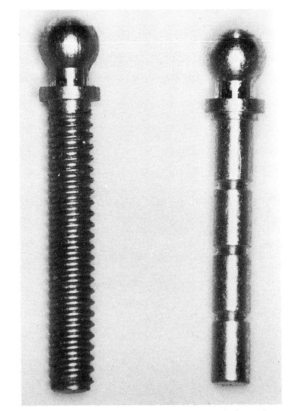

Fig. 442 Screw-retained stud attachment (left) and transfer unit. This transfer unit is placed in the impression so that it becomes incorporated in the master cast.

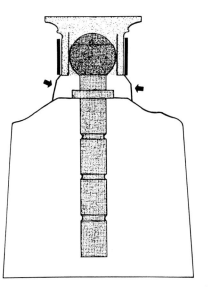

Fig. 443 The female unit is placed on the transfer unit, undercuts blocked with plaster, and the denture waxed up around it. The female unit is thereby incorporated with the denture base.

similar to those of complete dentures. Exceptions are comparatively rare but include situations where four or more teeth remain and comparatively rigid attachments are employed.

An adequately extended final impression is a prerequisite of any satisfactory prosthesis. For the denture to be stable, occlusal loads must be distributed as widely as possible and the forces of both adhesion and cohesion are developed to their maximum. To resist vertical loads, coverage of the buccal shelf area of the mandible is essential, whilst palatal coverage in the maxillae plays a similar role. If the impression features some mucosal displacement the impression surface of the denture will be contoured to the shape the mucosa will assume under load. The denture base will, therefore, need to make a scarcely perceptible movement before occlusal load and mucosal resistance reach equilibrium. Movement of the denture base around the roots will then be reduced to a minimum. Such an impression technique will also help in the development of a border seal necessary for the production of adequate retention.

The presence of roots presents problems and the final impression must include details of the roots, gingival margins and denture bearing mucosa. While slight displacement of the denture bearing mucosa is a necessary part of the impression procedure, no displacement of the gingival margins should take place (Fig. 444). Where muco-gingival surgery has been undertaken sufficient time must be allowed for healing before impression procedures are undertaken.

Correct extension of the complete lower denture base is not only essential if the retentive forces are to be developed to the best advantage, but is necessary for maximum stability. However, interpretations of what constitutes 'correct' vary widely, probably because much appears to depend on clinical judgement rather than anatomical criteria. Our terminology may be partly to blame.

'Over-extension' conjures up visions of a denture base projecting beyond the permitted anatomical confines, but otherwise satisfactory. In most regions of the mouth the directions in which denture flanges run are determined by the contours of the underlying bone, and by the extension of the soft tissues. In the posterior lingual region this does not hold true, since it is necessary to allow the mylohyoid muscle freedom of movement. In this area, the inclination of the lingual flange may be correct. For example, most people will have seen poorly-extended complete lower dentures that appear to balance precariously on the edentulous ridge. Commonly, the lingual flanges rest on the mylohyoid ridges where they cause trauma and subject the denture to a displacing force whenever the patient moves his tongue. The problem is not one of simple extension as the base is already over-extended in this region; nor will reduction of the flange help matters. The answer lies in a lingually-inclined, fully-extended, flange with a border seal, allowing the mylohyoid muscle freedom of movement underneath.

The mylohyoid muscle probable causes more difficulty in denture construction than any other single muscle. The posterior part of the mylohyoid muscle guards the entrance to the retromylohyoid fossa and it is this part that so frequently causes difficulty. The mylohyoid muscle forms the floor of the mouth. Anteriorly it is attached fairly low to the internal aspect of the mandible. However, in the premolar region the level of attachment rises sharply, and it is from this point to its posterior border that the mylohyoid is related to the denture base (Fig. 445).

When the mylohyoid is relaxed, its more posterior fibres run almost vertically downwards to the hyoid bone; when it contracts, the hyoid bone is raised and the direction of the fibres become more horizontal (Fig. 446).

A vertical denture flange adapted to the mylohyoid muscle at rest will be displaced as soon as the mylohyoid muscle contracts. This occurs however short the flange. The resulting trauma may be quite substantial, for if attachments are being used, these hold the denture firmly in place, and the occlusion of the teeth will press the denture back on to the contracted mylohyoid muscle. It is, therefore, necessary to swing the denture flange lingually around the contracted mylohyoid muscle so that it can move under the flange. Once the flange is behind the posterior border of the mylohyoid muscles it may be turned back into the retromylohyoid fossa (Fig. 447). It is true that a flange adapted to a contracted mylohyoid muscle may leave a potential space when this muscle is at rest, but as the seal is maintained in the reflection of the lingual mucosa, this potential space is unlikely to be of clinical significance. Figure 448 illustrates the denture base made for a patient with particularly prominent mylohyoid muscles.

Since one starts a primary impression procedure with a stock tray and hopes to finish with a well adapted impression it is hardly necessary to point out the importance of a good selection of correctly contoured metal trays. Impression compound is a convenient material for extending the tray to its correct boundaries but, in order for the compound to flow, it must be compressed between the tray and

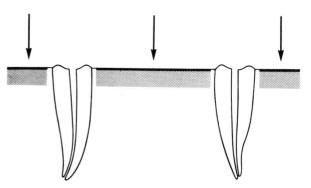

Fig. 444 Best results are usually obtained with an impression technique that provides slight displacement of the denture-bearing mucosa, but no load should be applied to the gingival margins.

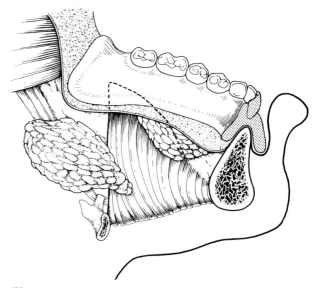

Fig. 445 Simplified diagram to show the relationship of the mylohyoid muscle to the denture base.

the mucosa. The distance it can flow beyond the tray is limited, while the direction in which it flows is influenced by the tray as well as the mucosa. One of the common faults of a stock tray is a short, straight lingual flange which directs the composition vertically downwards and does not guide it posteriorly into the retromylohyoid fossa. Quite frequently the compound is used in a viscous state, resulting in displacement of the mylohyoid muscle and distortion of the border structures (Fig. 449).

Another common mistake is to employ a stock tray that distorts the sulci, particularly the labial

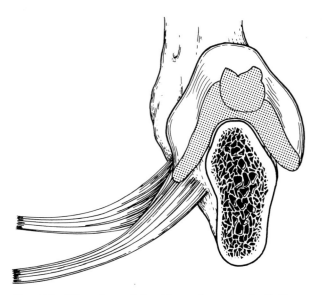

Fig. 446 When the mylohyoid muscle contracts, its fibres become more horizontal as the hyoid bone is raised.

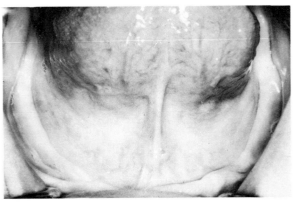

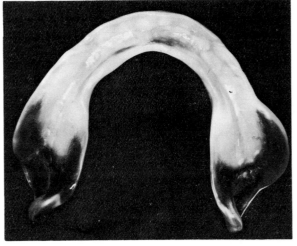

Fig. 448 *Above:* An edentulous patient with prominent, contracted mylohyoid muscle.
Below: The denture base constructed. Note the sweep of the flange allowing the mylohyoid muscle freedom of contraction.

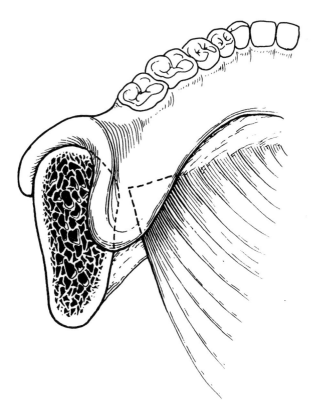

Fig. 447 The distal extension of the lingual flange, once clear of the mylohyoid muscle, should be turned into the retromylohyoid fossa.

sulcus (Fig. 450). The impression of the sulcus is bulky, but inadequately extended. The tray constructed to the cast will reproduce this error and the impression made in it can only follow these contours. As a result the denture will have a thick labial flange. Although this flange can be reduced, the extension will be inadequate and the border seal compromised.

A simple technique has been well described by Neill and Nairn (1973). The initial compound impression is made with the mylohyoid muscles contracted, and the patient's tongue firmly pressed forward against the anterior section of the palate. The impression is then removed, chilled, and the bulk reduced with a sharp knife. At least 2 mm of compound is removed from the surface overlying the mylohyoid muscles and from the surface over the buccal aspects of the roots. Compound is notoriously prone to displace soft tissues and fraenae, so that extra bulk must be carefully removed. The extension is then checked in the mouth and, when satisfactory, the surface is painted with adhesive and an alginate wash impression made. The cast from this impression provides details of the denture-bearing area and shows the position of the root preparations. A closely adapted acrylic resin tray can be made on this cast (Fig. 451). The lingual flange should be about 4 mm thick in the molar region so there is room available to relieve the impression surface from the mylohyoid muscles (Fig. 452). Posteriorly, the lingual flange may be thinned slightly and turned laterally into the retromylohyoid space. The tray must be completely rigid to eliminate any distortion when the impression is made. Three stub handles are useful; the anterior one for positioning the tray in the mouth, the posterior ones for holding the tray in place when the impression is made.

The rear stub handles should be placed slightly buccal to the midline of the ridge so that the impression load is taken by the buccal shelf area – one of the primary stress bearing regions of the edentulous mouth. The anterior stub handle is employed for positioning the tray in the mouth. Finger holds are placed in the handles as the tray can become slippery (Fig. 453). Ideally, the labial surface of the handle and tray should resemble the contour of the completed denture so that the labial sulcus is faithfully reproduced and not, as one often sees, with a large handle that displaces the lower lip and distorts the labial sulcus. Holes are cut over the roots slightly larger than the roots and their gingival margins.

Elastomeric impressions possess the advantage of recording details of post preparations, edentulous areas and of their relative locations at one attempt (Fig. 454). It is, of course, necessary that each of these separate factors is correct before the impression may be used. The setting time of the impression materials is considerably greater than that of zinc oxide eugenol pastes. However, there is little doubt that experienced operators can produce excellent results with these materials, the choice of which is a matter of individual preference.

Building the impression in stages allows the advantage of checking each step before proceeding. The impressions of the post preparations are made with the aid of copper bands and transfer copings constructed on the dies.

Metal transfer copings will not distort and give the most consistent results (Fig. 455). A hard resin such

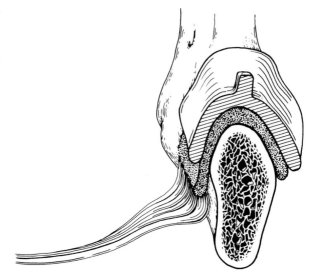

Fig. 449   A common mistake with a stock tray. A short straight lingual flange guides the impression material vertically downwards resulting in displacement of the mylohyoid muscle.

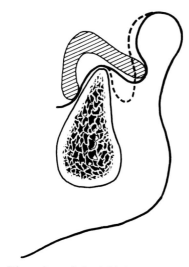

Fig. 450   Distortion of the labial sulcus by the tray will lead to the construction of a poorly extended and bulky denture base.

as Duralay may be substituted in expert hands with great care taken to ensure correct seating and application of excessive loads. It is essential they engage the antirotation slot and do not exhibit the slightest movement in the mouth. The shape of the transfer coping should include an undercut projection from the diaphragm.

The impression is best made with zinc/eugenol

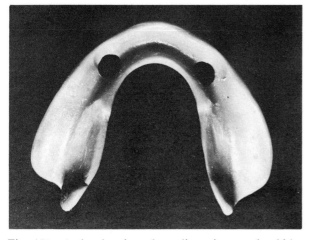

Fig. 451 A closely-adapted acrylic resin tray should be made on the cast of the primary impression. Holes should be cut over the roots, slightly larger than the roots and the gingival margins.

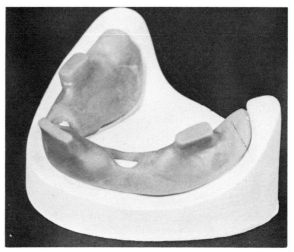

Fig. 453 The tray should be provided with three stub handles; the anterior one to be used for handling the tray; the posterior ones, in positions corresponding with the artificial molar teeth, for holding the tray in place when the impression is made.

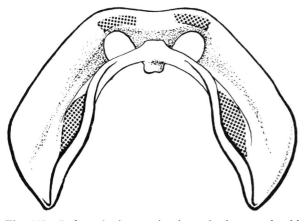

Fig. 452 Before the impression is made the tray should be relieved from the mylohyoid muscles and buccal aspects of the roots.

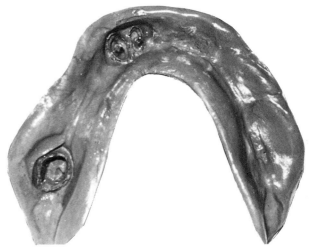

Fig. 454 If elastomeric impression materials are employed the tray is not perforated over the roots.

impression paste. Even with the greatest care, it is still unlikely that the first impression made with the tray could be used for construction of the denture base. The first attempt should be regarded as a diagnostic impression to correct the tray for minor discrepancies of adaptation of extension (Fig. 456). The extension of the base should have been decided at the primary impression stage, so it should be unnecessary to make major alterations at this stage. Border moulding may be carried out where necessary. If the tray shows through the impression paste over the mylohyoid muscle or buccal to the roots,

the tray should be further relieved and the impression repeated. On the other hand, the buccal shelf area, lying between the crest of the residual ridge and the external oblique ride, is well adapted to withstand load applied in a vertical direction.

Once it appears as though the next attempt will provide an adequate result, the metal transfer copings are placed on the roots (Fig. 457), the tray loaded with impression paste and inserted over the copings in the mouth. Excess zinc oxide that has

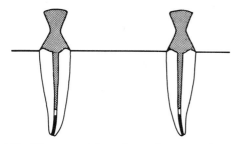

Fig. 455 Diagram to show the copings seated on the root preparation. The copings should have an undercut projection from the diaphragm.

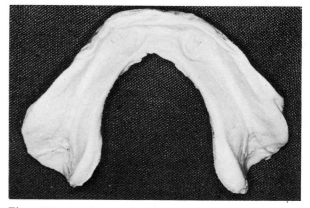

Fig. 456 An impression is made in the tray using zinc/eugenol paste. This impression is treated as a normal complete denture impression.

covered the projection of these copings is removed and the copings joined to the tray with auto-polymerizing resin (Fig. 458). The impression paste, by itself, is too weak to connect copings and tray. By placing the loaded tray over the copings, acrylic resin is kept away from the gingival margins and this critical area is reproduced with considerable accuracy by the impression paste. One practical tip is to allow adequate time for the polymerization of the acrylic resin that may be slowed by the eugenol of the impression paste. Once the resin has hardened the tray together with the copings can be removed. The dies are then carefully located on their respective copings before the impression is cast.

Once the master impression has been made (Fig. 459), the dies are positioned on their respective copings and the impression poured. The cast obtained for this impression, the master cast, is an accurate reproduction of the denture-bearing mucosa, the gingival margins, the root preparations, and the relation between these structures (Fig. 460). On this master cast the occlusal rims are made and the denture finally processed.

Correct jaw relation records are essential if the prosthesis and its supporting structures are to survive. The jaw relation records can be made in precisely the same manner as in complete denture construction. Since it is important to preserve the master cast, it is generally more convenient to use a hard wax base for the occlusal rims.* The wax can be laid down directly on the master cast but, while the base of the occlusal rim should be made of hard wax, the actual recording surface should consist of a soft wax. The hard base is necessary to prevent distortion in the mouth, but it is important that the centric relation record be made with the very minimum of load between the rims, so as to reduce any tendency to rock. As an aid to recording centric

* Moyco Extra Hard Beauty Wax.

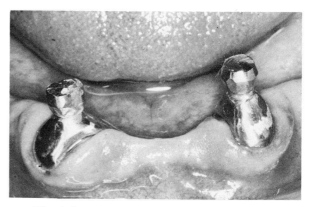

Fig. 457 Metal transfer copings in position.

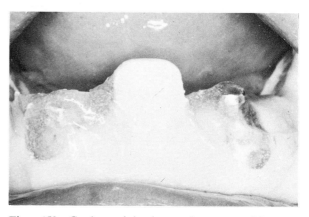

Fig. 458 Copings joined to the tray with auto-polymerising resin.

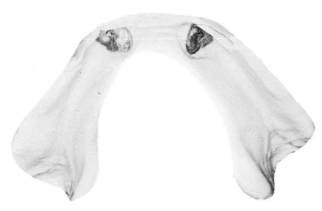

Fig. 459   The tray together with the attached copings now forms a master impression.

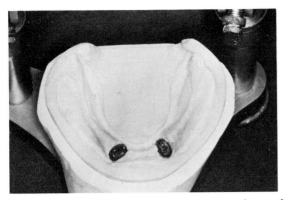

Fig. 460   The master cast accurately reproduces the denture-bearing mucosa, gingival margins, and root preparations.

relation, it is helpful to cut away the anterior section of the lower rim so that there is no anterior contact. It seems pointless making eccentric records until the centric relation record has been checked and found correct. A facebow record is conveniently made at this stage and used to mount the casts on an adjustable articulator (Fig. 461). The artificial teeth can then be arranged and set up with the articulator used as a hinge instrument. The initial trial insertion is concerned with ensuring that the vertical relation of occlusion and occlusal plane are correct, that the appearance is satisfactory, and that the centric relation record is correct. The centric relation record can be assessed quite accurately at this stage, for small errors can be felt, if not actually seen, due to cusps hitting an opposing incline instead of a fossa.

When the trial denture is satisfactory in all respects, eccentric records can be made and the

condylar guidances adjusted on the articulator. The posterior teeth can now be rearranged in the laboratory to provide a balanced occlusion. The attachments are only positioned in the denture at this comparatively late stage. Before this is done, the positions of the teeth are recorded with a plaster or silicone-based index.

The male units can then be aligned using the paralleling mandrel available with the attachments (Fig. 462). Placing the attachment slightly lingual to the root centres may help bucco-lingual space problems. The taller the attachment, the more critical bucco-lingual space becomes (Fig. 463). The attachments are soldered to their post diaphragms and the female elements positioned on them. With some attachments a metal spacer has to be incorporated between the two components. The teeth can now be replaced, the wax-up completed, and the denture processed. There is a minor problem associated with remounting the dentures on the articulator, as the master casts were articulated and the dentures processed on them. A remounting jig can be attached to the lower member of the articulator and a plaster indentation record made of the maxillary teeth, before the denture is processed. The denture is subsequently repositioned in this record. If this procedure is not followed, a new facebow record can be made when the dentures are first inserted.

When inserting the dentures there are several important checks to be made. The root caps with the male attachment units should be inserted, but not cemented, and their adaptation carefully examined. The retention apparatus of the female attachment should be slackened where possible and the denture

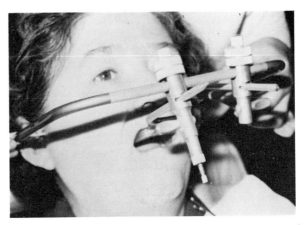

Fig. 461   It is convenient to make a facebow record together with the jaw relation records. The master casts are then mounted on an articulator.

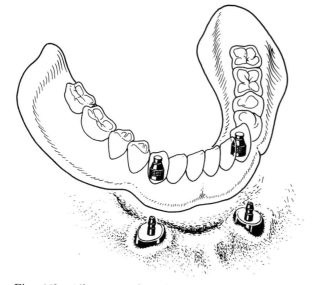

Fig. 462   Alignment of stud attachments is desirable. With the taller units it is essential.

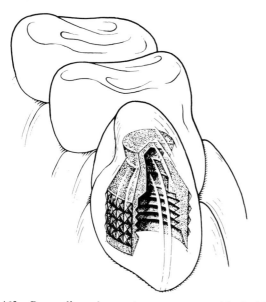

Fig. 463   Bucco-lingual space becomes more critical with the height of the restoration – a factor to consider when selecting attachments.

inserted. A correctly made denture will require firm seating pressure before the attachments engage.

The adaptation of the denture bases can now be checked with the aid of disclosing paste, ensuring that the opposing teeth do not contact during this procedure. Once the base extension and adaptation

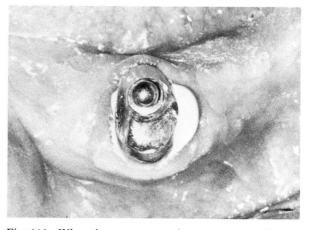

Fig. 464   When the post preparations are cemented, place the denture over them before the cement has finally hardened.

has been examined a check record will be required. The clinical procedures for a check record have been described in the previous chapter.

Once the occlusion and articulation of the dentures have been checked the post assemblies can be cemented (Fig. 464). The denture should be inserted immediately after the positioning of the post preparations and allowed to stay in place until the cement has hardened. A well-made post preparation should resist removal of the casting by the denture without the aid of cement. The degree of retention required through the attachment should produce a slight catch as it is inserted or withdrawn.

Overdentures should be inherently stable so that it is unnecessary to adjust the retention of an attachment to such a degree that the patient has difficulty in removing the denture. Overtightening the attachment forces the patient to exert a heavy extracting load on the roots each time he removes his denture. Apart from discomfort, this may result in damage to the periodontal structures, breakage of the denture, or dislodgement of the post preparations. The attachments are there merely to add to retention and stability that should be inherent in the denture itself. They do, however, allow the denture to seat home more securely than would otherwise be possible, and ensure that the border seal remains intact.

Inspection

All dentures require periodic inspection. When prefabricated attachments have been incorporated a six month recall should be used although this in general will need to be varied from patient to patient. The following examinations should be made.

Plaque control

Despite the greatest care possible with this essential therapy, some patients need a firm reminder. There can be few more annoying occurrences than finding the impression surface of the denture covered with calcified debris, an abundance of plaque around the roots, and the periodontal tissues in a disappointing state. In some situations the attachments themselves may become jammed.

There are two separate issues that must be appreciated. The first is good plaque control in the mouth, the second is adequate denture hygiene. One without the other is useless.

Despite claims to the contrary, mechanical removal of plaque from a denture is required. Soaking solutions are an adjunct not a substitute.

Infirm patients for whom difficulties with plaque control or denture hygiene may be anticipated require simplified constructions to ease the problems of this important task.

Periodontal condition of roots

The roots should be checked carefully for signs of gingival irritation, loss of attached gingivae, pocket formation, or increased mobility. Surveys of overdenture results show convincingly that it is in this area that problems can be anticipated.

Radiographical condition of roots

The roots should be examined for evidence of widening of the periodontal ligament or periapical pathology.

Oral mucosa

The oral mucosa should be examined for signs of irritation or ulceration arising from the borders of the denture, cheek biting, or occlusal errors.

THE DENTURES

Jaw relations

Changes in shape of the edentulous ridge may alter the manner in which the denture seats in the mouth. These changes may be seen as an error in the centric relation record. Absorption of fluid into the acrylic resin may have altered the dimensions of the denture bases. The original jaw relation may indeed have changed, as it may not have been recorded with accuracy during the original visits. Subsequent wearing of the denture accustoms the patient to posterior occlusal support and the return to centric relation.

Small errors of jaw relation may be corrected by alterations to the occlusal surfaces of the artificial teeth. If any rock or movement of the denture bases can be elicited, a rebasing procedure will be required as well.

Limitations of vision and mucosal displaceability preclude accurate spot-grinding in the mouth where complete dentures are concerned. A check record technique is therefore required. A plaster or wax interocclusal record is made with the teeth just separated. This record is used to mount casts on the articulator, and after removing the record the occlusion is examined. A routine check record should have been made when the denture was first inserted in the mouth. However, a further check record at the six-month recall is recommended.

Movement of the denture

The extension of the denture borders should be examined and the impression surface checked by disclosing paste. If there is any perceptible movement of the denture taking place, the denture should be rebased.

Since rebasing alters the position of the artificial teeth, a subsequent check record is necessary.

Retention adjustments

Most attachments incorporate an adjustment to allow for wear. The retention should be checked and adjusted if necessary, but only the minimal of adjustments made. Most broken attachments are due to incorrect or clumsy adjustments. Overtightened attachments may place excessive loads on roots and may also contribute to dislodgement of the root preparations.

Manufacturers of attachments usually provide detailed instructions for attachment adjustment. Since the male attachment is normally joined to the root, retention adjustments in these instances are usually carried out to the female section, embedded in the denture. Exceptions like the Conod and Battesti (Figs. 465, 466) feature a split male unit. An adjusting instrument with a screw allows the retention to be modified with precision. This arrangement allows the diameter of the entire unit to be

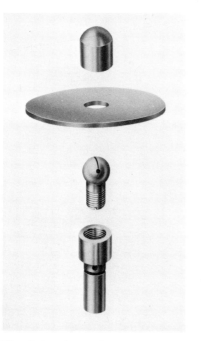

Fig. 465   The Battesti attachment incorporates a split male unit.

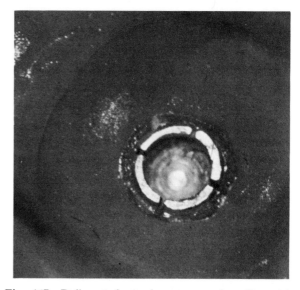

Fig. 467   Dalbo stud attachments may be adjusted by carefully bending the small engagement arms of the female unit.

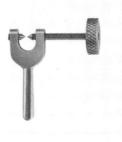

Fig. 466   The Battesti adjustment instrument. This tool is used for the Conod, which features a similar adjustment mechanism.

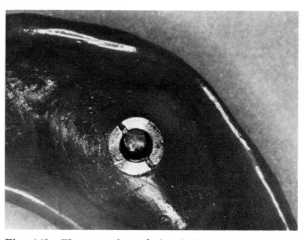

Fig. 468   The retention of the Gerber system may be adjusted by unscrewing the base of the female unit to gain access to the retaining clip.

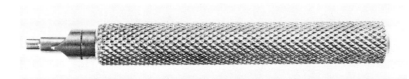

Fig. 469   The special screwdriver for gaining access to the spring clip of the Gerber system.

reduced to less than 2·5 mm but suffers from the problems of plaque removal from the depression in the male unit.

When employed as a stud attachment, Ceka units may be adjusted with a special device for separating the lamellae.

Stud attachments arranged in a conventional manner like the Dalbo attachments may be adjusted by carefully bending the small engagement arms of the female unit (Fig. 467), as may most other attachments of the ball and socket variety.

The retention of the Gerber system may be altered by unscrewing the base of the female unit and adjusting the retaining clip inside (Fig. 468). A special screwdriver is available for removing the base of the unit (Fig. 469). Adjustments of the retaining clip need to be carried out with care, and sharp bends avoided, if subsequent fracture of the clip is not to occur. Should the retaining clip break, a new one can be inserted quickly. It is essential, however, to ensure that all the pieces of the broken clip are removed before the new one is inserted.

Where the male unit is incorporated in the impression surface of the denture projecting into the post restoration, adjustments can be more difficult. In many situations the only way of increasing retention is to replace the male unit.

Spring replacement

Manufacturers of attachments containing springs often suggest they be replaced annually. The time taken before permanent deformation of the spring occurs varies as enormously as the loads applied. Since springs can be changed relatively quickly it seems sensible to change them at each recall. There is then less likelihood of overlooking this point. Wherever possible, it is more sensible to select an attachment without this complication.

In this chapter, methods of using attachments on remaining lower teeth have been considered, but the approach is virtually identical if they are employed on upper teeth. When an overdenture is opposed to natural teeth, it becomes more difficult to balance the articulation. However, in these circumstances it is particularly important to prevent errors of recording jaw relations, owing to the large displacing loads that natural teeth can place on dentures. Occlusal harmony can only be approached by careful reshaping of the natural teeth. In many instances this reshaping has to be carried out in two stages. The initial reshaping is planned on the diagnostic casts and should be completed before denture construction is begun. It is frequently necessary to narrow the teeth and to adjust their occlusal surfaces. The second stage is not always necessary. When setting the upper teeth in balanced articulation one may find small irregularities of the opposing natural teeth that make it impossible to obtain even contact in eccentric occlusions. If this occurs, the occlusal reshaping should be planned and carried out on the cast which is used as a guide to adjust the natural teeth. A new cast can be substituted for the previous one by remounting it on the articulator by means of an interocclusal record.

THE SELECTION OF ATTACHMENTS

The success of a prosthesis usually depends on careful treatment planning and attention to the prosthodontic problems; the mechanical ingenuity of the attachment is important, but must take second place. Large attachments are generally stronger than smaller ones, and also less prone to wear. As a rule one should, therefore, choose the largest attachment for which there is room. However, attachments must be surrounded by a reasonable thickness of acrylic resin, otherwise they will weaken the denture (Fig. 470). A metal lingual connector may be employed where bucco-lingual space is restricted. Apart from the size of the attachments, inadequate root preparations is the most common method of wasting precious space (Figs. 471, 472). If preliminary muco-gingival surgery has been performed, the level of attachment placement can be reduced (Fig. 473).

Inspection of manufacturers' catalogues will show the variety of different types of stud attachments available but it is only possible to describe a small number. The features discussed, however, will be typical of the group.

The space available will govern attachment selection but discussion still rages as to whether or not the comparatively rigid units should be selected as opposed to those that allow movement. The rigid units allow a neat, good looking and retentive restoration to be made where four or more widely spaced and secure abutments remain. In these situations tooth support plays an important role. The restoration replaces lost dental tissues and may take up little more space than the tissue it is replacing.

Where conventional overdentures are concerned, and these are largely mucosal supported, Mensor, quoting work by Fenner, Gerber and Muhlemann, (1956) has claimed that rigid or cylindrical stud

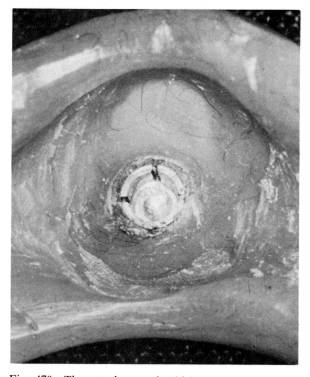

Fig. 470   The attachment should be surrounded on all sides by an adequate thickness of acrylic resin. This will minimise the dangers of weakening the denture.

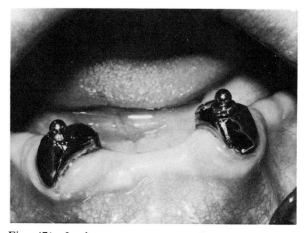

Fig. 471   Inadequate root preparation results in the attachments occupying unnecessary amounts of vertical space.

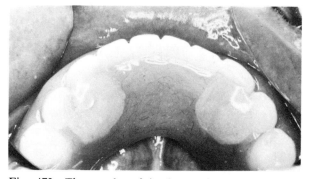

Fig. 472   The results of inadequate root preparation. Apart from the unacceptable bulge in the denture, this prosthesis would be prone to fracture even if tolerated by the patient.

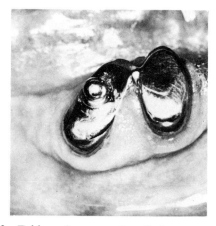

Fig. 473   Taking advantage of preliminary mucogingival surgery, the level of the attachment has been lowered as much as possible.

attachments produce no tipping action on the root; ball and socket designs are stated to produce four times as much tipping potential. A more recent laboratory study of Thayer and Caputo employed photoelastic stress analysis. They found that forces applied to a Dolder bar were resolved in an apical direction, whereas stud attachments engaging the post diaphragms (and presumably other similar devices) might produce tipping potentials. These tests illustrate the mechanical advantages of splinting roots.

Without laboratory tests, prosthodontic techniques would not improve. Nevertheless, laboratory tests cannot yet match the variables of the human mouth and of the different clinical techniques for dealing with individual situations.

The leverage effect upon the root must be an important factor. The movements will be influenced by the design of the attachment, but also by the level at which loads are applied. The more rigid attachments usually occupy more vertical space than the ball and socket variety: dome shaped

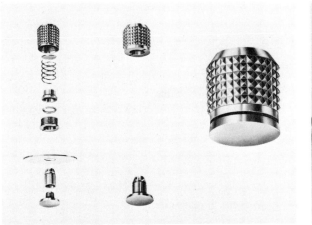

Fig. 474   The resilient Gerber unit allows vertical play. Two sizes of the attachment are produced.

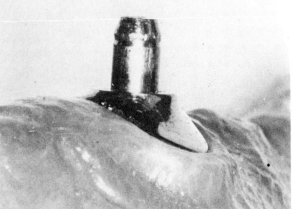

Fig. 476   Male section of resilient Gerber attachment in position.

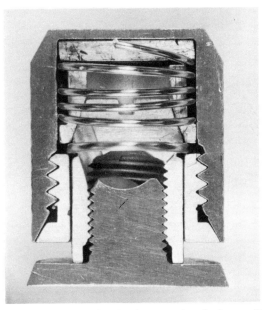

Fig. 475   Cross-sectional photograph of the resilient attachment. Note the coil spring controlling vertical movement and the encircling clip that determines the retention.

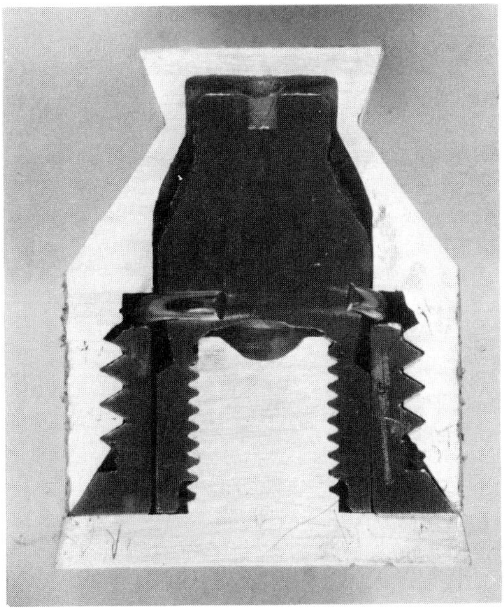

Fig. 477   Cross-sectional photograph to show close contact between the two parts of the rigid Gerber attachment when in place. This attachment is made in two sizes.

copings occupy the minimum of space and leverages applied must be relatively small.

Apart from leverage aspects, a major consideration in attachment selection must still be the space available for the unit and meticulous prosthodontic techniques.

The Gerber system of stud attachments is versatile and consists of two types of unit, one allowing some vertical movement (Figs. 474–476) the other almost rigid (Fig. 477). Each of these units is available in two sizes.

These well tried and tested units are among the largest of stud attachments. The larger of the resilient units is 5·2 mm high and the shorter one measures 4·7 mm. The diameters are 4·4 mm and 4·0 mm respectively. Bearing in mind these units must be covered by an adequate resin layer, space considerations must limit their application.

The retention of both types of Gerber attachment is obtained by a spring clip in the female unit engaging a peripheral groove in the male section. The spring clip may be removed for adjustment by unscrewing the base of the female unit (Fig. 478). Both types of male unit are screwed on to their soldering bases (Fig. 479) and prevented from unscrewing with a little resin cement. They may be unscrewed in the mouth with a heated screwdriver, leaving exposed a screw thread projecting from the base of the attachment (Fig. 480). This screw thread is identical with the Schubiger attachment. A specially manufactured nut is available to screw another attachment to the base. It will be seen later that this arrangement can be useful when the Schubiger base is used to join a bar to a root preparation. If a tooth should be lost, the bar can be unscrewed and a stud unit substituted.

The Gerber unit with the conical male part is the more rigid of the two types of attachment. The designer of this attachment points out that if two or more teeth are used, the most distal attachment should allow more vertical play than the anterior ones, as it is likely that greater displacing forces will be applied to the molar surfaces of the prosthesis. Gerber (1966) suggests that if one has canine and first premolar roots, the rigid attachments be used on the canines and the squarer, resilient unit on the premolars. Mechanics apart, there is more room for the larger unit on a premolar. In many ways, the mechanical features of the attachments receive undue attention. If the denture has been correctly designed and constructed there will be little need for elaborate systems of 'stress-breaking'. Furthermore there is very seldom need to use three attachments to retain a denture where two will suffice. The third attachment adds unnecessarily to the complexity of the restoration and the space it occupies weakens the denture. Where three roots remain the third root is normally best restored with a simple coping. Provided the denture is sound, the important factor is to choose an attachment strong enough to withstand the loads to which it will be subjected and one that can be accommodated within the contour of the denture.

The Battesti designs are worthy of note as the male unit is split and incorporates the adjustment for retention. The male unit may also be unscrewed from the base and replaced. This allows a comparatively neat female unit to be made reducing the overall diameter of the assembled unit to a remarkable 2·3 mm. Three designs of the unit are made. Two allow vertical translation of which one is a ball

and socket design, the other limits movement to the vertical plane (Fig. 481). The third member of the group is comparatively rigid (Fig. 482).

Dr Conod's rigid stud unit (Fig. 483), available in three heights, also incorporates a split male unit. This allows the diameter of the assembled attachment to be reduced to 2·4 mm.

Split male units require special instruments for adjustment while plaque control and removal of debris from the split is a complicating factor.

Of all the stud attachments produced, it is probably the Dalbo that is by far the most popular. Combining neatness with strength it has proved itself over many years. Although three types of design were produced, the ball and socket unit is the most popular (Figs. 484, 485). The rigid Dalbo attachment provides a firm connection between the two components (Fig. 486) but cannot match the versatility of the ball and socket unit.

The ball and socket Dalbo is the smallest of the series and is readily accommodated in most dentures (Fig. 487). Nevertheless, it is still 4 mm high. It allows limited vertical and rotational movement between the two parts of the attachment and has a spherical-shaped male section (Fig. 488) that is easy to clean. The fact that the attachments allow movement does not imply that this should occur. Sound denture construction will limit the movement that actually takes place. Adjustments are simple to carry out and if correctly aligned wear of the male unit is slight. The fingers of the socket are surrounded by a nylon ring that simplifies adjustments. With this series of attachments the female units need simply be buried in the acrylic resin of the prosthesis. Soldering to a sub-frame is unnecessary and may weaken the unit.

The Rothermann unit requires remarkably little vertical space. Rigid and resilient units are available. The design of the attachment has been modified and improved. The overall height of the rigid unit is only 1·1 mm and that of the resilient unit is 1·7 mm (Figs. 489–493).

The Rothermann is a button shaped attachment with the male unit incorporating a groove of uneven depth. The clip of the female section slides over the tapered upper edge of the male, with the free ends of the female engaging the deepest retaining groove (Fig. 490). The female clip is designed to be retained by the acrylic resin.

Apart from the minimal vertical space requirements, an additional advantage claimed is the tolerance for limited misalignment of attachments. This tolerance can be particularly useful where tilted teeth are involved.

Since the tapered area on the male unit is of

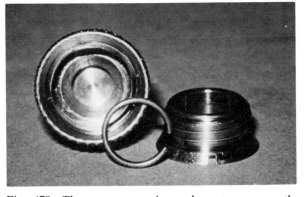

Fig. 478 The screw may be undone to remove the retention clip for adjustment.

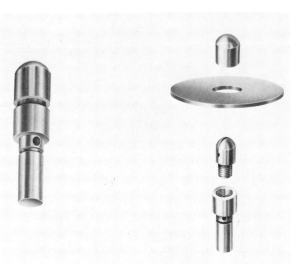

Fig. 481 The Battesti 'resilient' unit is remarkably compact. The rigid unit has no spacer but is otherwise similar.

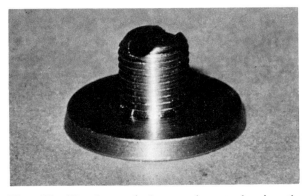

Fig. 479 The base of the attachment showing the projecting screw. Two sizes of screw are available and for each of these sizes an entire range of Gerber and other units is available.

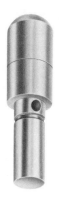

Fig. 482 The rigid Battesti unit.

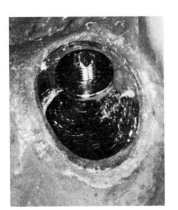

Fig. 480 The male sections of both types of Gerber attachments have a common screw base. It is therefore possible to unscrew them in the mouth, interchange attachments if required, or join the root to another type of attachment.

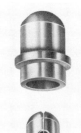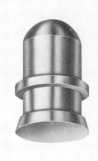

Fig. 483 The Conod attachment.

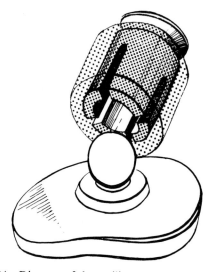

Fig. 484　Diagram of the resilient Dalbo stud attachment.

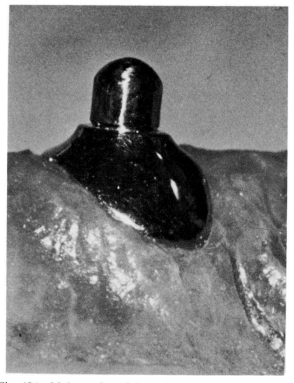

Fig. 486　Male section of the rigid Dalbo stud attachment in position.

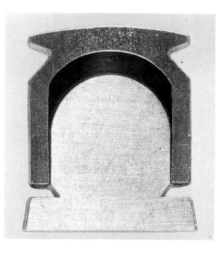

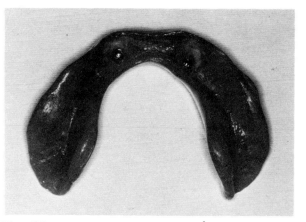

Fig. 487　Impression surface of the denture with two Dalbo stud attachments.

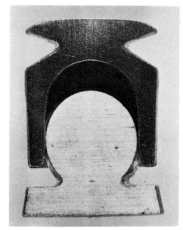

Fig. 485　Cross sectional photographs of (*top*) rigid and (*bottom*) ball and socket Dalbo units.

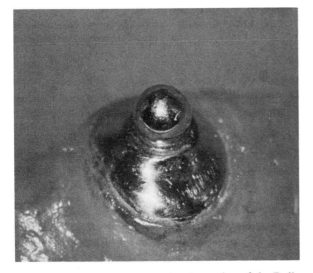

Fig. 488 The spherical shaped male section of the Dalbo stud unit is easy to clean.

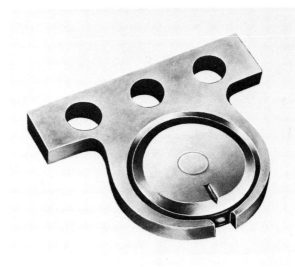

Fig. 490 The assembled rigid Rothermann attachment. Note the free ends of the clip engage in the deepest portion of the retaining groove. This point is marked by a line.

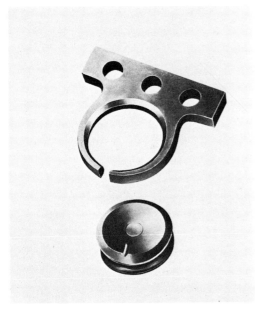

Fig. 489 The rigid Rothermann unit.

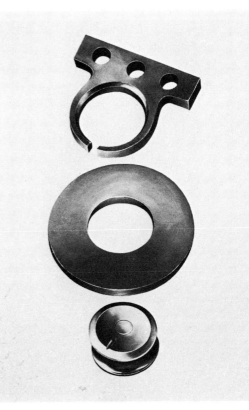

Fig. 491 Metal spacer used when curing acrylic resin around the resilient Rothermann attachment.

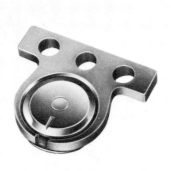

Fig. 492   The assembled resilient Rothermann attachment. Note the increased height of the male section allowing some play between the two components.

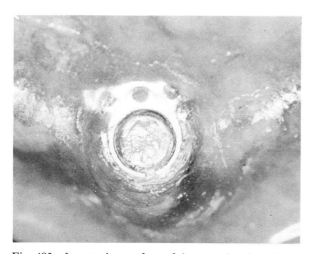

Fig. 493   Impression surface of denture showing a Rothermann unit.

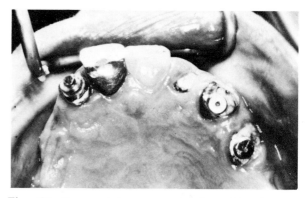

Fig. 494   Incorrect treatment planning with misuse of Rothermann attachments.

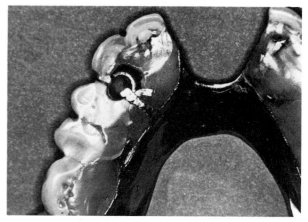

Fig. 495   The effects of inadequate vertical space and poor denture design and construction.

restricted size, the guidance available to aid the patient to find the correct path of insertion is similarly limited. This factor together with inadequate depth of surrounding acrylic resin must contribute to the number of denture fractures unfairly blamed on the attachment (Figs. 494, 495). Like most other stud units adequate bulk of acrylic is essential round the attachment. Once this is appreciated consistently satisfactory results can be obtained with the unit.

The Baer and Fäh units are interesting. Both are relatively rigid and require little vertical space (Fig. 496). However it is the unit with the rounded male section that requires the least space (2·2 mm) and not

the other way round. Both units are compact and robust. They require alignment and positioning procedures similar to other stud attachments (Fig. 497).

The Ancrofix (Fig. 498) is another compact unit with many worthwhile features. The small bubble on top of the male unit allows the female component to rotate. However, if this bubble is ground down, the female unit seats further down on the stud thereby restricting movement. Two thicknesses of spacers (0·25 mm and 0·4 mm) are provided, together with a useful range of ancillary devices. While the vertical space occupied is only 3·2 mm, the diameter of the flange is 4·2 mm.

The popular Ceka system has applications for overdentures. Rigid and resilient designs are available that share a common base (Figs. 499, 500). Unlike the Ceka extracoronal unit the female sections

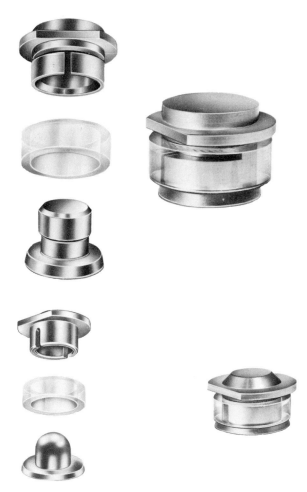

Fig. 496 The two Baer and Fäh units. The attachment with the rounded male section requires only 2·2 mm of vertical space.

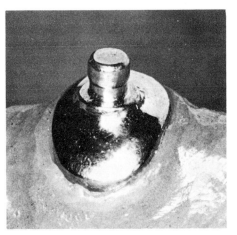

Fig. 497 The rigid Baer and Fäh attachment in position.

are not identical. It is not, therefore, possible to change resilient for rigid constructions merely by changing the retention pins as the female section will need to be changed as well. The vertical travel allowed by the stud unit is 0·4 mm (Figs. 501, 502), as opposed to 0·3 mm of the extracoronal unit. The retention pin or male section is screwed onto the base ring and the base soldered to the root diaphragm.

Like other Ceka attachments, they are a technicians delight to employ. A wide range of ancillary instruments are produced to simplify adjustments, changing attachments, and rebasing. A limiting factor is the vertical space required by the unit. The base is 1·4 mm high and, no matter how carefully it is positioned on the root some considerable proportion of this height must be added to the attachment, resulting in a 5 mm vertical space requirement for overdentures. Space permitting, the versatility of this unit must give it many applications.

The Zest Anchor system (Fig. 503a) is original in several respects. A nylon male element is incorporated in the denture base and projects downwards engaging a recess in the root preparation. The design reduces vertical space requirements and impairment of the strength of the denture. Two sizes are available, depending on the root length and diameter.

The system has been extensively modified and a comprehensive kit is now available (Fig. 503d). Vertical space requirements are similar to those required for the Rothermann Unit although the technical aspects are far simpler.

The tooth is cut down to just above gingival level and a root face prepared. The alignment of the attachment is decided by using a No. 6 round carbide bur and then a special diamond instrument is employed to prepare a precise cavity and root face for the stainless steel insert. Two sizes of inserts are available with matching burs differing in length only (Fig. 503b). The shorter unit is more difficult to employ and should be used where vertical space requirements dictate. The stainless steel insert can then be cemented into the root and its margins polished to blend with the root surface. This simple procedure avoids the technical and periodontal problems of root coping construction, but does leave exposed an area of dentine and cementum surrounding the stainless steel. This necessitates meticulous plaque control and creates an obvious problem of removing debris and plaque from the depression within the stainless steel. An additional problem can be caries of the root surface.

Given good patient motivation, together with

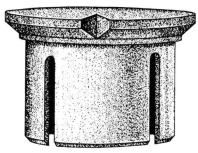

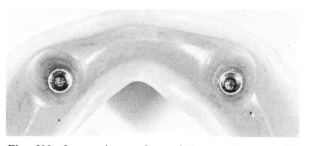

Fig. 500   Impression surface of denture incorporating two Ceka female units.

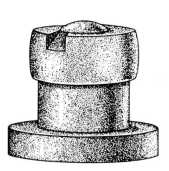

Fig. 498   The Ancrofix attachment. The movement potential can be reduced by grinding the bubble on top of the male unit.

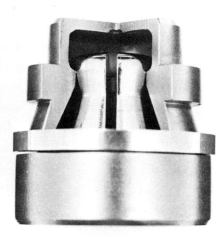

Fig. 501   Cut away model of resilient Ceka stud unit with washer in place.

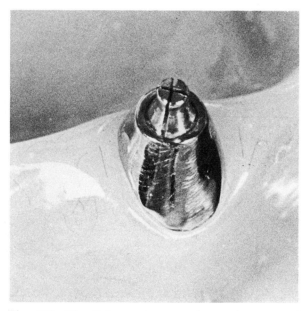

Fig. 499   The Ceka system may be used as a stud retainer. The retaining pin is screwed onto its base. Resilient and rigid units are available.

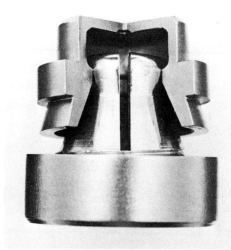

Fig. 502   Cut away model of resilient Ceka stud unit with washer removed showing vertical travel possible.

regular application of a fluoride-containing substance to the root face, caries may not provide the expected complication, although the danger exists. A nylon transfer unit is available for placement in the stainless steel during impression procedures. This transfer unit incorporates a centering sleeve to ensure correct relationship between the male and female elements during the impression procedure. Before casting the impression, a resin dummy female element is placed over the transfer unit and this dummy female section is incorporated in the master cast. The denture is processed ensuring that the acrylic resin does not impinge upon the root surface. The recommended procedure is to incorporate the nylon retentive male element in the mouth using self-polymerising acrylic resin. The nylon retentive element is produced with its own centering sleeve which must be in place during this procedure (Fig. 503c). Another feature of the retaining element is a slight flattening of the ball retainer in two places thereby facilitating escape of air and providing a better seating. With this technique, as with others involving locating procedures in the mouth, best results are usually obtained by cutting a vent so that excess acrylic resin flows onto the external surface of the denture. The centering sleeve is then removed. Replacement of the nylon section should produce little problem and this design can be expected to provide a limited degree of retention and stability for an overdenture. Thayer and Caputo have pointed out the tipping potential on the root but it is up to the operator to ensure that the denture constructed does not apply these forces.

Modifications of the Zest system allow it to be used with a gold root coping. It can be seen that this versatile attachment system has particular application to the retention of transitional prostheses. The technical work is minimal and a considerable amount of it can be carried out at the chairside.

The Ginta attachment is another unit featuring the male element in the impression surface (Fig. 504). However, it differs from the Zest Anchor in several ways.

A root preparation for a coping is required and a precious metal hollowed out female post attachment is incorporated. This is achieved by reaming the canal with a Para-Post system drill to at least 6 mm. A plastic post is placed in the canal and removed with the impression. The special female unit is then fitted into the die and the coping waxed up and cast onto it, the centre of the unit being prelocated with a graphite rod. The male section is metal and the manufacturers suggest that it is located in the mouth with the aid of a spacer and self-polymerising resin.

Like the Zest system this attachment may provide a degree of retention and some stability.

It is only possible to describe a small number of attachments and these have been chosen as typical of their group. The shape and size of the unit is normally the overriding consideration although the ancillary devices that accompany the attachment must influence the choice.

The importance of a correct vertical space assessment is hard to over-emphasize, and it is for this reason that mounted diagnostic casts are so useful. The precise space requirements may be checked after the trial insertion stage and an occasional change of attachment may be required. There is, however, little excuse for finding inadequate space for any attachment at this late stage. It is this type of casual treatment planning that leads to a frantic search for the smallest attachment that is surrounded with a minute thickness of acrylic resin. The fractured denture is an inevitable result.

Attachment movement is generally over stated. The rigid units, due to their small size, are not entirely immovable; other categories, however, frequently allow more movement than should ever be required.

Ball and socket, together with other attachments that allow movement, do no harm provided the potential movement is regarded as a safety valve and not as a means of anchoring an unstable denture to a rigid root. They do, of course, possess a tendency to cause tilting forces to be applied to the roots, but that depends on the overdenture. It must be apparent, therefore, that the prognosis of the restoration is influenced more by the planning, biological, and prosthodontic aspects, rather than the ingenuity of individual attachment mechanics.

Extra bracing of the retaining roots may be obtained by joining the diaphragms with a highly polished gold bar in right contact with the mucosa (Fig. 505). Bracing action apart, this connection may result in resolution of forces applied in a more apical direction. It is naturally essential that this bar be cleaned well by the patient and that the design and construction facilitate plaque control.

Most attachment manufacturers provide excellent technical information with their products. Attachments allowing a limited degree of play between male and female units are often provided with metal spacers for use during processing. Sharp edges of acrylic should be removed from the impression surface but no specific area should be cut away in this region. The important feature is that the base should be well adapted and easy to maintain plaque free.

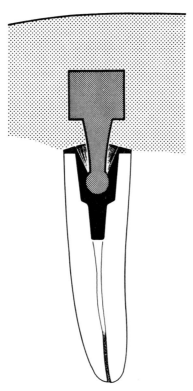

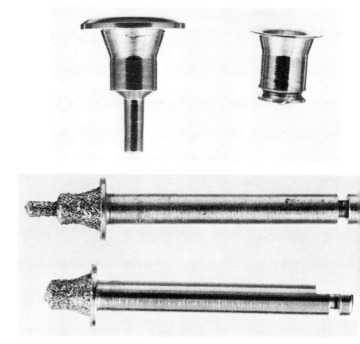

Fig. 503b Regular (*top left*) and miniature Zest stainless steel female units (*top right*). The corresponding reamers are shown below.

Fig. 503a The Zest Anchor System. A nylon male element is incorporated in the denture base and occupies minimal vertical space.

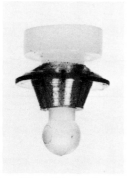

Fig. 503c The nylon male unit incorporates a centering sleeve to ensure the correct relationship between the components during locating procedures. The sleeve is subsequently removed.

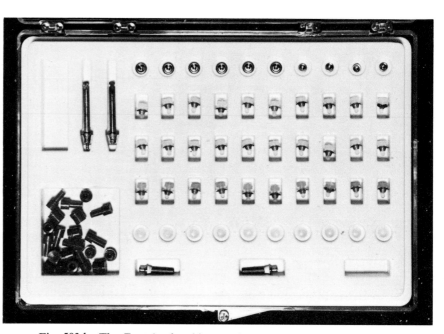

Fig. 503d The Zest Anchor kit contains numerous ancillary devices.

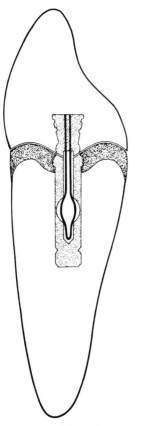

Fig. 504   Diagram of the Ginta attachment.

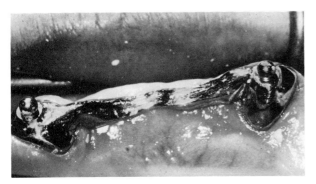

Fig. 505   Extra bracing of the retaining roots may be obtained by joining the diaphragm with a highly polished gold bar in light contact with the mucosa. This connection will resolve forces in a more apical direction.

Soldering attachments to a metal sub-frame in the denture may be an ideal way of ensuring that the location remains undisturbed. However, the majority of stud attachments cannot be attached in this manner and must simply be buried in the acrylic

resin. In this case, curing of the base must not take place unless a locating dowel or similar device is employed to prevent any movement of the attachment.

REBASING ATTACHMENT-RETAINED OVERDENTURES

Most complete dentures require periodic readaptation of their impression surfaces to the underlying mucosa. Care taken in denture construction is usually rewarded by a long time interval before rebasing is necessary. The technique of rebasing a complete overlay denture appears perfectly straightforward. Unfortunately, it is one of those procedures easy to carry out, but difficult to carry out well.

In theory, and occasionally in practice, the rebasing procedure can be treated as a complete denture. The peripheral adaptation of the denture border is examined and adjusted if necessary. Border moulding is carried out at this stage when indicated. Undercuts should then be removed from the acrylic resin of the denture impression surface, and a zinc-oxide impression made within the denture. Where applicable, a spacer should be put between the two units and the denture held in place by finger pressure with the opposing teeth out of occlusion. If the teeth are allowed to contact when the impression is made, it will superimpose occlusal errors onto the impression surface of the denture. An impression of the opposing dentition is also made together with a facebow record. This stage will not be necessary if the original 'check-record' casts have been kept. Processing dowels (dummy male attachments) should be placed in the female units of the denture before the impression is cast.

After processing, the denture is inserted to ensure that it seats firmly in the mouth and that the attachments engage. This is where trouble is frequently encountered. If the denture seats correctly, a check record is made and the occlusion adjusted on the articulator before the patient leaves. Unfortunately, the localisation between the roots and the mucosa can be disturbed by processing. As a result, the dentures may seat back in the mouth but the attachments may not engage. This mishap rarely occurs if locating dowels are employed.

No processing of the denture base should be carried out without locating dowels (Figs. 506, 507). Most manufacturers provide these valuable ancillary devices. If one cannot be obtained, an improvisation can be made by soldering tagging to the base of a corresponding male unit and using this as the

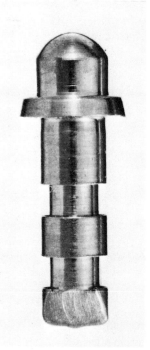

Fig. 506   Modified Dalbo attachment for incorporation within the artificial stone of the master cast. This ancillary device is essential for rebasing procedures.

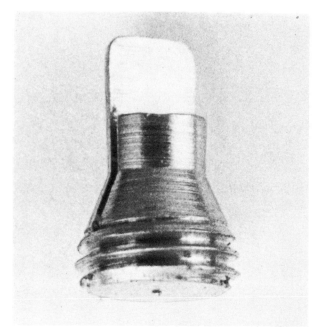

Fig. 508   The retaining pin of the Ceka stud unit can be replaced in the mouth with this locating dowel. An impression is then made over it.

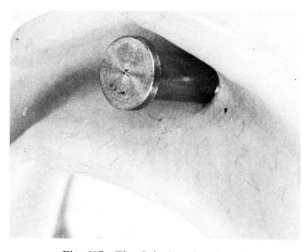

Fig. 507   The Ceka locating dowel.

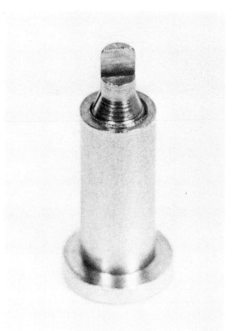

Fig. 509   The locating dowel with its removable base.

locating device. An alternative method with the Ceka is to unscrew the retaining pin and substitute a locating dowel on the diaphragm (Fig. 508). An impression is then made over the dowel. Subsequently the dowel is unscrewed and placed with its base in the impression before casting (Fig. 509).

Correction of a locating accident may be achieved by cutting the female attachments out of the denture and relocating them with self-polymerizing resin in the mouth, a difficult and demanding procedure. Prevention is far simpler than cure. Removal of the attachments from the denture base needs to be carried out with a fine fissure bur handled with care. It is easy to damage the facings, denture, and attachments in this process. Having removed the attachments, place the female units over their corresponding males using spacers when indicated. Insert the denture over the attachments ensuring that it now seats correctly and does not bind on one or both attachments. If it does bind then extra acrylic resin must be removed around the offending unit.

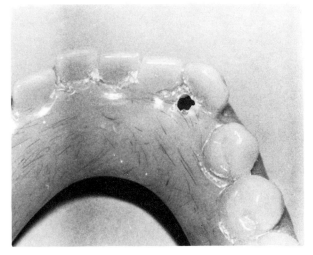

Fig. 510 Having removed the attachment ensure a lingual or occlusal vent is present to allow escape of excess acrylic resin.

Once the denture can be seen to seat correctly remove it together with the female attachments from the mouth. Protect the gingivae with petroleum jelly. Drill a hole through the lingual aspect of the denture to aid excess material to escape rather than flow under the impression surface of the denture (Fig. 510). Place the female units over their respective attachments with spacers, if required, insert a small amount of denture base coloured self-polymerizing

resin in the attachment site in the denture (remarkably little is required) and insert the denture ensuring that it is correctly seated. Err on the side of using too little resin as small defects are simple to restore. Excess resin flowing under the impression surface is difficult to remove and will spoil the accuracy of the base adaptation.

Errors in the relocating procedure may show up in several ways. One or both attachments may fail to engage. The denture may have a pronounced tendency to rock around the attachments, or an apparently well-seating denture may demonstrate an error in jaw relations.

If persistent difficulties are encountered, the entire impression surface of the denture will need to be stripped away and the attachments located in the impression, but secured with resin to the denture base. The attachments are secured by placing resin through a lingual window cut in the denture. Bearing in mind that some of the artificial teeth may need to be changed if there is a large subsequent error in jaw relationships, the magnitude of the task may not be far short of remaking the denture.

REMAKING ATTACHMENT-RETAINED OVERDENTURES

The procedure is identical to that of remaking a complete denture with one complication, the male attachments and related diaphragms. The problem is overcome by placing the female sections over their male counterparts in the mouth, with spacers when required, and incorporating them in the impression. The female units are joined to the tray with self-polymerizing resin rather like transfer copings.

A great deal of time can be saved by employing a denture duplicating technique.

Sticky wax sprues are attached to the denture which is placed in a container of molten agar. Once the agar has gelled, it is removed from the container, divided in two, and the denture taken out. The agar can now be replaced in the container and forms a mould. Tray resin is poured into the mould and when polymerized duplicates the form of the existing denture.

The 'duplicate' denture of tray resin is now employed as a tray. First of all, a hole is cut through the tray around the attachment, allowing female attachments to be placed over their male units with a small space around them. Having removed undercuts from the tray, border moulded it, and placed the female attachments in the mouth, a zinc oxide-eugenol impression is made. The attachment is connected to the tray with self-polymerizing resin. Since the tray shows the position of the artificial teeth, it is possible to make the facebow record, and centric relation record at this one visit.

Casting the impression should follow the procedures already laid down, with locating dowels in position. One has therefore achieved a master cast with adequate information to proceed directly to the trial insertion stage.

OTHER USES OF STUD ATTACHMENTS

Because of their apparent simplicity, stud attachments are often prescribed for non-vital partial denture abutments. The loads applied in these circumstances can be considerable and for this reason one of the larger, and stronger, units is recommended. Space requirements might be a complicating factor here.

Another application is for the retention of a small, tooth supported restoration with non-vital abutments. In theory, a neat well retained prosthesis could be constructed, with little more bulk than a fixed prosthesis yet including all the advantages of a removable prosthesis. In practice, the rigidity of

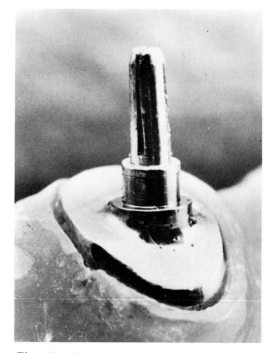

Fig. 512   The Introfix attachment in position.

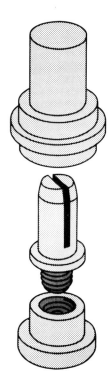

Fig. 511   The Introfix attachment. A robust and rigid unit with a removable male section.

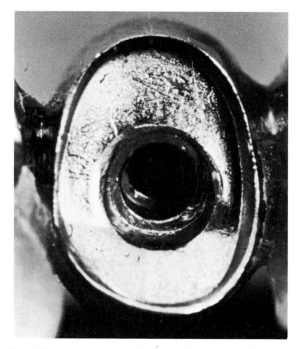

Fig. 513   Impression surface of the prosthesis demonstrating the Introfix attachment.

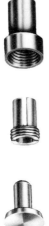

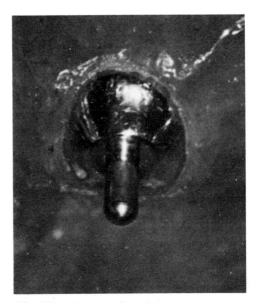

Fig. 514   The Gmur attachment showing the retaining collar of the female undone.

Fig. 517   Male section of Gmur attachment.

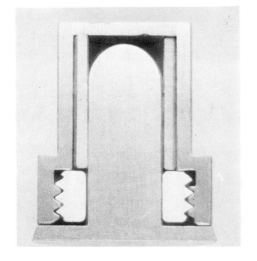

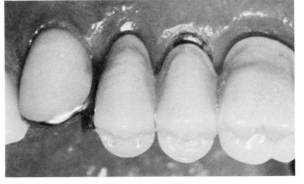

Fig. 518   Prosthesis being inserted.

Fig. 515   Cross-sectional photograph of the Gmur attachment.

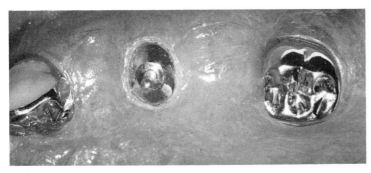

Fig. 516   Intermediate abutment root with Gmur attachment.

even the larger stud attachments cannot match that of an intracoronal attachment, so that as a general rule the use of stud attachments in these circumstances is limited to that of an intermediate abutment restoration. An example of this use would be for a root lying in a span to be restored by an attachment-retained prosthesis. This type of restoration is primarily tooth-borne and the stud unit will to some extent be protected by the other retainers when the prosthesis is removed and inserted.

Almost any rigid stud attachment with sufficiently long parallel sides can be employed. The Gerber and Battesti units have been described already. The Introfix is another robust unit (Figs. 511–513). The Gmur (Figs. 514, 515) is a similar unit that provides good support while occupying the minimum of vertical space. It is one of the few attachments that can be used on a lower incisor root. An example of the application of this attachment is illustrated (Figs. 516–518).

The apparent simplicity of stud attachments can be deceptive. Space requirements and load distribution require very careful consideration thereby placing careful treatment planning and meticulous prosthodontic techniques at a premium.

REFERENCES AND FURTHER READING

BARRETT, S. G. and HAINES, R. W. (1954) The structure of the mouth in the mandibular molar region. *J. prosth. Dent.*, *9*, 692

BARRETT, S. G. and HAINES, R. W. (1962) The structure of the mouth in the mandibular region, and its relation to the denture, *J. prosth. Dent.*, *12*, 835

BOUCHER, C. O. (1958) Fundamental approach to the problems of impressions for complete dentures. *Dent. Practit.*, *8*, 162

BOUCHER, C. O. (1970) *Swenson's Complete Dentures*, 6th edn. C. V. Mosby, St Louis, Mo.

BRILL, N. (1967) Factors in the mechanism of full denture retention – a discussion of selected papers. *Dent. Practit.*, *18*, 9

BRILL, N., SCHÜBELER, S. and TRYDE, G. (1962) Aspects of occlusal sense in natural and artificial teeth. *J. prosth. Dent.*, *12*, 123

DE VAN, M. M. (1952) Basic principles in impression taking. *J. prosth. Dent.*, *2*, 26

EDWARDS, L. F. and BOUCHER, C. O. (1942) Anatomy of the mouth in relation to complete dentures. *J. Amer. dent. Ass.*, *29*, 331

FENNER, W., GERBER, A. A. and MUHLEMANN, H. R. (1956) Tooth mobility changes during treatment with partial denture prosthesis. *J. prosth. Dent.*, *6*, 520

FISH, E. W. (1948) *Principles of Full Denture Prosthesis*, 4th edn. Staples Press, London

GERBER, A. (1966) *Retentions Zylinder und Retentions*

Puffer für Brücken und Prosthesen mit verdeckten Verankerungen. Cendres et Metaux, Biel, Bienne, Switzerland

HANNAM, A. G., MATHEWS, B. and YEMM, R. (1968) The unloading reflex in masticatory muscles of man. *Arch. oral Biol.*, *13*, 361

KURER, H. G., COMBE, E. C. and GRANT, A. A. (1977) Factors influencing the retention of dowels. *J. prosth. Dent.*, *38:5*, 515–525

KURER, P. F. (1979) A press stud denture retainer. *Brit. dent. J.*, *146*, 4, 119–122

LAWSON, W. A. (1965) Retention of full dentures. *Dent. Practit.*, *15*, 199

MENSOR, M. C. (1977) Attachment fixation for overdentures, Part I. *J. prosth. Dent.*, *37:4*, 366

MENSOR, M. C. (1975) Attachments for the overdenture. In *Overdentures*, by Brewer, A. A. and Morrow, R. M. C. V. Mosby, St Louis, Mo.

MILLER, P. A. (1958) Complete dentures supported by natural teeth. *J. prosth. Dent.*, *8*, 924.

MORROW, R. M., FELDMAN, E. E., RUDD, E. D. and HOWARD, H. J. (1969) Tooth-supported complete dentures. An approach to preventive prosthodontics. *J. prosth. Dent.*, *21*, 513

NAIRN, R. I. (1964) The posterior lingual flange of the complete lower denture. *Dent. Practit.*, *15*, 4

NEILL, D. J. and NAIRN, R. I. (1973) *Complete Denture Prosthetics*. John Wright, Bristol

PREISKEL, H. W. (1967) Considerations of the check record in complete denture construction. *J. prosth. Dent.*, *18*, 98

PREISKEL, H. W. (1967) Prefabricated attachments for complete overlay dentures. *Brit. dent. J.*, *123*, 161

PREISKEL, H. W. (1967) Anteroposterior jaw relations in complete denture construction. *Dent. Practit.*, *18*, 39

PREISKEL, H. W. (1968) An impression technique for complete overlay dentures. *Brit. dent. J.*, *124*, 9

PREISKEL, H. W. (1968) The posterior lingual extension of complete lower dentures. *J. prosth. Dent.*, *19*, 452

SCHWEITZER, J. M., SCHWEITZER, R. D. and SCHWEITZER, J. (1971) The telescoped complete denture: a research report at the clinical level. *J. prosth. Dent.*, *26*, 357

TALLGREN, A. (1967) The effect of denture wearing on facial morphology. *Acta odont. scand.*, *25*, 563

TALLGREN, A. (1969) Positional changes of complete dentures – a 7-year longitudinal study. *Acta odont. scand.*, *27*, 539

TAYLOR, R. L., DUCKMANTON, N. A. and BOYKS, G. (1976) Overlay dentures: philosophy and practice I. *Australian Dent. J.*, *21:5*, 430

THAYER, H. H. and CAPUTO, A. A. (1977) Effects of overdentures upon remaining oral structures. *J. prosth. Dent.*, *37:4*, 123

CHAPTER 11

Bar Attachments

Bar attachments act as splints, joining teeth or roots and spanning the edentulous regions between. There is little new about splinting bars; Carr (1898) described one at the end of the last century, and in 1913 Goslee published a comprehensive article on the subject. About this time Gilmore (1913), Fossume (1906) and Bennett (1904) had designed similar attachments as substitutes for fixed restorations; their names are still applied to various forms of bars. The results obtained with many of these attachments were disappointing, mainly because of failure of the swaged crowns it was necessary to use with them, for they were the only available abutment restoration. Their demise was also hastened by the focal sepsis scare. Nowadays one can, perhaps, make a more critical evaluation of these devices.

Since the bar is positioned close to the alveolar bone supporting the teeth, forces applied to those teeth through the bar exert a far smaller leverage than those applied through an occlusal rest of a partial denture (Fig. 519).

Thayer and Caputo's work suggests that the joining bar resolves forces applied to the teeth into a more apical direction than would be the case if the teeth remained unconnected.

It is often claimed that connecting a group of teeth reduces the mobility of the unit. From the mechanical point of view there is little doubt about the argument. The long-term biological advantages are not so clear cut although the load sharing possibilities can only be beneficial.

On the other hand, the bulk of the bar and related structures raises several problems. Vertical and bucco-lingual space requirements will limit applications in many instances (Fig. 520). Plaque accumulation around the bar is another important consideration. No matter how well the prosthesis is designed and executed, bar attachments require more plaque removal skill on the part of the patient than most others. Their use cannot be recommended for arthritic patients with limited manual dexterity, nor for those whose motivation is in the very least suspect.

All bar attachments require adequate and approximately equal retention for abutment retainers if cementation failures are to be avoided. The prognosis is best when mobility patterns of abutments do not reach Grade II.

Like stud attachments, bar attachments fall into two groups, those allowing slight-movement – the bar joints – and the comparatively rigid bar units.

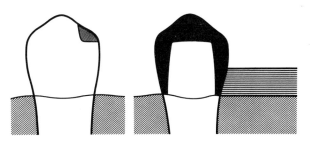

Fig. 519 Leverages applied to teeth through the bar are considerably less than those applied through an occlusal rest of a partial denture.

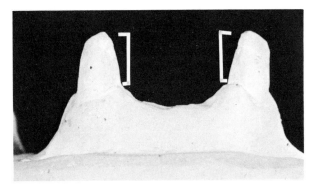

Fig. 520 Assessment of both vertical and labiolingual space is essential if bar attachments are to be employed. The contact of the base of the bar with the edentulous ridge needs to be planned at this stage.

209

BAR JOINTS

Bar joints are those attachments allowing movement between the two components. They have their main application in overlay denture construction where two, three, or possibly four teeth remain. The advantages of preserving roots in this situation have been discussed.

The bar is usually attached to diaphragms on root filled teeth, locking the roots together and improving the crown/root ratio. Augsburger (1971) has described endodontic stabilization to reduce mobility still further. A common path of insertion for the retaining posts is desirable although divergences can be overcome by mechnical means. Alternatively the abutment teeth may be crowned and these crowns connected by the bar. This arrangement can be useful where natural teeth are in opposition or where a long undercut precludes the use of a flange.

Bar joints can be subdivided into:
1. Single sleeve bar joints.
2. Multiple sleeve bar joints.

Single sleeve bar joints

The Dolder Bar Joint is an excellent example of this type of attachment. This well tried bar is produced from wrought wire, pear shaped in cross-section and running just in contact with the oral mucosa between

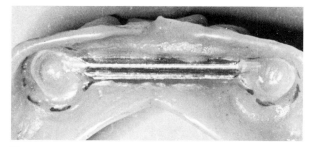

Fig. 522 Impression surface of denture showing the open-sided sleeve of the Dolder Bar Joint. Note the inadequate denture borders that may contribute to a subsequent fracture.

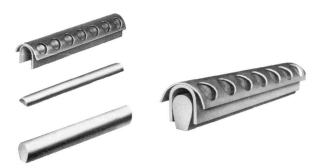

Fig. 523 The components of the Dolder Bar Joint. Two sizes of this attachment are produced and each size is available in various lengths.

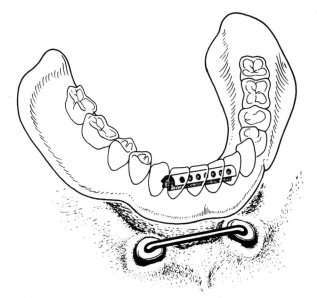

Fig. 521 The Dolder Bar Joint, a well tested and popular example of a single sleeve attachment.

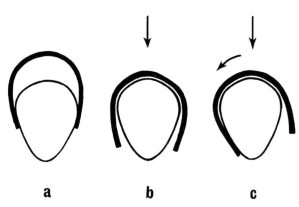

a   b   c

Fig. 524 The original aim of the Dolder Bar Joint design was to allow a wide range of movements under load. (A) The sleeve at rest. (B) The sleeve subjected to vertical load. (C) The sleeve subjected to rotational forces.

the abutments (Fig. 521). An open-sided sleeve is built into the impression surface of the denture (Fig. 522) and engages the bar when the denture is inserted.

Two sizes of Dolder Bar Joint are produced with heights of 3·5 mm and 4·55 mm. The cross sections are 2·3 mm×1·6 mm and 3·00 mm×2·2 mm respectively. Apart from the artificial teeth, a sufficient bulk of acrylic resin must cover the sleeve to prevent fracture, although a lingual metal plate may be used where space is restricted. A spacer is provided with this Bar Joint (Fig. 523) to allow a degree of movement potential. The spacer is removed after the acrylic resin has been cured. The retention tagging forms part of the sleeve ensuring excellent adherence to the surrounding acrylic resin.

The original aim of the Dolder Bar Joint design was to allow a considerable measure of both vertical movement and rotation around the long axis of the bar (Fig. 524). The spacer used for the larger bar allowed over 1 mm of vertical play – far more than should ever be necessary for an overdenture. The bar allows some side to side tilting but lateral loads are well resisted. Dolder (1961) has pointed out the transitional nature of these restorations but excellent results can be obtained if the bar is used with care and discretion.

As a single sleeve bar has to run straight, it cannot follow the antero-posterior curvature of the alveolar ridge, nor can it be adapted to small vertical contours. This type of bar therefore lends itself to square arches where the remaining roots or teeth can be joined by a straight line (Fig. 525). Where possible the bar should be aligned perpendicularly to a line bisecting the angle between two lines drawn along the crests of the posterior edentulous ridges (Fig. 526). If the roots lie in a curved arch the space for the denture base will be restricted lingual to the bar and the denture may break unless a metal lingual plate is employed. In some circumstances, two connecting elements can be used to join the roots to a straight bar, but only the straight bar can be used for retention (Fig. 527). However, this is not usually an arrangement to be recommended in view of the unfavourable leverages that may fall upon the roots, descriptively known as the 'bucket-handle effect'. Where the arch is markedly curved, the bar may occupy too much tongue space so that it is generally better to select a different attachment system.

Due to the irregular shape of the mucosa small spaces may be left under the base of the bar (Fig. 528). Unless all the surfaces of the bar are kept plaque free, the resultant irritation causes these small spaces to fill by mucosal proliferation. At one time it was an accepted procedure for the technician to adapt the bar to minor mucosal irregularities by soldered additions to the undersurface of the bar. These soldered additions are particularly difficult to maintain plaque-free as they are irregularly shaped and scratch easily. Again they result in irritation. (Fig. 529).

Another method that has been tried is to employ a modified bar that includes a skirt (Fig. 530). This skirt, unfortunately, simply provides additional surface area for plaque accumulation.

Where there are marked irregularities of the mucosa and mucogingival areas preliminary minor surgery usually gives the best results. A thin wedge of tissue is removed from the area to be covered thereby taking away more from the high areas than from the low ones. The technique not only provides for better adaptation but usually contributes more space for the attachment unit (Figs. 531–533).

Where a large depression is found the bar can be cranked into it with two connecting elements, thereby reducing the space it occupies. Plaque control would be simplified by providing a large cleansable space of more than 4 mm between bar and mucosa. Unfortunately there is seldom adequate space for this arrangement unless across a cleft palate or an area of gross resorption. For the majority of patients the bar needs to be placed in even contact with the mucosa.

So far, the bar has been described as if it were positioned approximately at right-angles to the saggital plane. This is the position in which it works best. However, Dolder has suggested that his bar be used where there are just two teeth or roots on the same side, such as a canine and first molar. In this case, the bar joins the two roots and runs along the crest of the ridge. Any rotation allowed is sideways.

Space problems have been mentioned already, an aspect that can be critical in the lower anterior region. Space is required for the bar and sleeve, a thickness of acrylic resin and for the artificial teeth. Placing the bar slightly lingual to the crest of the edentulous ridge may help make room for the necks of the lower teeth. However, the reduced lingual thickness may weaken the denture and a metal lingual plate will then be necessary.

One of the more common mistakes associated with bar-joint prostheses arises when an inexperienced operator attempts to push out the necks of the lower anterior teeth in an effort to make room for the bar. This gives the patient an unpleasant

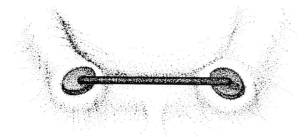

Fig. 525 The Dolder Bar works best where the remaining teeth or roots are in a square arch and can be joined by a straight line.

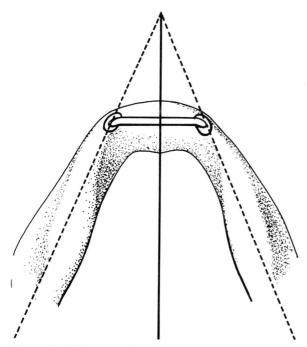

Fig. 526 Where possible, the bar should be aligned perpendicularly to a line bisecting the angle between the posterior edentulous ridges.

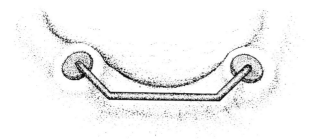

Fig. 527 Although a straight bar may be used to join roots on a curved arch, this arrangement commonly occupies too much bucco-lingual room anteriorly, and can also result in unfavourable leverages applied to the abutment roots.

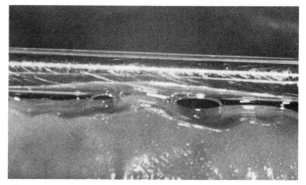

Fig. 528 Small spaces left under the bar tend to be filled by mucosal proliferation.

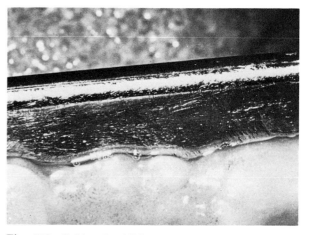

Fig. 529 Soldered additions to the bar are difficult to clean and scratch easily. The adherence of plaque leads to mucosal irritation.

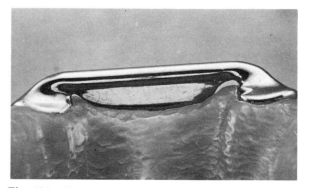

Fig. 530 The addition of a metal skirt simply provides additional surface for plaque accumulation.

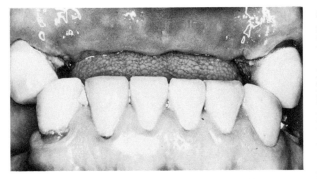

Fig. 531 Anterior edentulous span. Apart from poor periodontal tissues, there is inadequate vertical space for a Dolder Bar.

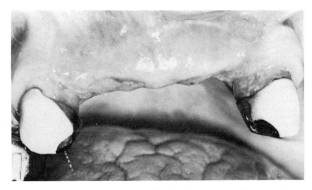

Fig. 532 Following mucogingival surgery, ridge contour is improved, and more vertical space provided.

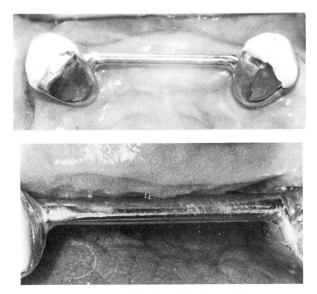

Fig. 533 Dolder Bar Joint in position.

appearance, as though he has a swollen lip and a mouth perpetually full of food. Appearance apart, the lip will exert a displacing action on the denture.

Dolder (1964) followed up 270 patients with bar joint prostheses and found that after 6–18 months 95% of his patients had lost the small space allowed between the sleeve and bar. This small space is provided by processing the denture with a metal spacer between the bar and sleeve and the spacer subsequently removed. The most likely cause of this space becoming obliterated would be alveolar resorption, for this would allow the bases to sink slightly. Dolder found that as a result of this subsidence the denture was now rocking about the bar and subjecting the abutment roots to a heavy occlusal load. Dolder recommended that the sleeve should then be repositioned in the denture. This is accomplished by cutting out the sleeve from the denture base, clipping it over the bar with the metal spacer in place, and then seating the denture over it. The sleeve is reunited to the denture base by self-polymerising acrylic resin. Cutting out the sleeve from the denture base can be difficult and requires care to avoid damage to the artificial teeth or breakage of the denture. Careless handling can damage the retention tagging of the sleeve. Soft wax or impression plaster should be placed between the bar and the mucosa to prevent acrylic resin flowing under the bar. However, repositioning the sleeve is only half the answer, for if the denture bases have moved they will have carried with them the occlusal surfaces of the teeth. A subsequent check record is required and in some cases replacement of the posterior teeth will be necessary.

A more satisfactory approach is to rebase the denture with the spacer inserted. After all, it is loss of support to the impression surface of the denture that has resulted in this subsidence. However, when this impression is made no load should be applied distal to the bar, for this might cause the denture to rotate around the bar. The rebasing procedure will have altered the relationship of the occlusal surfaces to the mucosa and a check record will be required.

Quite apart from damage caused to the mucosa and edentulous ridge, it is obviously unsatisfactory to construct a denture that requires frequent re-basing or frequent relocating procedures in the mouth. As with all other prostheses, the main object must be to gain support from the maximum possible area, and reduce to a minimum any displacing loads falling on the denture. When used for retaining overdentures the principles of complete denture construction must take precedence over mechanical considerations of attachments. The main object must be to gain maximum support and reduce displacing forces to a minimum.

Despite the potential for movement the manner in which the denture has been constructed should make it unnecessary to cut away areas of the impression surface around the gingival margins. The removal of sharp edges is, of course, another matter. A denture that moves perceptibly in the mouth requires attention. It may require rebasing, a relocating procedure, or remaking, but if a continuous movement is allowed to take place unchecked it will cause damage to the denture supporting structures.

Apart from overdenture construction the Dolder Bar Joint may be used to connect small groups of teeth. In these circumstances, as with with overdentures, the bar can be cut and soldered to follow ridge contours bearing in mind the problems previously discussed. The sleeve is inserted on a straight section or it may be cut in two and applied to more than one part of the bar. Once sleeves are no longer in the same plane, they will prevent rotation, which should not occur in any case with a partial denture retainer. Provided adequate vertical space exists, the Dolder Bar Joint combines the splinting efficiency of a fixed prosthesis with many of the advantages of a removable restoration. It is particularly useful for spanning anterior edentulous spaces where there is adequate room (Fig. 534).

Incorporating guide planes on the distal abutments will help prevent the tendency for the partial denture to rotate around the bar while providing rest seats will ensure adequate occlusal support.

Excellent results can be obtained if the restoration can be kept simple and readily cleansable. Problems arise when attempts are made to connect tilted abutments by means of screw connectors that are difficult to clean. The debris around these devices can lead to gingival and mucosal problems of surprising extent.

A bar joint that has become popular in the United States is known as the Baker clip. It is available in a 12 or 14 gauge bar size. The sleeve requires roughening to provide retention for the acrylic resin as, rather like the earlier Dolder Bar Joints, no retention tags are provided. The sleeve can be sectioned if the bar is not run in a straight line.

Multiple sleeve joints (Fig. 535)

If several short sleeves are substituted for the continuous one, there is no need for the bar to run straight and it can be bent to follow the vertical contours as well as the antero-posterior curvature of the ridge. Gilmore's original design was an attachment of this type and is still available today. Ackermann's bar is almost identical (Figs. 536–539). It can be obtained in various shapes of cross-section, but it is the bar with the circular cross-section that lends itself to bending in all planes. As this unit has a small cross-section and can be bent, it can frequently be positioned with a cleansable space under the bar, yet the bar does not interfere with the positioning of the artificial teeth. The small sleeve units can be placed at the most convenient sites.

The circular cross section is fairly simple to keep clean, but the results of poor plaque control can be anticipated (Fig. 540). It is interesting to note that the mucosa is relatively healthy midway between the abutments.

More rigid bars with pear-shaped and oval cross-sections are available, while a wax pattern of the bar is produced as well. This wax pattern can be contoured to the correct shape and then cast in gold. The diameter needs reduction to about 1·8 mm after the casting process.*

If it were considered important to have movement between the two sections of the attachment, bending the bar to an antero-posterior curve would prevent hinge rotation and might substitute a rocking motion. This is of slight clinical significance provided the denture is soundly constructed. When using this type of unit it is recommended that a short extension of the bar be carried 5 mm behind the most distal root (Fig. 541). The sleeve positioned on this section will prevent any tendency for the distal part of a lower denture to rise when sticky foods are

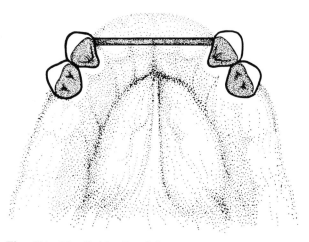

Fig. 534 The Dolder Bar Joint may be used to connect groups of teeth.

* Dr H. Ackermann, personal communication.

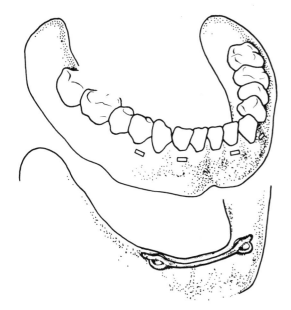

Fig. 535 The Ackermann bar. This unit closely resembles the original Gilmore attachment and is a good example of a multi-sleeve bar joint.

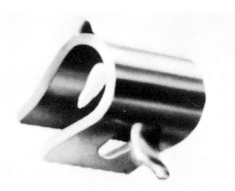

Fig. 537 The sleeve of the Ackermann bar. Note the retention tags at right angles to the long axis of the bar.

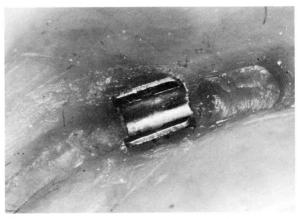

Fig. 538 Impression surface of a denture showing one of the small metal sleeve units.

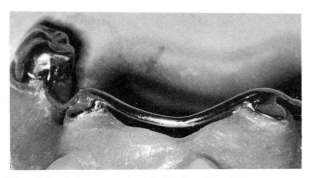

Fig. 536 Ackermann bar following the ridge contour, yet with a cleansable space under the bar.

chewed. Multiple sleeve bar joints are more versatile than the single sleeve units, but the bars seem to have slightly less rigidity.

Augsburger's development (1971) of the original Gilmore bar may well prove useful for splinting certain canine teeth. The required hinge action, however, could be obtained only when the bar has not been bent antero-posteriorly.

The sleeves of the Ackermann bars incorporate retention tags for the acrylic resin that project bucco-lingually. This positioning requires the removal

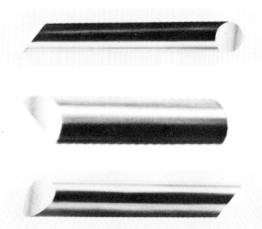

Fig. 539 The Ackermann bar: *top*, circular section; *middle*, the spacer; and *bottom*, oval section.

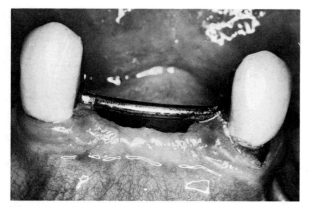

Fig. 540   The results of inadequate planning and poor plaque control.

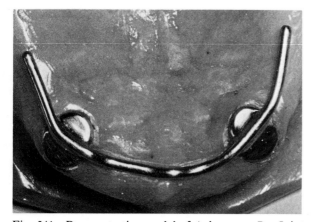

Fig. 541   Demonstration model of Ackermann Bar Joint to show the 5 mm extension behind the most distal abutment. The sleeve fitting on this extension prevents sticky foods displacing the distal part of the base away from the mucosa.

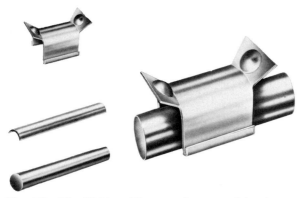

Fig. 542   The CM bar. The retention tags of the sleeves are aligned with the long axis of the bar, a feature that simplfies relocation procedures.

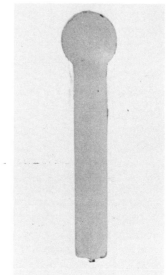

Fig. 543   Plastic pattern for the Hader Bar Joint.

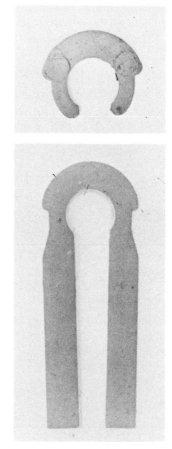

Fig. 544   Two heights of plastic sleeve are available for the Hader Bar Joint.

of considerable amounts of acrylic resin during relocating procedures. The Ackermann systems are well tried and tested and provide excellent results.

The CM bar is similar in profile to the circular Ackermann bar (Fig. 542). The diameter is 1·9 mm and the similarity is close so that the CM sleeve can be used on the Ackermann bar. The CM bar is produced in precious and semi-precious alloys, the latter recommended for long spans. The retention tags of the sleeve project in the long axis of the bar and this simplifies relocating procedures should they be required. Two types of sleeve are manufactured, the most popular with short flanges that do not project below the base of the bar. The longer flanges are employed where the bar has to be bent in the vertical plane over a short distance.

The Hader Bar Joint is interesting in that the manufacturers provide prefabricated plastic patterns that are adapted to the master cast and then cast in the alloy of choice (Fig. 543). While the versatility is apparent the mechanical properties of laboratory casts cannot possibly match those of wrought bars of specially formulated alloys. The plastic form allows considerable versatility in adapting the bar to the ridge contour. Sleeves produced for the system made of plastic have a drawback in that retention adjustments can be achieved only by replacing the sleeves (Figs. 544, 545), but it is possible to substitute metal sleeves.

Remaking a bar joint denture

The main problem is reproducing the bar now firmly in the patient's mouth. With regard to the Dolder bars and similar structures that run in a straight line the procedure is as follows.

A primary impression is made with compound in a stock tray this impression being made over the bar. It is then trimmed and an alginate wash made in the same way as for a stud-retained denture. The distance between the abutments should be measured and a length of bar and sleeve obtained some 4 mm longer.

A closely adapted acrylic resin tray is then made on the cast of the primary impression and a slit cut in the tray overlying the bar. This slit should be wider than the sleeve that is to be fitted over the bar.

The new sleeve should now be placed over the bar in the patient's mouth incorporating the spacer. Gaps between the base of the bar and the mucosa should be blocked out with soft wax or impression paste and inserted into the mouth. When the material has set, excess paste that has flowed

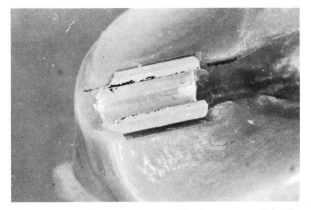

Fig. 545 Plastic sleeves are easily incorporated in the denture but their retention cannot be adjusted. In these circumstances they need to be replaced.

through the slit is removed while the tray is still in position. The sleeve is thus exposed and the slit filled with self-polymerizing acrylic resin that unites the sleeve to the tray. When the tray has been removed, the sleeve will be locked in the impression. The spacer is now placed in the sleeve followed by the spare bar. When the impression has been cast, the bar will be held in the artificial stone and the denture constructed upon it. Under no circumstances should the impression be cast without the bar in place as the artificial stone will flow into the sleeve and result in the cast breaking when the impression tray is removed.

Crowns joined by a bar cannot be covered by the resin tray. In these circumstances the tray is cut away from the crowns which then project through the tray. The tray is then removed in an overall alginate impression covering both crowns and the acrylic tray.

Multiple sleeve bars or simple sleeve units that have been bent are more difficult to reproduce as a spare bar cannot be placed in the impression. A closely adapted resin tray is made and the impression made without the sleeve in place. Gaps under the bar should have been obliterated however. The cast of the impression will show the position of the bar although the reproduction will not be exact. The sleeves with spacers are placed on the cast and the denture waxed up around them. The sleeves are not incorporated in the acrylic resin of the denture base, but are just used to ensure that an adequate space is left for them.

The location of the sleeves to the denture is carried out in the mouth – a difficult and exacting task. With the spacers and sleeves in place it is essential to establish that the denture is correctly seated and does not rotate around the sleeves.

The next vital step is to ensure that all the gaps and undercut under the bar are adequately obliterated with wax or plaster. Even the slightest amount of resin flowing into such a space will lock the denture firmly to the bar and make removal both painful and difficult: the denture may even need to be cut away completely from the bar.

Small holes should be drilled through the lingual aspect of the denture over the sleeves so that excess resin flows through onto the lingual aspect of the denture rather than onto the impression surface.

Once the locating of the sleeves has been established the free ends of the sleeves should be cleared of resin with a hot instrument and the retention adjusted. The occlusion must then be checked and a check record procedure carried out.

CLINICAL PROCEDURES

When used to retain overdentures, the clinical procedures of using a bar joint are similar to those of stud attachments. However, the site of the bar must be examined critically and preliminary mucogingival surgery carried out when necessary.

Impression procedures vary according to the type of construction. If the bar is to be run between two surfaces the impression technique is identical to that of stud attachments.

Where the restoration is opposed by natural teeth it is better to modify the design and run the bar between two crowns rather than build the denture over the roots (Fig. 546). In this way, some of the lateral loads will be borne directly by the teeth rather than transmitted through the denture. This approach is recommended where there are large buccal undercuts around the roots preventing a satisfactory denture base extension.

Most operators today prefer elastomeric impression materials for these situations. Speedy and accurate results can be achieved if the impression tray is made correctly. The tray requires to be close fitting over the edentulous areas but spaced with two thicknesses of wax around the abutments. A correctly extended border is essential. When polysulphide, polyether, or even some silicone impression materials are applied in this tray displacement of the denture bearing area will be achieved together with an impression of the abutment preparations and a good border seal. Failure of one part of the impression does require another attempt using expensive materials with relatively slow setting times.

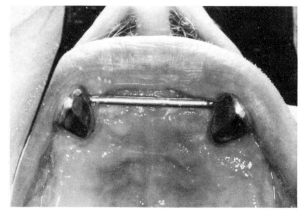

Fig. 546 When natural teeth oppose the denture it is often better to employ two crowns as abutments provided their root support is adequate. Some lateral loads are then borne directly by the teeth instead of being transmitted through the denture.

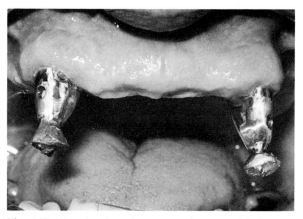

Fig. 547 Despite the advantages of elastomeric impression materials, transfer coping techniques still have application.

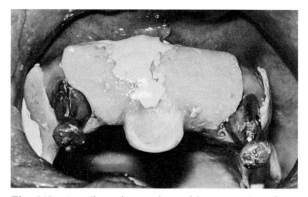

Fig. 548 Acrylic resin tray in position around copings.

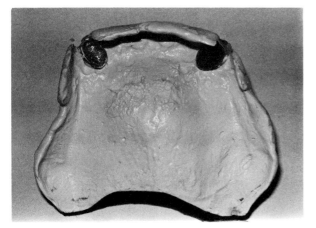

Fig. 549 Master impression with copings joined to the special tray.

For this reason transfer copings are still employed by some (Fig. 547). It is certainly the recommended technique when there are particular problems of border seal anticipated. A close fitting acrylic resin tray is constructed. When large buccal undercuts are present the tray buccal to the roots is cut away (Fig. 548). The resin tray is border moulded and an impression of the edentulous area made with zinc oxide eugenol impression paste. The transfer copings are then located to the tray in the mouth with acrylic resin and the tray removed (Fig. 549). In some situations it may be necessary to remove the impression tray and transfer copings with the aid of an overall impression.

Once the master cast is obtained the recording of jaw relationships and trial insertion are conventional. Where two crowns are used as abutments, the occlusal rims and artificial teeth are set around them and the preparations kept out of occlusion.

Where overdentures are concerned the insertion of bar joint prostheses closely resembles the procedure employed for stud retained dentures. The bar structure is placed in the mouth uncemented and the diaphragms checked for correct location and adaptation. The engagement of the denture to the bar can then be examined and the retention of the two sections adjusted.

A check record is now made and the prosthesis remounted on the articulator. The check record is complicated if abutment crowns are employed, rather than diaphragms, as these crowns form part of the occlusal surface. The abutment crowns should, therefore, be removed with the check record so that the entire occlusal surface can be mounted on the articulator and adjusted.

Technical considerations

Insufficient space for the attachment is a most common problem. While hardly technical, it is a problem that may first become apparent in the laboratory. Measurement of vertical and buccolingual space should have been part of the preliminary treatment but carelessness at this early stage may become obvious comparatively late in the therapy when the bar is set up on the master cast after the final trial insertion.

The wax up of the trial insertion is conventional, and when the position of the teeth has been decided, the position of the anterior artificial teeth is recorded with a plaster overcast. This overcast (Fig. 550) allows the teeth to be removed and subsequently replaced in exactly the same position. If at this late stage insufficient room is available a smaller bar attachment will have to be selected. The multisleeve bar joints are useful in this respect. Where the space problems do not allow this, the treatment plan may need to be reviewed. Raising the level of the occlusal plane or pushing forward the necks of the anterior teeth as last minute attempts to position the attachment seldom succeed. They result in prosthodontic problems of even greater magnitude that require remaking the restoration.

Like most other attachments, bar joints dictate the use of acrylic resin teeth due to space considerations.

Spacers are provided with most bar joint systems to ensure that a small gap is preserved between the sleeves and bar during processing. The spacer is then removed. The Dolder Bar Joint spacers are usually too large. It is usually more convenient to employ the spacer for the smaller bar when the larger bar is used; when the smaller bar is employed the spacer is thinned slightly.

The free edges of the sleeve should be just clear of acrylic resin to enable them to have a slight clip action, but the amount of relief required is small. If a large relief is allowed, it creates a space when the denture is in position. The original sleeve of the Dolder Bar Joint was prone to separate from the denture if insufficient retention was provided (Fig. 551). The latest version incorporates a retention plate which is far superior (Fig. 552). Rotation around the long axis of the bar can be restricted by incorporating distal guide planes in the abutment crowns (Fig. 553).

Prefabricated bars, like the Dolder Bar, may be cranked to adapt to certain vertical contours of the ridge. A small connecting section can also be

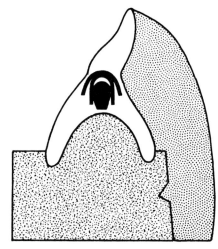

Fig. 550 After the bar and sleeve have been set up, the anterior teeth are repositioned with the plaster overcast and the denture waxed-up.

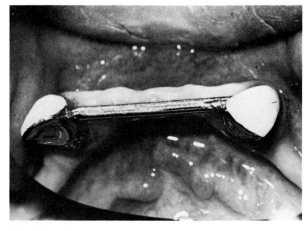

Fig. 553 Rotation around the long axis of the bar can be restricted by the use of distal guide planes on the abutment crowns.

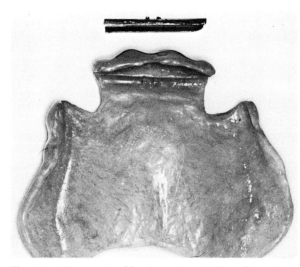

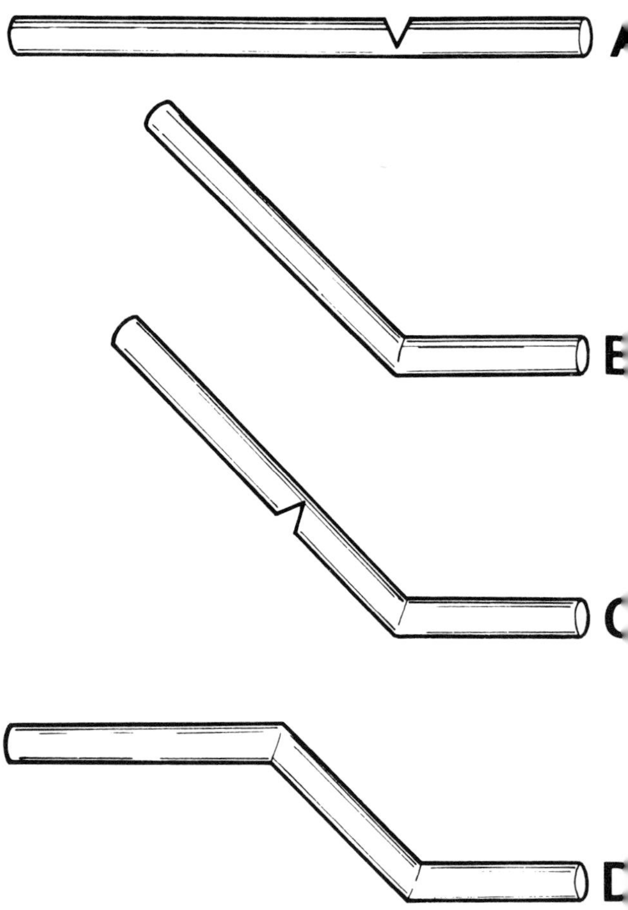

Fig. 551 The result of inadequate retention of the sleeve within the acrylic resin. This type of design is prone to fracture around the sleeve.

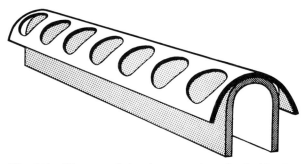

Fig. 552 Diagram of the sleeve section of a Dolder Bar Joint incorporating a retention plate.

Fig. 554 Stages in the bending of a Dolder bar. After soldering, the bar should be annealed before further adaptation is attempted.

employed to approximate it to antero-posterior curvatures of the ridge, but the dangers of using other than small connections have been mentioned.

A section of bar, longer than the edentulous space, is softened by heating to dull red and plunging in water. A V-shaped cut is made into the bar and the cut closed by bending the bar. The joint is then fluxed and joined with a high fusing solder (Fig. 554). After soldering, the bar should be annealed before further adaptation is attempted.

Multisleeve bars are usually easier to adapt to the master cast although annealing will be required. Both single and multisleeve bars will need to be soldered to the abutment crowns.

The soldering of any bar prosthesis requires a great deal of experience and care, particularly when a wrought bar is to be joined to a highly platinised gold crown. No matter what alloy is employed, some distortion can easily arise and the effect of a comparatively small distortion is greatly magnified when the span of the prosthesis is long and may give rise to a pronounced rock on the master cast. All sections need to be annealed (usually 5 minutes at 700 °C) before assembly for soldering. After soldering, full heat hardening treatment is necessary.

SCREW CONNECTORS FOR BAR JOINTS

Since bar joints are commonly soldered to the diaphragms of the post preparations, it is necessary for all the posts to have a common path of insertion. Where roots diverge, it will not be possible to insert the whole structure as one unit. A similar problem arises when crowns with divergent paths of insertion are employed as abutments.

Instead of soldering the bar to the root diaphragms, it is possible to screw the bar to one or more of the diaphragms in the mouth. Another method is to separate the root diaphragms from their posts, solder the bar to the diaphragms, and screw the diaphragms down to their respective posts in the mouth. This approach requires large posts and has limited application. It is also possible to screw the diaphragm directly to the root using a threaded post. Screw-retained telescopic crowns can be employed when the abutments are crowns.

The Schubiger attachment

This attachment uses the base of the Gerber stud unit and is given a fuller description in the next chapter. A threaded stud projects from the root diaphragm and a matched sleeve is slid over the thread and held in place by a cylindrical nut (Figs. 556–558). The bar is soldered to the sleeve. Although there is no need for the root posts to be aligned, the threaded studs have to be parallel to allow the sleeves at either end of the bar to be slid over them. A special mandrel is supplied for correctly aligning the screw projections before they are invested and soldered to the diaphragm of the post preparation (Fig. 559).

Two sizes of screw base are manufactured. The smaller has a diameter of 3·0 mm and the larger 3·2 mm. For each of these bases is available an entire range of accessories, including Gerber stud units. If several roots are involved and one is lost, the bar can be unscrewed and Gerber stud units substituted.

The main drawback to this unit is bulk, for the bar is now attached just above the highest point of the diaphragm, instead of being soldered to the lowest part. The bar may, therefore, occupy a considerble amount of interalveolar špace. Where the bar is to span a cleft palate the extra height of the connector is of little consequence. In these situations divergence of the roots can be marked and the connector particularly useful (Fig. 560).

It is more common to find that raising the bar is an embarrassment, as vertical space is so often restricted. This effect can be minimised by using two small connecting elements to crank the bar (Fig. 561).

By the very nature of its design this type of attachment and its connecting elements has several small external projections that will be difficult to clean. Bar joints have their own plaque control problems but where connectors are employed one must be doubly sure of the patient's plaque control.

Other connectors

A neater, but less versatile, system can be used in conjunction with a thick post. A modified post is used, with a threaded screw hole tapped in the gingival portion (Fig. 562). The posts are cemented and the diaphragms with the connecting bar then screwed onto their posts in the mouth. The bar is soldered to the edge of the diaphragm so that there is virtually no encroachment upon vertical space. It may, however, complicate plaque control. A modification of this approach is to pass the screw through the bar (Fig. 563).

To safeguard the restoration it is wise practice to incorporate antirotation components for both post and sleeve. When the diaphragm is inserted it is recommended that it be cemented in place and the screw inserted before the cement has set.

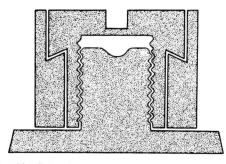

Fig. 556   The Schubiger screw system showing the sleeve to which the bar can be soldered. Two sizes of screw are available.

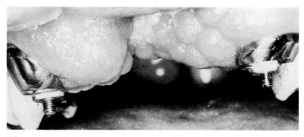

Fig. 560   Schubiger screw projections either side of a cleft palate.

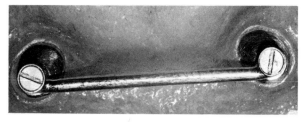

Fig. 557   The Schubiger threaded screw unit allows the bar to be screwed to the post diaphragms in the mouth. Divergence of the post preparations is allowed, and the bar may be removed if necessary.

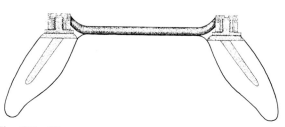

Fig. 561   The screw connector tends to raise the level at which the bar runs above the mucosa. This disadvantage can be overcome by cranking the bar with two small connecting sections.

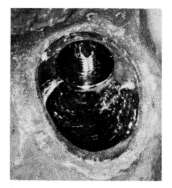

Fig. 558   The bar can be unscrewed to leave the threaded screw projection. This projection is identical with the base of the Gerber stud unit.

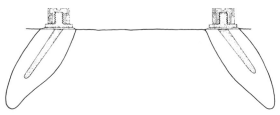

Fig. 559   Although the post preparations need not be aligned, the threaded screw projections should be parallel. A special mandrel is supplied for this purpose.

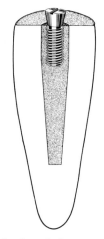

Fig. 562   Post with threaded screw hole allowing the diaphragm to be joined to the post in the mouth. The bar is soldered to the diaphragm.

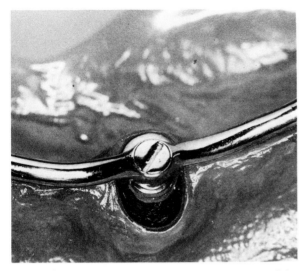

Fig. 563   A modified approach, passing the retaining screw through the bar.

The Kurer screw retained post is another method of connecting diverging roots. The bar is soldered to the diaphragms and the stud screw or screw assembly passes through them. The method of use has been described in the previous chapter.

Where tilted abutment crowns are concerned, the application of intracoronal attachments and extra-coronal screw connectors are discussed further on. Both require considerable vertical space. It is, however, possible to join the bar to the external surfaces of telescopic crowns. This is a particularly neat arrangement. Apart from the space required for the connector some skill is required to ensure that the screw head is flush with the surface of the crown when it is finally tightened. Unless the screw passes through a coping at right angles to its long axis, turning the screw will alter its seating against the surface of the crown (Fig. 564). For this reason the screw should not be trimmed and polished until it has been finally tightened.

BAR UNITS

Bar units are comparatively rigid allowing no movement between the sleeve and bar. Although some load may be distributed to the mucosa, these prostheses are mainly tooth-borne. Bar units may be useful where:

1. There are four or more abutment teeth and large edentulous spaces.
2. The number and distribution of the teeth does not allow construction of a satisfactory clasp-retained partial denture.
3. There are edentulous areas with considerable resorption.
4. Rigid splinting is required of the remaining teeth or roots.
5. The appearance of the remaining natural teeth requires post preparations.

Bar units provide excellent retention and stability for a denture while rigidly splinting the abutments. Artificial mucosa can be provided by the denture flange and the removable section can be rebased or repaired like a clasp retained prosthesis (Fig. 565). While combining many of the advantages of fixed and of removable prostheses, they have drawbacks as well.

The bar provides a medium for the accumulation of plaque and great care is necessary in the planning and execution of the prosthesis to ensure the patient can maintain a good standard of plaque control and denture hygiene. Infirm patients with poor manual dexterity cannot be expected to cope with such restorations. Other contra-indications are those in which there is limited vertical or bucco-lingual space. Bar prostheses are difficult to construct where heavy occlusal forces may be applied. There are also considerable technical difficulties in spanning a gap of more than four units with a bar unit owing to distortions that can occur. Despite those limitations the wide range of prefabricated and laboratory produced bars available gives the operator considerable latitude in his treatment planning.

Abutment preparations

All types of bar prostheses require a common path of insertion for the fixed section of the restoration, unless an auxiliary system has been incorporated. The retention of an attachment is often severely reduced in an effort to align it with others, and consequently the abutment restoration may subsequently loosen under load applied by the removal of the prosthesis. Tilted posterior abutments with short clinical crowns are notorious in this respect, as are tapered post preparations of limited length (Fig. 566).

Employing auxiliary devices for tilted molar abutments is second best to uprighting them with orthodontic therapy. Even the most ingenious auxiliary devices require considerable clinical crown length. Intracoronal attachments may be soldered to bar units connecting them to the tilted abutment (Fig. 567). The problem here is vertical space for the

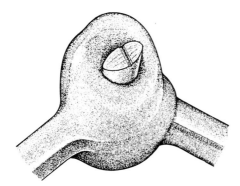

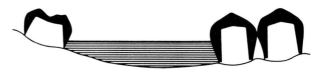

Fig. 566   Crowns cemented to tilted posterior abutments are prone to loosen as the retention from the preparation is reduced by aligning it with anterior crowns.

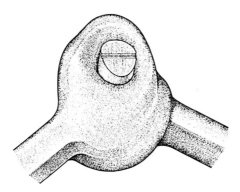

Fig. 564   Turning the screw alters its seating against the surface of the crown. The head should not be trimmed until final tightening.

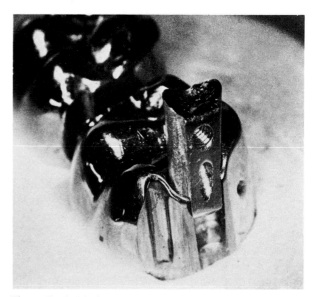

Fig. 567   Soldering the bar to an intracoronal attachment sometimes overcomes misalignment problems of posterior abutments.

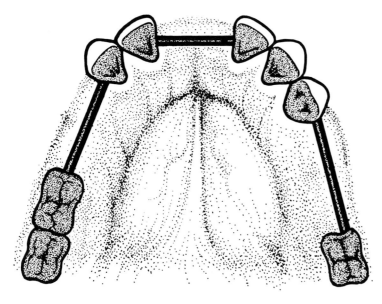

Fig. 565   Bar units provide the splinting action of a fixed prosthesis while allowing the provision of an extremely stable removable restoration. Used with discretion they combine the advantages of fixed and of removable restorations.

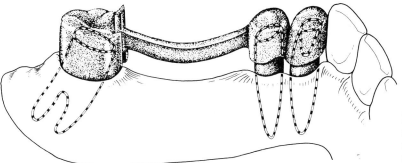

Fig. 568 Considerable vertical space and a non vital abutment is usually required if this arrangement is not to result in overcontouring.

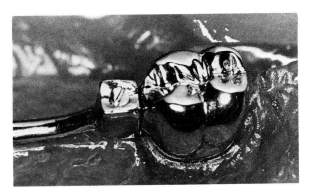

Fig. 569 Malalignment overcome by screw connector joining bar to crown.

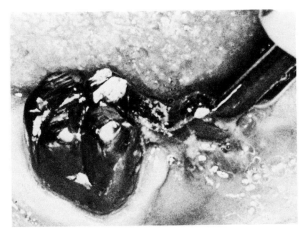

Fig. 570 Results of poor plaque control around screw connector.

intracoronal attachment. Secondly, if the gingival section of the attachment is within the crown contour the occlusal section may be well into the pulp chamber if the tooth is markedly tilted (Fig. 568). Connectors that screw the bar to the crown in the mouth overcome the pulpal problems but often raise an insuperable plaque control problem where lack of vertical space exists (Figs. 569, 570). It is tempting to consider a telescopic crown in which the outer section is soldered to the bar to solve this problem. Unfortunately this does not solve the vertical space problem as the proximal contour of the inner coping would be an unacceptable plaque trap if it were to correct a tilted abutment. Mechanical solutions to the tilted molar may be considered where clinical crown height exceeds 5 mm. If orthodontic therapy is not feasible, the short tilted abutment should be considered a contraindication to the bar unit. The only way to prevent cementation mishaps is to plan the retention available from each abutment.

Dislodging forces applied through the bar to the abutment crowns may cause distortion of the restoration, and for this reason partial coverage retainers, when employed, need to be planned with great care. Since the bar is soldered to the crowns, a sufficient bulk of metal is required near the margins. A shoulder or chamber preparation adjacent to the bar is recommended, for this will contribute to the strength of the crown margin. Knife-edge finishes contribute to weak crown margins which are then prone to damage under load (Figs. 571, 572).

PREFABRICATED BAR UNITS

The Dolder Bar Unit is a well established and reliable unit. The bar has parallel sides, unlike the pear-shaped profile of the bar joint. Retention for the sleeve is entirely frictional, provided by the parallel vertical surfaces of both sections. The sleeve fits the top and sides of the bar precisely (Fig. 573). Two sizes of bar unit are available 3·5 mm and 2·7 mm high from the base to the top of the sleeve (Fig. 574). Although the larger attachment is stronger and provides greater retention, there is seldom room for it anteriorly in the mouth. Before using either of

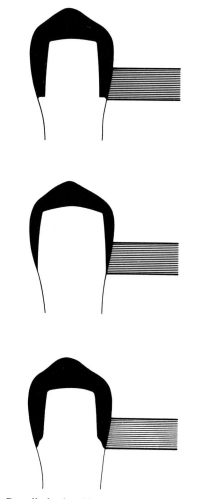

Fig. 571 Bevelled shoulder (*top*) or chamfer edged (*bottom*) preparations are desirable. Knife-edged crown margins may be weak and liable to damage under load.

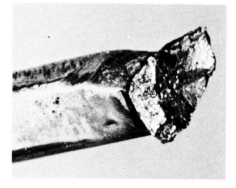

Fig. 572 Fracture of a crown margin adjacent to the bar.

these attachments it is important to assess not only the contour of the mucosa between the abutments, but the amount of bucco-lingual and vertical space available for the prosthesis.

In view of the wide base of these attachments and the long spans commonly traversed, careful planning is needed to blend the bar with the contours of the underlying ridge. The bar can be soldered to the diaphragm of a post preparation or the proximal surface of a crown (Fig. 575). However, as the bar cannot be bent it is necessary to negotiate a curve with a series of joined straight sections. These sections can be connected at suitable points, such as over a root diaphragm, or they may be soldered on either side of a crown (Fig. 576). Since the parallel sides of the bar require a precise path of insertion of the denture, the various sections of the bar must be carefully aligned. This is carried out on a rigid surveyor using a special mandrel supplied by the manufacturer (Fig. 577).

The technical requirements are similar to those of a bar joint. It is, however, usual to join the sleeve of this unit to the metal framework of the denture and this is best carried out by surrounding the sleeve with an extension of the major connector (Fig. 578). The manufacturers do not recommend soldering the sleeve to the major connector as it is thin. The sleeve is identical to that of the bar joint and incorporates retention tags for the acrylic resin.

These bar units provide a denture with excellent support, stability, and retention. Furthermore the abutments are rigidly splinted, while the retainers of the denture are entirely buried in its impression surface and therefore do not show (Fig. 579). The attachments are also strong and have a high resistance to wear.

After posterior tooth loss it is occasionally necessary to convert a rigid bar unit to a bar joint. The bar can be adapted by grinding the vertical sides of the bar to resemble the pear-shaped cross-section of the bar joint (Fig. 580). This is a valuable first aid measure after tooth loss, but a prosthesis designed primarily as a tooth-supported denture cannot be expected to function long in this new role. The extension of the denture base will be far too short and its impression surface will not be adapted to the shape of the ridge.

A subsequent complete denture incorporating a sleeve for the bar unit should, therefore, be made as soon as possible. If postponed, movements of the original denture may well cause damage to the denture-bearing area.

The technique of remaking the denture is similar to that described for bar joint prostheses.

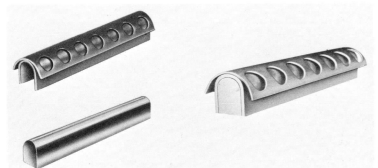

Fig. 573 The sleeve of the Dolder Bar Unit is common to the Dolder Bar Joint.

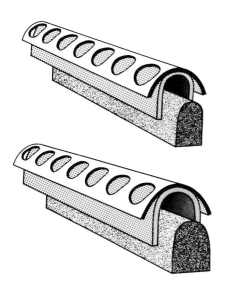

Fig. 574 The Dolder Bar Unit. Two sizes are available.

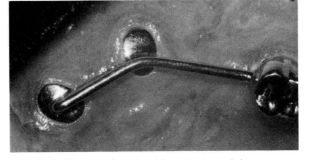

Fig. 576 Since the bar should not be bent, it is necessary to negotiate a curve with a series of straight sections. They may be joined over a root diaphragm or attached either side of a crown.

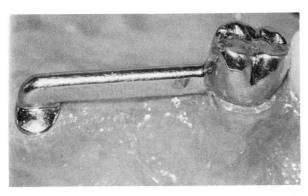

Fig. 575 The bar can be soldered to the diaphragm of a post preparation or to the proximal surface of a crown.

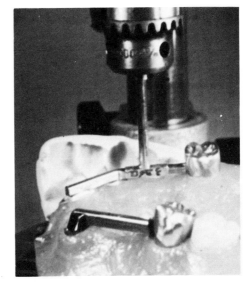

Fig. 577 The various sections of the attachment must be carefully aligned so that the sides of the bars are mutually parallel.

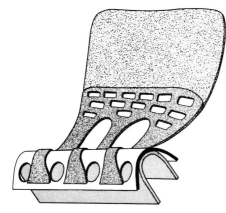

Fig. 578   The sleeve should be surrounded by components of the connector. They should not be soldered.

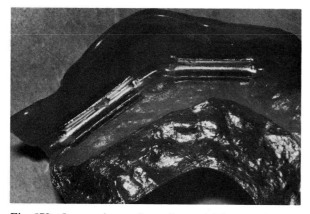

Fig. 579   Impression surface of a partial denture showing the sleeve units of a Dolder Bar assembly.

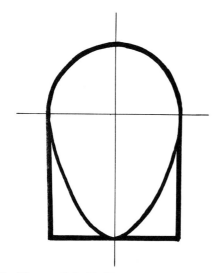

Fig. 580   The parallel-sided bar can be altered to resemble the bar joint by careful grinding of its sides.

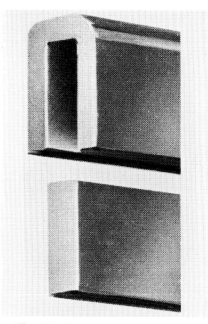

Fig. 581   The MP Channel System comprise a series of matching gold bars and sleeves.

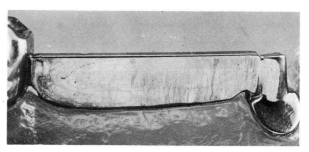

Fig. 582   Demonstration model of MP Channel System.

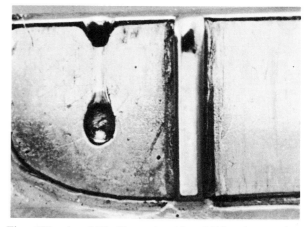

Fig. 583   An MP Channel with additional retention provided by a plunger attachment. Note the guiding flange on the bar.

Another prefrabricated bar unit is known as the MP Channel system, consisting of matching wrought gold bars and sleeves (Figs. 581, 582). The bars are only 1·1 mm wide and have a rectangular profile 6 mm or 3 mm high. Two heights of sleeves are available. The sleeve for the smaller bar may be fitted to the taller unit so that this bar may be cut away from the base to follow vertical contours of the edentulous ridge. The sleeves may be contoured in a similar fashion. The sleeves have no retention tags for acrylic resin and will need to be roughened, preferably with retention notches. Additionally, pieces of wire can be soldered to them.

These MP channels are extremely slim and save the operator and technician the problems and expense of milling. Additional retention between the two sections of the unit can be provided by incorporating a plunger in the sleeve (Figs. 583, 584). Guiding flanges should be incorporated to prevent rotation around the plunger and to obtain maximum retention.

LABORATORY PRODUCED BARS

Producing one's own bar has the advantage that it can be made to follow precisely the contours of the mouth, and its dimensions chosen in relation to the amount of room available. The retention and stability provided by the unit is influenced by the parallel vertical sides of the bar, so there is every advantage in making the bar as high as possible consistent with the space available. Moreover, the bar can be comparatively narrow so that mucosal coverage is reduced to a minimum (Fig. 585). The minimum width of the bar should be about 1·5 mm. If reduced below this figure it will be extremely difficult to produce a well fitting sleeve because of the restricted bulk of investment material.

This type of bar prosthesis illustrates the necessity of correctly mounted diagnostic casts, for the amount of vertical and bucco-lingual room available for the bar and denture can be readily assessed. The parallel sides to the wax bar are obtained with a wax trimmer mounted in a surveyor, and the procedure is usually carried out on a duplicate master cast. Where possible, the best results are obtained by finishing the casting on a paralleling milling device (Fig. 586).

The CM bar (Fig. 587) may be helpful in reducing laboratory time. It is a parallel sided precious metal bar 1·8 mm wide, 10 mm high and 100 mm long. A copper template is provided for adaptation on the master cast. This template is then placed over the bar and the outline scribed on to it so that the bar can be cut to the correct shape.

In preparing the bar, the contours of its base against the mucosa must be planned with care. The aim must be to prevent accumulation of debris and to facilitate plaque control. For this reason, comparatively narrow cross sections have advantages while a wide base that overhangs the ridge crest should be avoided (Fig. 588). The laboratory produced bar has therefore considerable advantage over its prefabricated counterpart. Unfortunately one cannot expect the mechanical properties of a laboratory cast bar to match those of a specially wrought prefabricated unit. For this reason, the design of the sleeve and bar component requires careful thought. The dimensions cannot be reduced excessively and the design must not only minimise the tendency for wear, but also provide some allowance for any wear that does take place.

Guiding flanges (Fig. 583) on the bar increase the surface area of contact, prevent rotational displacements of the sleeve and thereby improve stability

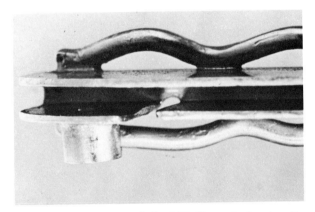

Fig. 584 The sleeve of the MP Channel showing the recess for the guiding flange.

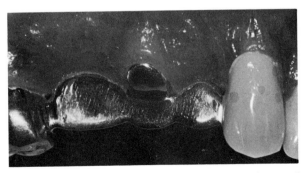

Fig. 585 A simple laboratory-made bar waxed up and cast to follow the contours of the mucosa. Maximum height should be used to gain the best retention and stability for the prosthesis. Minimum width should be about 1·5 mm.

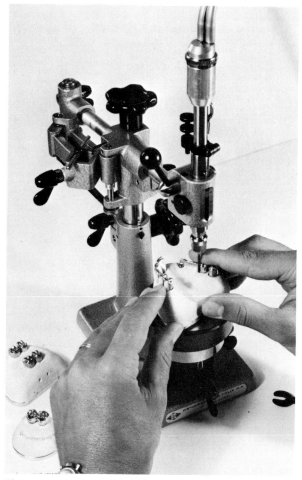

Fig. 586   Milling a laboratory-produced bar to produce parallel sides.

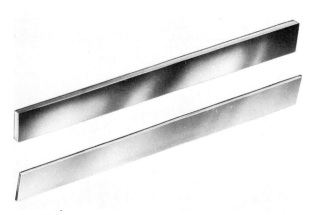

Fig. 587   The CM bar, a useful aid to reducing laboratory time. The copper template (*below*) is adapted to the master cast. The bar is subsequently trimmed with the aid of the template.

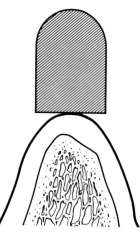

Fig. 588   Unsatisfactory bar profile relative to the ridge contour.

and retention of the assembly. During the final milling, grooves may be prepared on the adjacent crowns before the sleeve is waxed up and cast. These grooves augment the action of guiding flanges.

Provided the sleeve has been given a precise path of insertion and withdrawal, additional retention can be provided by plunger-type attachments.

Plunger-type attachments, described in more detail in the next chapter, provide a simple means of increasing the retention available. The attachments consist of a spring loaded plunger located in one section engaging a slot in the other part. In most cases it is simpler to incorporate the plunger unit in the removable section of the prosthesis, mounting the attachment lingually (Figs. 589, 590). In addition to grinding a retention slot or dimple in the bar for the plunger to engage, a small guiding recess should be ground in the occlusal edge of the bar to retract the plunger when the denture is inserted. If there is insufficient lingual space for mounting the attachment, a modified unit is obtainable for mounting in the bar, which has to be thickened to accommodate it (Fig. 591). The plunger should point buccally in this case and the retention slot and guiding recess should be ground in the removable section (Fig. 592). All these attachments can be taken to pieces quite easily and the activating spring or cartridges changed.

An alternative arrangement is to employ the Ceka attachment for additional retention. The female section may be incorporated in the bar (Figs. 593, 594) or used as a stud attachment over root diaphragms (Fig. 595). The OL series is available with straight or curved resin bars that can be trimmed and moulded on the master cast. The OL pattern incorporates a special notch for engagement of the

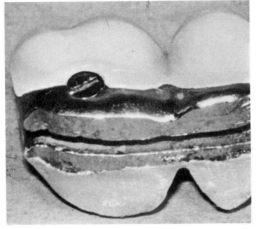

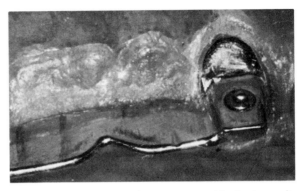

Fig. 591   A plunger attachment mounted in the bar unit.

Fig. 589   Extra retention can be provided by a plunger type of attachment. Where there is sufficient room, it is usually more convenient to mount the attachment lingually in the removable section of the prosthesis.

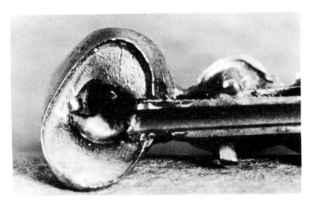

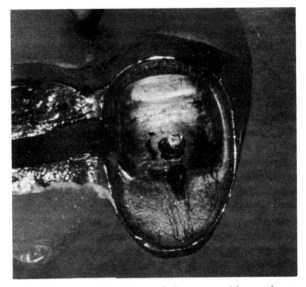

Fig. 592   Internal surface of the removable section to show retention slot engaged by the plunger and the guiding recess to retract the plunger as the denture is inserted.

Fig. 590   Pressomatic plunger unit in removable section of the crown. Note the guiding groove.

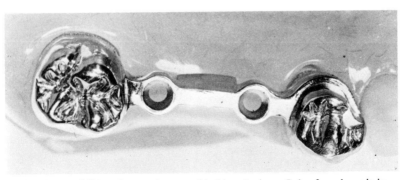

Fig. 593   Additional retention provided by placing a Ceka female unit in the bar.

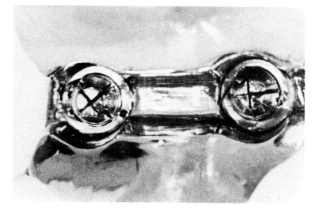

Fig. 594   Removable section of the prosthesis.

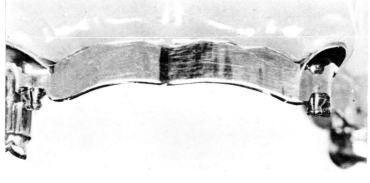

Fig. 595   Additional retention provided by Ceka attachments used as stud units.

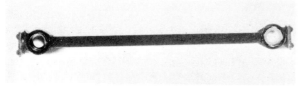

Fig. 596   The OL series can be used with a plastic pattern to form a bar with built-in retainers.

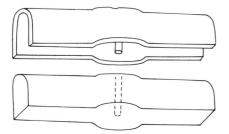

Fig. 597   The Steiger and Boitel bar. This laboratory-produced bar has additional retention provided by parallel-sided pins in the sleeve engaging holes in the bar.

resin bar (Fig. 596). It is, therefore, possible to cast one's own bar incorporating Ceka retainers.

The Steiger and Boitel bar is a well established bar unit. Bulges in the side of the bar ensure a precise path of insertion for the sleeve, while strengthening the components as well. Since there is no possibility of rotational displacement of the sleeve, additional retention can be provided by a series of parallel-sided pins in the sleeve, engaging holes in the bar (Fig. 597). The bar is waxed-up around stainless steel pins that act as spacers, so that on removal from the casting they leave a hole. The pins are aligned with the aid of a surveyor, and around each hole the bar should be strengthened by a lateral bulge on both sides of the bar. Where space is limited, a retention groove may be substituted for a retention hole, so that only one lateral bulge is necessary. The bar is cast in gold, trimmed, polished and then fitted back on the master cast. These pins are removed, or dissolved after casting. The sleeve may be waxed-up around it with stainless steel pins inserted through the holes in the bar, and the sleeve cast. These stainless steel pins are subsequently replaced with wrought gold pins. The outer surface of the sleeve should be roughened to gain retention in the acrylic resin of the denture saddle. As with most bars, it is necessary to use acrylic resin anterior teeth and first premolars. More posteriorly there may be sufficient room to use porcelain teeth.

Where distal extension prostheses are concerned, it is essential that the denture base covers the maximum possible area. In this way the distal extension section of the prosthesis is virtually self-supporting. The retaining pins may be protected by some form of hinged connection between denture base and framework although seldom necessary in practice (Figs. 598–601). This restoration also demonstrates how the splinting efficiency of a fixed

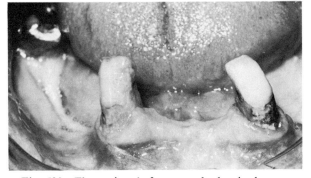

Fig. 598 The patient before prosthodontic therapy.

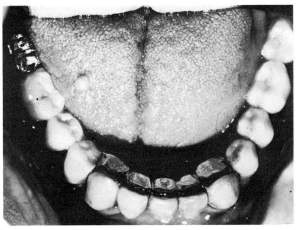

Fig. 601 The completed restoration.

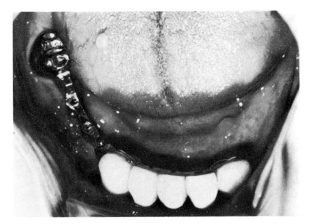

Fig. 599 The fixed section in place. Some of the parallel-sided pinholes are visible.

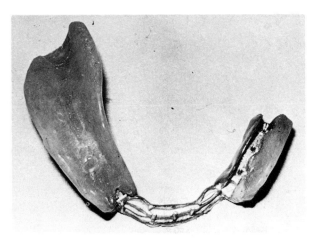

Fig. 600 The removable section of the prosthesis. Note the retaining pins, and the extension of the denture base.

prosthesis may be combined with all the advantages of a removable restoration.

Like other bar units the Steiger and Boitel unit requires careful planning and a great deal of technical skill. Particular care must be paid to heat treatment, polishing, and soldering if distortion is not to occur. Text books by Steiger and Boitel (1959) and by Gaerny (1969) provide useful information about many of the technical aspects of these prostheses.

The design of laboratory produced bars

The rigidity of the bar itself can be a limiting factor in the length of span that can be crossed, as it is seldom possible to increase the cross-section as the span becomes longer. Furthermore, the longer the span, the more sensitive the restoration becomes to the minute dimensional changes that may accompany soldering, heat treatment, and polishing (Fig. 602).

Introducing a series of curves into the lateral surfaces helps increase the rigidity of the bar. It also increases the area of contact between the bar and sleeve and can dictate a precise path of insertion and withdrawal for the sleeve (Fig. 603). If designed with care additional retaining elements may be unnecessary.

In designing the bar adequate provision must be made for plaque control. The traditional method of bar design maintained the bar base in even contact over the mucosa and gingival margins (Fig. 604). This approach has obvious mechanical advantages and the close adaptation over the entire area was felt necessary to prevent accumulation of debris under

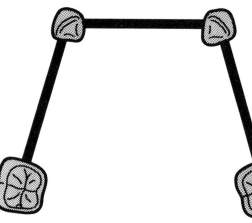

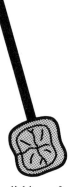

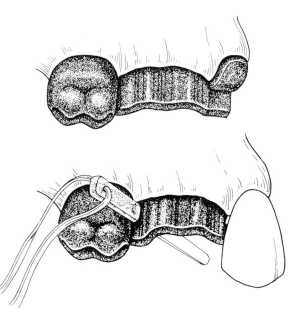

Fig. 602   Soldering, heat treatment, and polishing of large-span bar prostheses requires attention to small detail if distortion is to be avoided.

Fig. 605   Allowing space for the insertion of floss complicates the design and requires more vertical space than the traditional method (*top*).

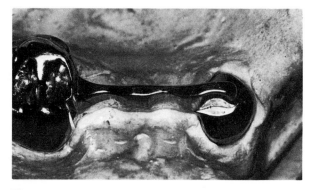

Fig. 603   The curved lateral surfaces of the bar prevent rotational displacements of the sleeve. The area of contact is increased and additional retention may be unnecessary.

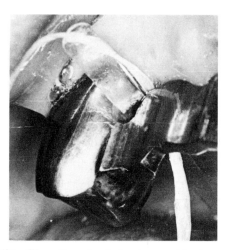

Fig. 606   Floss threader being inserted in the mouth.

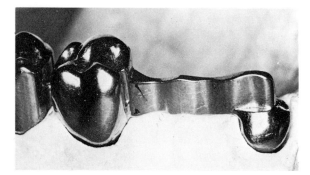

Fig. 604   The traditional bar design maintained the base in contact with the mucosa and gingival margins. It is mechanically efficient but complicates plaque control. Note the guiding groove on the molar crown.

the bar. Some even went so far as to suggest it would prevent plaque accumulation but at best this can only be described as wishful thinking. Provided the patient can maintain the bar and surrounding area plaque-free there will be few problems. However, it can be difficult to insert floss under the base of a closely adapted bar. It is for this reason that the design should include provision for the insertion of such a device despite the mechanical and space problems that will result.

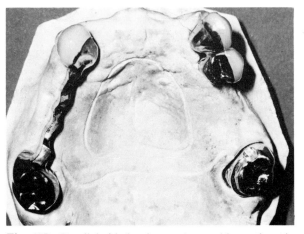

Fig. 607   Parallel sided units can be used in conjunction with intracoronal attachments provided the bracing arms of the attachments are of similar height to the bar.

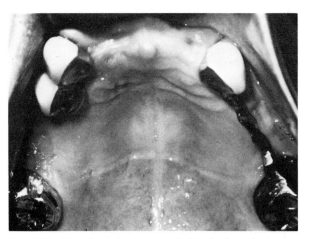

Fig. 609   Prosthesis in the mouth. Lack of vertical space precluded connecting the anterior abutments with the bar.

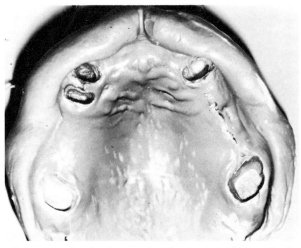

Fig. 608   Locating impression for removable prosthesis, withdrawing bar and abutment crowns. The adaptation of the bar to the mucosa can be clearly seen.

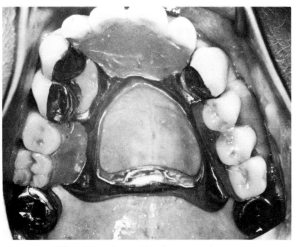

Fig. 610   Assembled restoration.

Providing a cleansable space adjacent to an abutment crown complicates the design and requires additional vertical space (Figs. 605, 606). The advantages are generally worthwhile.

Curved bars with parallel sides are remarkably efficient retainers. They can be employed in conjunction with intracoronal attachments on the other side of the arch provided the bracing arms of the attachments are no shorter than the height of the bar (Fig. 607).

Since the construction of the abutment crowns usually requires sectioning of the original cast a subsequent impression will be required. This impression is made with the bar and other components in the mouth, withdrawing the entire assembly in the impression. This overall impression is useful for checking the adaptation of the abutment retainers and also for examining the contact between bar and mucosa (Fig. 608). The rigidity of polyether materials make them useful for this purpose. The dies are then placed on their respective crowns and a new master cast prepared. The sleeve together with the other components are waxed and cast, and the removable prosthesis subsequently assembled and completed (Figs. 609, 610).

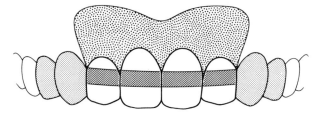

Fig. 611   Diagram to show a milled bar used to retain an anterior removable prosthesis.

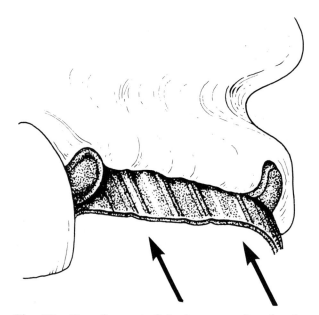

Fig. 612   The alignment of the bar must allow for the insertion of the labial flange.

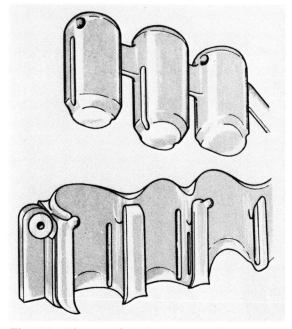

Fig. 613   Diagram of the Gaerny retention system.

THE GAERNY BAR

This retention system has been modified from the Channel Shoulder Pin concept. Retention is provided by precise contact between the virtually parallel surfaces of the inner and outer copings, and the similar contact between the connecting bars and sleeves (Fig. 613). Pins are not employed. In order to provide an adequate contact area, a crown length of about 5 mm is usually required. The demanding technical procedures are described at length in Gaerny's interesting textbook (1969).

Gaerny believes that the interdental spaces should be obliterated by small connecting bars between the fixed inner copings. By so doing, he feels the deposition of plaque will be restricted to the overlying removable section and thus easily displaced when that part of the prosthesis is taken out. This connection at gingival level contributes to the rigidity of the substructure and allows generous vertical space for the removable unit.

In commenting upon milled precision bars, Gaerny points out the advantage of using plunger type units, particularly when there is limited frictional surface area. Wherever possible parallel abutments are soldered. Screws are used as seldom as possible, in view of the problems of plaque control around the screw heads, and the small niches around the screws. Screws are used only where the pattern of

Given adequate space and plaque control, milled bars can be provided for a variety of edentulous spaces. The bar may be useful in restoring missing anterior teeth, where loss of bone requires the provision of a labial flange (Fig. 611). Unlike intracoronal attachments large box preparations in the abutments are unnecessary while the abutments either side are effectively splinted. Anterior bars require careful analysis of the space available, and alignment to allow for the insertion of the labial flange (Fig. 612).

The splinting efficiency of bar units can be useful in other quadrants of the mouth involving considerable spans.

insertion of the matrix with markedly tilted abutments leaves no other choice. Intracoronal attachments are employed on distal tilted abutments. Gaerny in fact favours home made units incorporating a locking screw. Gaerny comments that earlier on he used to construct bridges with multiple screw retention in an attempt to make it easier to remove a single intermediate abutment should this be necessary. He points out, however, that this has seldom been required over twenty five years which pays testimony to his excellent treatment planning.

Current opinion favours neither the encroachment of the interdental space, nor the bulky assembled restoration of limited contour, but extremely successful long term results have been claimed and demonstrated. The patient's plaque control must naturally play an important role in the prognosis as indeed it does for any prosthesis.

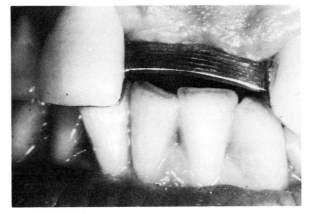

Fig. 614 The Andrews Bar. It occupies less space and provides greater retention than most conventional precious metal bars.

THE ANDREWS BRIDGE

An interesting development in bar prostheses has been devised by Andrews and has been used since 1966. Unlike other bar systems these prefabricated units are made of stainless steel and not of a gold alloy. Very high tensile and yield strengths are claimed for this material so that the bar is thin and occupies minimal vertical space as well. The bars are precision machined rather than cast. Retention is provided by the adaptation of the sleeve to the bar and resistance to wear is high.

Two types of bar are manufactured: a single bar for use anteriorly (Fig. 614) and a twin bar for posterior gaps (Figs. 615–617). These bars are available in three lengths of three different curvatures. Each curve is a segment of a circle and the combinations available allow its adaptation to most clinical situations. Since the bar is on the arc of a circle it simplifies reconstruction should a patient lose or damage the removable section.

The Andrews Bar has several apparent advantages over most other prosthesis. Reduced bulk is probably its greatest attribute while the curved section allows the use of bars anteriorly where the usually straight section could not be employed (Figs. 618–620). For any given situation Andrews recommends using the bar with the greatest possible curvature, for this allows maximum length, hence more friction and less wear. It also results in a more critical path of insertion reducing the chance of accidental dislodgement of the prosthesis. The posterior bar provides greater retention and resistance to all dislodging forces than a single

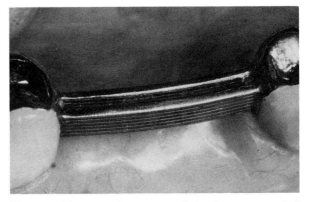

Fig. 615 For posterior gaps a twin bar is recommended. It provides greater retention and resistance to dislodging forces than a single bar of the same height.

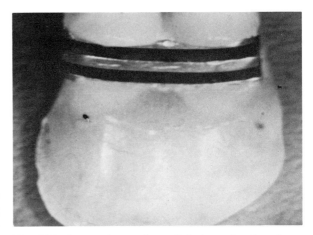

Fig. 616 Impression surface of denture showing sleeve of the posterior twin bar.

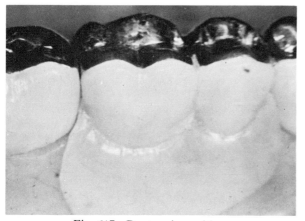

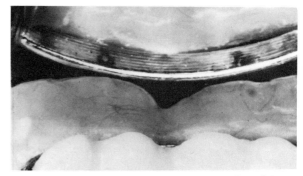

Fig. 620   Palatal view showing close adaptation of the bar to the mucosa.

Fig. 617   Denture in position.

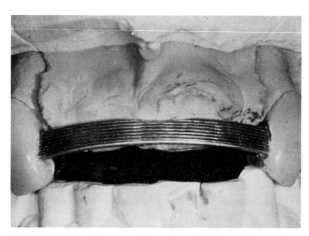

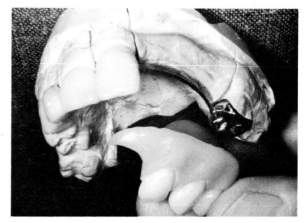

Fig. 621   A single bar can be used for posterior restorations provided there is sufficient vertical space for the bar without seriously reducing its height.

Fig. 618   The thin, curved section of the bar allows close adaptation to the edentulous ridge contour with minimal coverage of the mucosa, yet provides excellent retention.

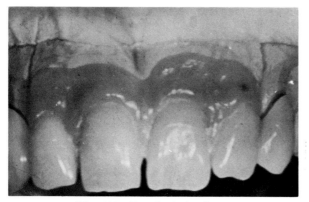

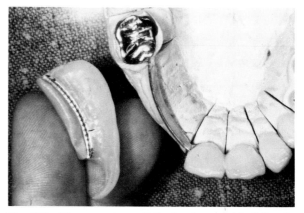

Fig. 619   Prosthesis in place.

Fig. 622   The curvature of the bar is useful in following the edentulous ridge, and provides additional retention and stability for the prosthesis. Several splinted anterior teeth are required as an abutment in view of the loads that may be transmitted by the bar.

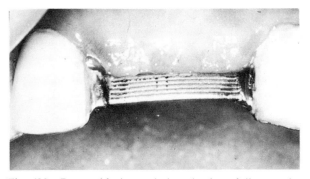

Fig. 623 Poor soldering technique leads to failure at the bar/crown junction (upper right central incisor).

bar occupying the same vertical space. Smaller versions of both anterior single and posterior twin bars are available where vertical space is limited.

As with all other bar prostheses careful planning is required, which should include an assessment of the vertical and bucco-lingual space available, and an examination of the mucosa to be covered by the bar. Preliminary treatment to remove small irregularities of the mucosa may be necessary, but the small cross-section of the bar keeps this to a minimum, especially as the base of the bar may be ground to follow the mucosal contours on the master cast. The small cross-section also simplifies plaque control.

Adjustment for wear is another unusual feature of the unit for the bar is adjusted, not the sleeve. Only the very slightest distortion of the bar will produce a significant improvement of the retention.

There is no reason why a single bar should not be used for a posterior restoration, provided there is sufficient vertical space for the bar without seriously reducing its height. It may be useful when bucco-lingual space is limited and when the anterior abutment is well forward in the arch (Figs. 621, 622). The value of the curve in the bar lies not only in its ability to follow the shape of the edentulous ridge, but also in the retention and stability that it provides for the prosthesis. However, it is important that several splinted anterior teeth be used as an abutment.

The manufacturers supply special transfer sleeves for each of the bars produced, so that a duplicate removable prosthesis can be quickly made in case of accidents. Maximum advantage appears to have been made of the mechanical properties of this new material. While it is claimed that soldering the bar to a gold restoration does not interfere with its corrosion resistance or mechanical properties, the soldering process itself seems more complicated than usual (Fig. 623). Where posterior restorations are concerned a recessed occlusal rest seat is recommended for the abutment teeth to reduce loads applied to the solder joints. In order to strengthen the junction, a mechanical lock should be cut in the bar to rest within the contour of the abutment crown. Wherever possible a box should be cut in the preparation to prevent overcontouring of the crown although this presents difficulties in the case of a lateral incisor. In spite of this drawback it can be seen that the Andrews Bridge system has several worthwhile advantages over conventional bar units. For further details readers are recommended to study the specially produced Laboratory Manual.*

REFERENCES AND FURTHER READING

ACKERMANN, H. (1957) Ein Neuer Halter Für Steg Prostheses. *Schweiz. Mschr. Zahnheilk.*, *67*, 1013

ACKERMANN, H. (1964) Uber Stegprothesen und neue Prothesenhalter Zahnärztl. *Welt/Reform*, *65*, 644

ADISMAN, I. K. (1962) The internal clip attachment in fixed-removable partial denture prosthesis. *N.Y. J. Dent.*, *32*, 125

ANDREWS, J. A. and CARLSON, A. F. (1976) *The Andrews Bridge–Laboratory Technique Manual.* Institute of Cosmetic Dentistry.

AUGSBURGER, R. H. (1966) The Gilmore attachment. *J. prosth. Dent.*, *16*, 1090

AUGSBURGER, R. H. (1971) Abutment stabilization through endosseous and cross-arch splinting. *J. prosth. Dent.*, *26*, 406

BELLOCQ, P. (1951) Attachement ruptueur des forces pour bridges amovibles en extension. *Inform. dent.* (Paris), *33*, 1591

BENNETT, A. G. (1904) The vertical half-cap or bridge-work anchorage. *Dent. Cosmos*, *46*, 367

BIAGGI, A. and ELBRECHT, H. J. (1951) *Gelenkige Prothesen und Ihre Indikation.* Zahnarzliche Welt, Konstanz

BOITEL, R. H. (1954) A new bar attachment for removable bridges and partial dentures. *Trans. Amer. Dent. Soc.* (Europe)

BRILL, N. (1955) Adaptation and hybrid prosthesis. *J. prosth. Dent.*, *5*, 811

CARR, C. M. (1898) Anchored adjustable dentures. *Dent. Cosmos*, *40*, 219

CENDRES et MÉTAUX (1972) *Attachments and Components for Prosthetic Dentistry.* Cendres et Métaux S.A., Biel-Bienne, Switzerland

DOLDER, E. J. (1953) Die steg-gelenk-prosthese im unterkiefer. *Schweiz. Mschr. Zahnheilk*, *63*, 339

* Institute of Cosmetic Dentistry, Box 487 Amite, Louisiana 70422 USA.

DOLDER, E. J. (1961) The bar joint mandibular denture. *J. prosth. Dent.*, *11*, 689

DOLDER, E. J. (1964) Bar dentures. *Int. dent. J.*, *14*, 249

DOLDER, E. J. (1966) *Steg-Prothetik. Die Steg-Gelenk-Prothese und die Steg-Geschiebe-Prothese.* Hüthig, Heidelberg.

DOLDER, E. J. (1971) *Steg-Prothetik, Die Steg-Gelenk-Prothese und die Steg-Geschiebe-Prothese. Ein Lehrbuch für die Praxis.* Hüthig, Heidelberg. S. 31, 62, 100

FOSSUME, F. L. (1905) A new method of removable bridge work. *Conn. St. dent. Ass. J.*, pp. 49–53

FOSSUME, F. L. (1906) Removable and stationary bridges. *Dent. Cosmos*, *48*, 859

GAERNY, A. (1961) Closure of interdental spaces with removable anterior bridges. *Dent. Abstr. (Chic)*, no. 9

GAERNY, A. (1969) *Der abnehmbare Interdentalraum-Verschluss (I.R.V.).* Quintessenz, Berlin

GILMORE, S. F. (1913) A method of retention. *Council of Allied Dental Societies*, 8, 118

GOSLEE, H. J. (1912) Removable bridgework. *Dent. Items Interest*, 34, 731

IGARASHI, Y. (1975) Selection of retainers in lower overlay denture in relation to the abutment tooth mobility (a laboratory study). Bull. *Tokyo Med. Dent. Univ.*, 22, 207–220

MARQUARDT, G. L. (1976) Dolder bar joint mandibular overdenture: a technique for nonparallel abutment teeth. *J. prosth. Dent.*, 36:1, 101

MATSUMOTO, M., MIZUTANI, H., IGARASHI, Y. and SHIBUYA, T. (1974) A case report on a mandibular removable partial denture with bar attachment. *J. Japanese Prosthodontic Society*, 17:2, 138–143

MILLER, P. A. (1958) Complete dentures supported by natural teeth. *J. prosth. Dent.*, 8, 924

OSIAS, M. (undated) *Baker Internal Snap-on Attachment.* Englehard Inc., Baker Dental Division, East Newark, N.J.

POUND, E. (1955) The problem of the lower anterior bridge. *J. prosth. Dent.*, 5, 543

PREISKEL, H. W. (1967) Prefabricated attachments for complete overlay dentures. *Brit. dent. J. 123*, 161

PREISKEL, H. W. (1968) An impression technique for complete overlay dentures. *Brit. Dent. J. 124*, 9

PRINCE, I. B. (1965) Conservation of the support mechanisms. *J. prosth. Dent.*, 15, 327

SCOTT, J. and BATES, J. F. (1972) The relining of partial dentures involving precision attachments. *J. prosth. Dent.*, 28, 325

STEIGER, A. A. (1952) Progress in partial denture prosthesis. *Int. dent. J.*, 2, 542

STEIGER, A. A. and BOITEL, R. H. (1959) *Precision Work for Partial Dentures.* Stebo, Zürich

THAYER, H. H. and CAPUTO, A. A. (1977) Effects of overdentures upon remaining oral structures. *J. prosth. Dent.*, 37:4, 374

VIG, R. G. (1963) Splinting bars and maxillary indirect retainers for removable partial dentures. *J. prosth. Dent.*, 13, 123

CHAPTER 12

Auxiliary Attachments

This large group of miscellaneous attachments has applications in many branches of restoration dentistry. Only the more common types can be described. Since many such devices can be used with some form of telescopic prostheses, thought should be given to the principles governing telescopic restorations in general.

TELESCOPIC PROSTHESES

Larger span telescopic prostheses are often employed to splint groups of teeth but the practice of connecting teeth as an aid to periodontal therapy is controversial. Rateitschak (1963) found that removable splints contributed little to periodontal health, but the efficiency of fixed splints is seldom doubted. Although fixed splinting is an established method of tooth immobilisation following periodontal therapy, it has been suggested that the rationale underlying the method is based on purely subjective criteria, as there is no scientific evidence to show that splinted teeth have a longer life than those left alone. Waerhaug's observation (1969) that over decades mobile teeth function satisfactorily without splinting and without bone loss is also subjective, but he makes valid points in stressing the overriding importance of preventive measures and the damage that can be caused by the crowns retaining the fixed splint. Crown margins carried below the gingival margin have been termed 'advanced bases from which the bacteria can attack the periodontium', and poorly adapted margins and incorrect crown contours have been indicted as well. There are, however, few restorations that are entirely harmless if poorly constructed.

While loose teeth may survive for a period of time, it is apparent that these teeth could play more active roles if their mobility were reduced. Irrespective of these controversies it is necessary to join the teeth to provide adequate abutments where edentulous areas are to be restored. The prosthesis may provide cross-arch bracing as well. Most prostheses, however, are constructed to improve the appearance or restore lost occlusal surface; a considerable number achieve both these aims.

Fixed splints usually consist of a series of linked partial or full crowns. A prosthesis depending on such crowns requires a common path of insertion for the abutment restoration unless intracoronal attachments have been employed. Loss or damage to one of the abutments may, therefore, jeopardise the entire prosthesis, and a more flexible type of treatment is often to be desired.

Telescopic prostheses are made in two layers and union of the teeth can be achieved by joining the inner sections or outer sections of the restorations (Fig. 624). The diagrams show the substantial tooth reduction necessary for both types of prosthesis. Vertical space for two thicknesses of gold is required while additional room for facings must be provided on the buccal and labial surfaces. Palomo and Peden (1976) have pointed out the importance of adequate proximal spaces. Overcontouring in these regions, particularly posteriorly, will displace the papillae or interfere with plaque control. Telescopic prostheses are particularly prone to this type of mishap and adequate tooth preparation is vital.

Joined inner sections

Joined inner sections provide a rigid substructure which can be covered by individual crowns. The disadvantages are that a common path of insertion for the entire restoration has to be provided by the abutment preparations, and the junction between the inner copings needs to be kept close to the gingivae. In many instances, the proximal spaces may be virtually obliterated so that the subsequent difficulties of maintaining oral hygiene may cause deterioration of the periodontal tissues. In the anterior parts of the mouth, appearance dictates that

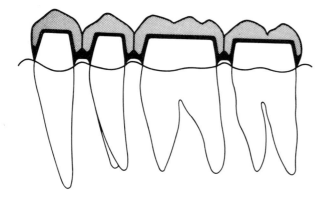

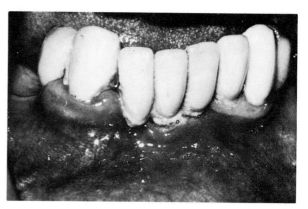

Fig. 626   Fracture of an unsatisfactory prosthesis as a result of the inadequate strength of the substructure.

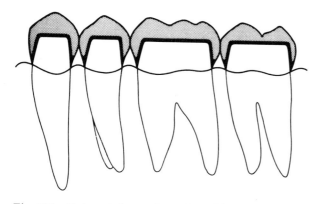

Fig. 624   Union of the teeth can be achieved by joining the inner sections of the outer sections of the telescopic prosthesis. Note the proximal spaces.

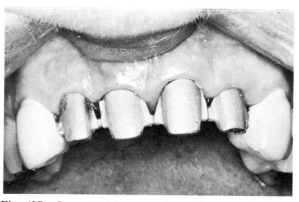

Fig. 627   Connected inner copings. The strength of the aluminous porcelain allows the junction to be clear of the gingivae.

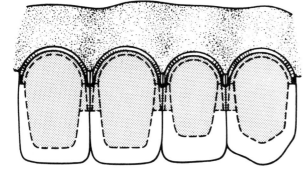

Fig. 625   The outer crowns need to cover the inner copings, this may lead to square unattractive crowns, with restricted proximal spaces.

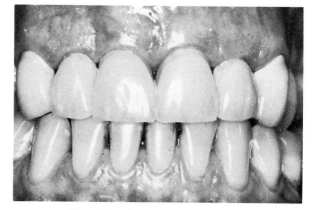

Fig. 628   The crowns in position.

this junction between the copings be covered by the outer crowns. These outer crowns therefore, although constructed individually, need to be of a somewhat square and unattractive form (Fig. 625). Attempts to thin the junction between the copings may well lead to fracture (Fig. 626).

The introduction of alumina-reinforced porcelain now allows considerable freedom of proximal spaces (Figs. 627, 628) due to the strength of the material.

Crown preparations providing a common path of insertion can be relatively straightforward for small-span prostheses, but difficulties increase with the size of the restoration and are accentuated by tilted, overerupted, or migrated teeth.

Cementation problems of individual crowns have received attention and the difficulties of cementing accurately individual crowns are well known. Lange and Jorgensen found the average discrepancy caused by cementation to be 0·91 mm and the hydraulic pressures built up in the cement during crown seating caused a separation effect with virtually pure phosphoric acid in the areas of greatest pressure. Providing vent-holes in the occlusal surfaces of the crowns reduced the average gingival discrepancy to 0·375 mm and pressure separation of the cement constituents did not occur.

Simultaneous cementation of multiple crowns magnifies the seating difficulties, although poly-carboxylate cements may reduce the problem of acidity. It seems, however, a wise precaution to provide vent-holes in the copings to allow excess cement to flow out. Subsequent restoration of the vent-holes is unnecessary as there is an outer, cemented restoration to cover it.

The rigid substructure provided by this system has several worthwhile advantages, provided that the proximal spaces can be kept clear and a common path of insertion provided for the joined copings. When this is impossible, some other form of connection should be employed.

Joined outer sections

Connecting the outer sections of the crowns allows the inner copings to be treated virtually as individual restorations. The crown preparations do not therefore have to conform to one common path of insertion (Fig. 629), as it is only the frictional surfaces of the copings that require to be waxed-up to a common path. Since the solder joint connects the outer crowns, larger interdental spaces can be left. Easily cleansable pontics can be employed to span posterior gaps.

While the advantages are apparent when slightly tilted posterior teeth are considered, markedly proclined incisors cannot be joined in this manner due to the bulk required to build out the inner copings to align them with the posterior teeth. Unless intracoronal attachments are used, it will be necessary to devitalise the anterior teeth in these circumstances and to cut them down to gingival level. Alignment can then be achieved by posts and cores (Figs. 629–631). Devitalisation may also be required of overerupted or tilted posterior teeth.

There are three ways in which the outer structure may be joined to the inner copings:

1. It may be cemented permanently in place.

2. It may be held in place by screws allowing the dental surgeon to remove the prosthesis for periodic inspection.

3. It may be removable by the patient.

1. Permanent cementation

Permanent cementation is a straightforward and effective method of obtaining a lasting union between the various sections of the prosthesis. Hydraulic pressure may prevent the final seating of the outer structure, but since this is a gold-to-gold union with bevelled margins, this effect is unlikely to result in leakage. It will, of course, complicate plaque control. Minute corrections of the occlusal surfaces may be necessary but it is debatable whether these are entirely caused by the slightly increased cement film thickness. With zinc oxyphosphate cements, this effect can be reduced further by using a thin mix of cement, as the acidity is of little importance when cementing two gold structures. The majority of restorations will be made in this manner.

The main drawback of cementing lies with its very permanence, for with the outer section joined, the necessity to extract one of the abutments, or even repair a facing, could result in major and costly reconstruction. With experience, the difficulties of making a large span fixed restoration become more apparent. Surprisingly, the demand for large-span splints seems to be increasing and it is difficult to argue with the need to incorporate some safeguard should there be a subsequent accident. One simple safeguard is to cement the outer unit with a 'non-setting' or temporary cement. There are, however, several serious drawbacks. The film thickness of most of these zinc-oxide-based cements is considerable and prevents the complete seating of the outer crowns. The cements themselves tend to deteriorate and give an unpleasant odour. While this odour can be overcome by the incorporation of antibacterial

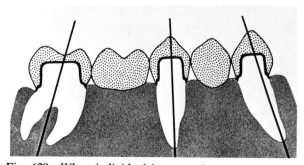

Fig. 629 When individual inner copings are employed the abutment preparations do not have to be precisely aligned. The frictional surfaces of the inner copings can be constructed to provide a common path of insertion for the outer section.

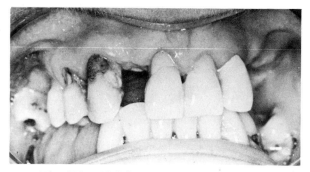

Fig. 630a Malaligned teeth before therapy.

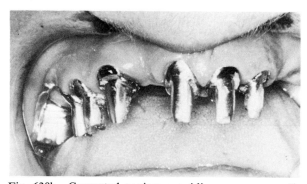

Fig. 630b Cemented copings providing a common path of insertion for the superstructure.

substances, there is one practical difficulty which most operators have experienced to their cost – the unpredictability of the cement. There is a fine line between a cement that allows the prosthesis to come loose, or loose in places, and one that sets and prevents its removal. Accidents of either kind are not uncommon. More predictable results can be obtained by using attachments.

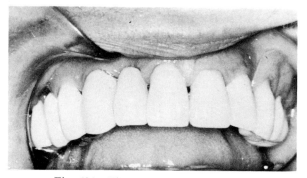

Fig. 631 The assembled restoration.

2. Prostheses removable by the patient

One of the most common arguments against large span splints is the relatively poor access available for routine cleansing, a drawback overcome by making the outer crowns removable by the patient. The outer, removable secton, must be sufficiently strong to resist handling by the patient and the greater wear and tear to which it may be subjected. The splinting action of such a restoration cannot possibly match that of a fixed restoration.

Since the outer section of the restoration is removable by the patient it may be treated as a partial denture with coverage of the edentulous areas.

Whereas loads falling on the teeth can be minimised by support from the denture base, the prostheses described in this section require more tooth support than overdentures.

Distal exension prostheses can be made together with others in which the mucosa may play a considerable part in the support of the restoration. This allows telescopic restorations where isolated molar or other abutments are to be found (Figs. 632–635). In the event of tooth loss, additions can be made to the restoration.

An important feature is that the design and construction of the restoration permits the patient to clean thoroughly both the fixed and removable section. The retention and stability provided by the crowns depends primarily on the taper of the thimbles, the size of the preparations and the accuracy with which the outer crowns fit the thimbles.

Yalisove (1966) advocates well tapered thimbles with the outer sections ground to allow a small amount of movement. It is comparatively simple to make use of misaligned abutments but the prosthesis constructed is basically an overdenture. Lateral

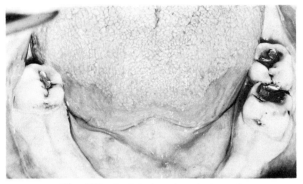

Fig. 632   Isolated molar abutments.

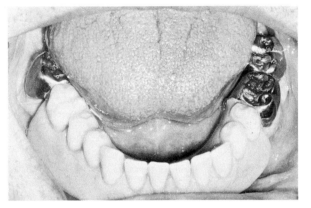

Fig. 635   The assembled restoration.

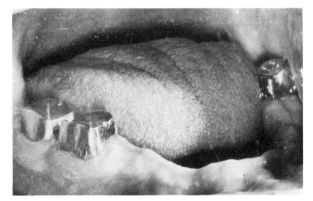

Fig. 633   Inner copings in place.

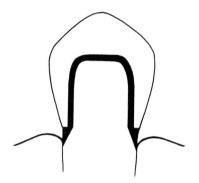

Fig. 636   The occlusal two-thirds of the coping should have a slight taper while the surfaces of the gingival third should be almost parallel.

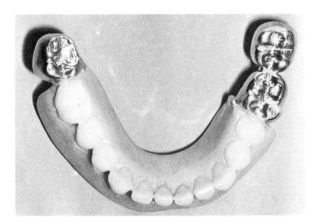

Fig. 634   The removable telescopic prosthesis.

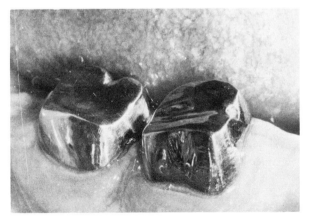

Fig. 637   Rotation around the inner coping (thimble) is prevented by the double abutments, the flattened proximal surfaces, and the small guiding grooves.

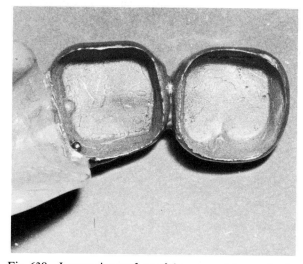

Fig. 638   Impression surface of the removable prosthesis. Note the plunger attachment.

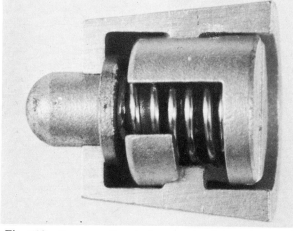

Fig. 639   Cross sectional photograph of Ipsoclip attachment. The spring-loaded plunger mechanism may be dismantled by undoing the bayonet clip at the opposite end to the plunger. This type of attachment is generally buried lingually in the outer, removable section of the prosthesis.

loads applied to the teeth are close to the occlusal surfaces and there is little retention provided. Most operators would therefore favour a more rigid type of construction that provides greater retention and stability.

Technical aspects of the coping will be considered later, but as the preparation of the tooth governs what can be achieved in the laboratory, the operator must be aware of the ideal shape of the coping. It is apparent that the tooth preparation must provide adequate resistance to the forces that will be applied.

A small taper is best incorporated on the occlusal two-thirds of the thimble, while the surfaces of the gingival third should be almost parallel (Fig. 636). The small taper simplifies insertion of the prosthesis, for it can be placed well over the thimbles before contact is made. The inclined planes then guide it into place.

The design of the inner coping is important. Apart from minimal taper, the design should normally incorporate some component to prevent rotation in the horizontal plane between the two sections of the crown. Flat proximal surfaces will normally suffice, but guiding grooves may be incorporated where the crowns are small (Figs. 637, 638). Guiding grooves, essential when the outer crown is of partial coverage, complicate plaque control. They do, however, increase the surface area of contact and increase the rigidity of the restoration.

Constant removal and insertion may cause wear of the frictional surfaces. Correct coping design and

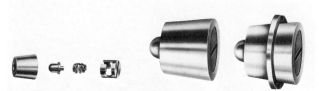

Fig. 640   Ipsoclip units. The attachment with the collar is for use with platinised golds. Releasing the bayonet clip releases the plunger mechanism.

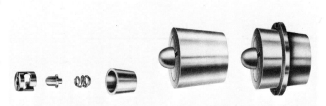

Fig. 641   Ipsoclip units designed for incorporation within the inner, fixed sections of the prosthesis. The dismantling clip is around the plunger.

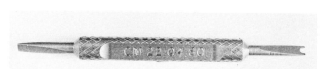

Fig. 642   Ipsoclip screwdriver for dismantling both types of unit.

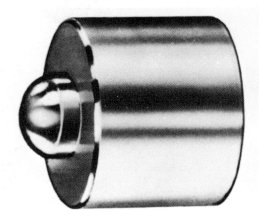

Fig. 643   The Pressomatic Unit.

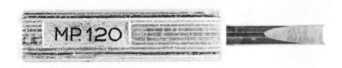

Fig. 646   Exploded view of the Mini-Pressomatic Unit. A small spring tensions the plunger.

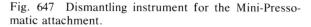

Fig. 647   Dismantling instrument for the Mini-Pressomatic attachment.

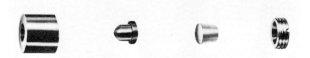

Fig. 644   Exploded view of the Pressomatic Unit to show resin cartridge that activates the plunger.

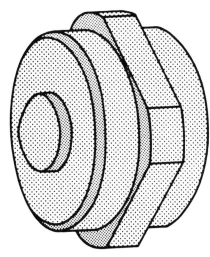

Fig. 645   The Mini-Pressomatic Unit. This neat attachment is only 1·75 mm long.

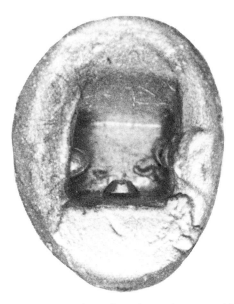

Fig. 648   Internal view of a telescopic crown. Note the guiding grooves and plunger.

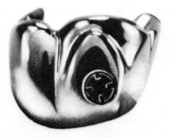

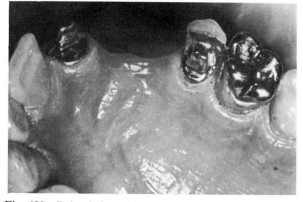

Fig. 650 Palatal view of inner copings. Note the retention slot on the palatal surface of the incisor coping.

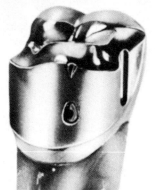

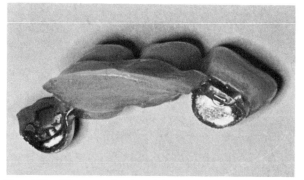

Fig. 651 The prosthesis with mucosal coverage. The engagement flange can be seen within the incisor crown and the plunger is visible in the premolar.

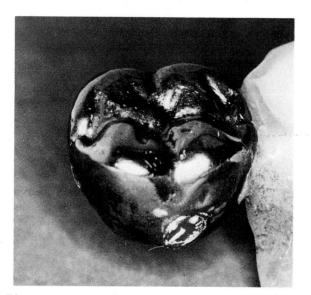

Fig. 649 Partial coverage telescopic crown containing Mini-Pressomatic attachment (*top*); full coverage telescopic crown with Mini-Pressomatic Unit (*bottom*).

selection of materials will help overcome this problem but, even so, wear will occur.

A simple yet effective method of improving the retention of the crown is to incorporate a plunger-type attachment between the two halves of the crown. These attachments have been mentioned already in connection with bar units. They consist of a flange or plunger in one section, engaging a depression in the other. The plunger is spring-loaded in the case of the Ipsoclip attachments (Figs. 639–642), while the Pressomatic units employ a plastic cartridge (Figs. 643, 644). The smaller Mini-Pressomatic unit (Figs. 645, 646) employs a stainless steel retention spring. These types of attachment can be dismantled easily for incorporation in either the removable or the fixed section of the prosthesis. A special instrument is produced for the purpose (Fig. 647). When incorporated in the inner, fixed section an attachment with a dismantling screw around the plunger should be used; attachments placed in the removable section should have the dismantling screw at the opposite end to the plunger where possible.

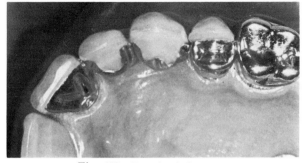

Fig. 652 Prosthesis in place.

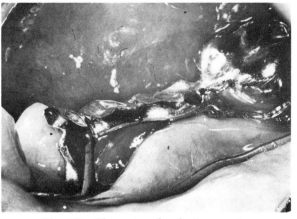

Fig. 655 The restoration in the mouth.

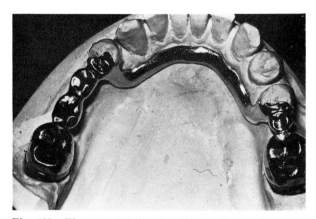

Fig. 653 The assembled restoration on the master cast.

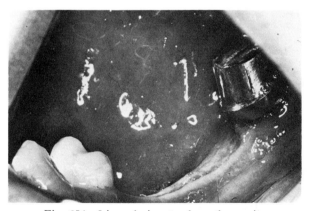

Fig. 654 Lingual view to show the coping.

It is usually simpler to incorporate the plunger mechanism in the removable section, for it simplifies construction and makes subsequent adjustments more convenient (Figs. 648, 649). A small, removable prosthesis is illustrated with the flange type of Pressomatic unit mounted palatally in the central

incisor and the rounded plunger mounted palatally in the premolar (Figs. 650–652).

A removable prosthesis allows the use of a major connector, with its advantages of load distribution and cross-arch stabilisation.

Figures 653, 654 and 655 illustrate the construction of a removable telescopic prosthesis. Tooth preparation was reduced to two teeth and a relatively economical restoration was made.

Technical considerations of the coping

The design and construction of the coping is dependent upon the shape and size of the preparation. It is for this reason the operator should be familiar with the problems involved.

The technical procedures are straightforward given adequate space and retention from the preparation. It is important to provide a precise path of insertion for the outer crown. Where there is a large area of contact and adequate vertical space relatively simple antirotation devices can be employed (Fig. 656). Where smaller teeth are concerned, guiding grooves will need to be incorporated. The coping is waxed-up, cast, and polished to a satin finish. The crown is then waxed-up around it, incorporating the attachment casing. The casing is then removed with warm tweezers and the wax pattern cast. The plunger casing is subsequently inserted into the hole and soldered to the crown. Before reassembling the plunger mechanism the crown should be slid over the thimble and a scratch made in the spot the plunger will touch. A small depression is then ground in the thimble just below (gingival to) this mark, using the mark as the uppermost level of the depression (Fig. 657). If the

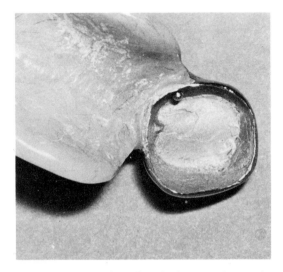

Fig. 656   Simple antirotation devices can be employed where there is a large area of contact and adequate vertical space.

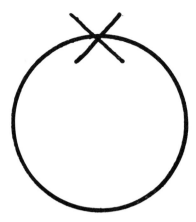

Fig. 657   A small scratch should be made on the inner coping at the point the plunger will touch. A small depression should then be ground gingival to this mark. If the depression is ground around the mark the outer crown will feel loose.

depression is ground around the mark, the outer crown will feel slightly loose. A small notch should be cut on the occlusal edge of the thimble to retract the plunger when the coping is inserted (Fig. 658). This retraction slot is unnecessary if the occlusal third of the coping is tapered.

Where smaller teeth are involved a parallel-sided coping with retraction slot and guiding grooves will be necessary. Figure 659 shows the method suggested for deepening the recess for the plunger.

Where guiding grooves are employed, they should be as long as possible with their depth from the coping surface greater than their radius (Figs. 660, 661). Guiding grooves complicate plaque control but can be useful to prevent movement between the two sections of the crown. Any movement that does occur will render the plunger ineffective.

It is now possible to obtain plunger mechanisms made of a highly-platinised gold alloy, and when these attachments are used the crown can be cast around the plunger casing. Plunger and spring should be removed when casting around the attachment or soldering to it.

If the attachment has to be buried within the outer crown, the crown must be thick enough to contain the plunger mechanism. There is not always space for this arrangement, especially anteriorly so that some other form of retention has to be found. If there is a devitalised abutment tooth, the plunger mechanism can be incorporated within the inner section (Figs. 662–664). It will be necessary to make

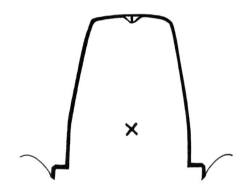

Fig. 658   The retraction slot for the plunger is unnecessary if the occlusal third of the coping is tapered.

a post and core to accommodate the attachment. With this arrangement, the attachment does not increase the bulk of the restoration, but the retention slot and guiding notch have to be incorporated in the removable sections. The places to be ground can be found by coating the inner surfaces of the coping with graphite and then inserting it over the thimble with the attachment in place. The plunger makes a track through the graphite that can be easily seen.

The springs or rubber cartridges that keep the plunger under tension should be changed at six-monthly intervals and the design of these attachments simplifies this procedure. The only point that may be difficult at first is deciding on the depth of the retention slot, for this directly affects the retention of the mechanism. It is advisable to start

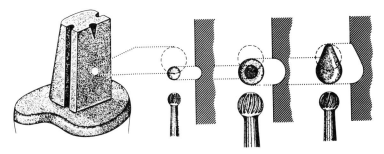

Fig. 659 Smaller preparations require parallel-sided copings, guiding grooves and retraction slots. The illustration shows a method of developing the indentation for the plunger.

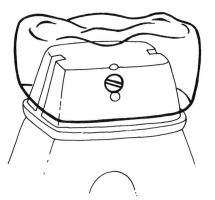

Fig. 660 Retention grooves complicate construction and plaque control. They are useful to prevent movement between the crown components where space is limited.

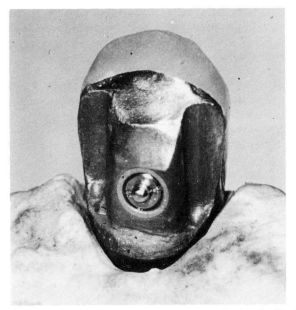

Fig. 662 The attachment placed lingually in a devitalised abutment. Note the substantial locating grooves.

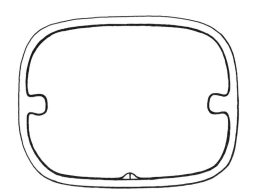

Fig. 661 Where possible, retention grooves should have a greater depth from the surface of the coping than their radius.

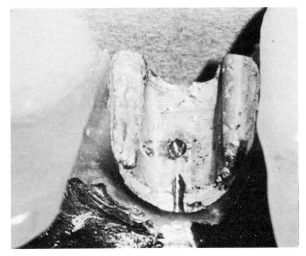

Fig. 663 The removable section of the prosthesis.

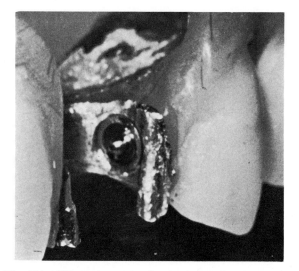

Fig. 664   Where space permits, incorporating the plunger in the removable section of the prosthesis will simplify maintenance.

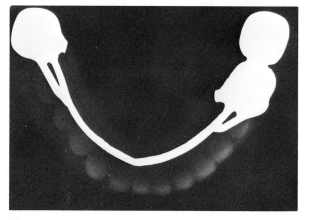

Fig. 665   Radiograph of denture to show the outer crowns connected by a metal sub-frame.

with a shallow depression; this indentation can be deepened subsequently if more retention is required.

One point, easily overlooked, is the method of connecting the outer crowns to the partial denture. Where there is a gold major connector the crowns should be soldered to it. Small tags buried in acrylic resin are insufficient and the outer crowns become loose. Where there are isolated molars to connect the crowns they should be joined to a metal sub-frame that spans the restoration (Fig. 665).

The Guessen attachment is a development of the Ipsoclip unit. This attachment is designed to allow the patient to remove the labial flange of a fixed bridge. Buried in the acrylic resin of the artificial mucosa is a metal flange. This metal flange engages a slot, incorporated in the pontic, and the retention of the flange to the slot is secured by means of a modified Ipsoclip unit (Fig. 666).

Removable labial sections of bridges will normally be connected by two attachments and it is therefore essential that they be aligned with one another (Figs. 667–671). Servicing of the Ipsoclip sections can be carried out in the normal way, as the servicing screws can be removed from the palatal aspects of the pontic teeth.

This particular type of attachment holds great promise as it may allow the construction of a fixed prosthesis in situations where appearance would otherwise dictate the use of a removable restoration.

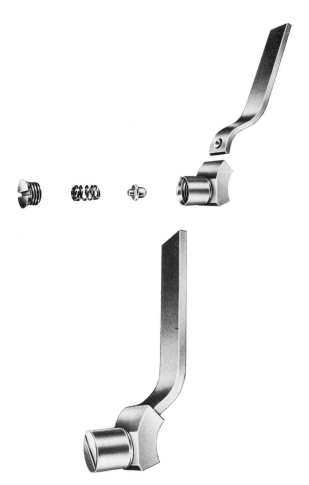

Fig. 666   The Guessen attachment. The metal flange is buried within the artificial mucosa. The modified Ipsoclip unit forms part of the pontic. The attachment is shown assembled below.

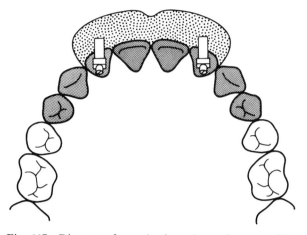

Fig. 667   Diagram of prosthesis to show alignment of the attachments.

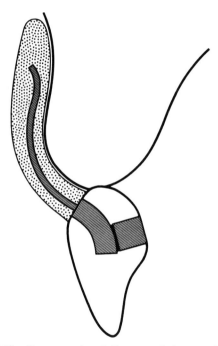

Fig. 668   Cross-sectional diagram of the prosthesis.

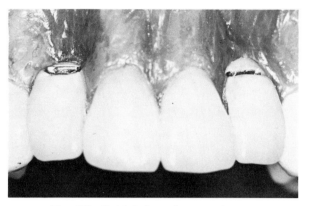

Fig. 669   Labial view of restoration.

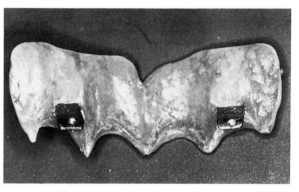

Fig. 670   Removable labial flange.

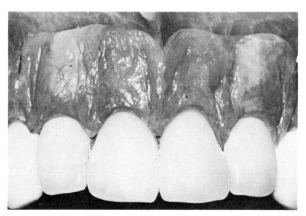

Fig. 671   Assembled restoration.

3. Screw-retained telescopic prostheses

If the outer structure is retained by small screws, the prosthesis can act as an effective splint between the abutments, but still allow its removal by the dental surgeon. The idea is by no means new (Fig. 672).

The advantages of having the crowns removable are several. It allows a flexibility of treatment since additions, repairs, or modifications of the prosthesis can be carried out in the laboratory; examination and cleaning are also simplified (Figs. 673–676). Acrylic resin facings can be replaced and their use overcomes the bulk, contraction and other associated problems of porcelain/gold restorations.

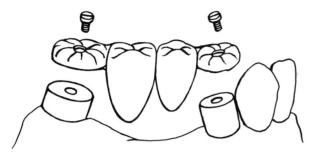

Fig. 672   An example of a screw-retained prosthesis described at the beginning of this century.

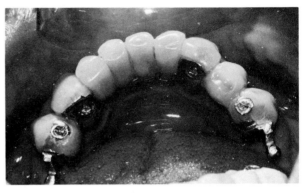

Fig. 675   Screw-retained section of the prosthesis in place.

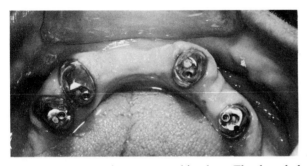

Fig. 673   Inner copings cemented in place. The threaded sleeves have been positioned for maximum length, bearing in mind ease of access for tightening the screws in the mouth.

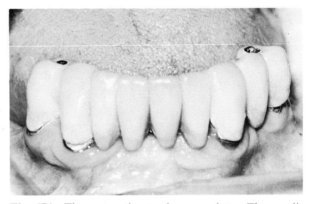

Fig. 676   The restoration twelve years later. The acrylic resin facings were changed after ten years.

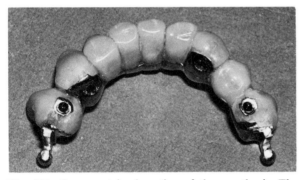

Fig. 674   Screw-retained section of the prosthesis. The Dalbo extracoronal attachments are retainers for a bilateral distal extension partial denture.

Screw retainers for vital teeth

These components usually consist of a threaded sleeve of precious metal embedded within the inner copings, and a matched screw that passes through the outer section (Figs. 677, 678). With some units a precious metal collar is provided for incorporation

within the outer section, thereby ensuring the best possible fit between screw and crown. The effectiveness of the screw unit depends on its size, but the length and diameter of the retainer is decided mainly by the height of the clinical crown, the crown contour, and pulp. Careful positioning and alignment of the sleeve unit within the waxed-up coping is thus essential (Fig. 679). It is wise to position the sleeves so that they are completely surrounded by the gold of the copings, rather than attempt to gain additional length by placing the sleeves on the edges of the copings (Fig. 680). Sleeve diameters range from 1·7 mm to 2·9 mm so that the preparation will need modification to provide adequate space for them.

Bearing in mind that the screw units are placed off-centre and need to be kept small, it might be wondered whether or not adequate retention could be provided. The answer lies in the design of the inner copings, for these should be virtually

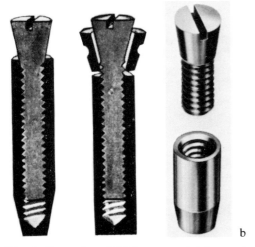

a

b

Fig. 677 (a) Examples of CM screw retaining systems available in different sizes and configurations. (b) the MP screw and sleeve.

parallel-sided. The outer section is therefore a precise friction fit and the screws are employed to maintain effective union.

The screws are aligned close to the path of insertion of the outer section, so that minute repositioning of the roots can be accommodated by tensioning the screws. However, the screw and the sleeve around it form parts of the occlusal surface of the restoration so that adjustments or fine contouring in this region are extremely difficult (Figs. 681–683). The positioning of the screw head and surrounding sleeve is critical. If the edge of the screw is in occlusion it is possible for it to become burnished into the sleeve, making the subsequent removal of the restoration impossible. The screw head itself must also be protected from the forces of occlusion.

Other screw-retained systems, employing screws at nearly right-angles to the occlusal surface do not suffer from this drawback, although considerable bucco-lingual space may be required for some of them (Fig. 684). With these systems the screws do not assist to the same extent with the final tightening of the prosthesis, and their popularity has been limited.

Designing the prosthesis

Finding space for the components is the greatest practical problem in constructing telescopic prostheses. Room has to be found for two layers of gold on the occlusal surfaces, while buccally and labially,

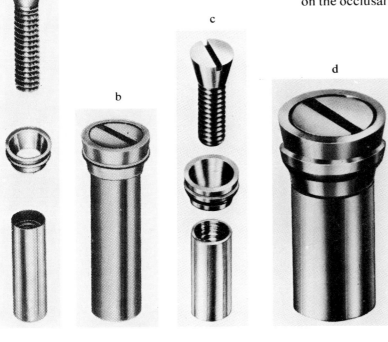

a

b

c

d

Fig. 678 (a) Components of the CM screw, collar, and threaded sleeve retaining unit. (b) Assembled unit. (c) The comparable MP system. (d) Unit assembled.

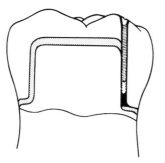

Fig. 679 Diagrammatic view of a screw-retained telescopic crown.

facings often need to be provided as well. Inadequate abutment preparations may lead to increased vertical dimensions and overcontoured teeth. A considerable amount of care needs to be taken in planning the preparations.

Teeth with particularly short clinical crowns do not normally lend themselves to telescopic prostheses, neither do teeth of limited bucco-palatal or labio-palatal dimensions. Telescopic prostheses are not therefore recommended for patients with class II division 2 malocclusions although, in exceptional circumstances, they may be constructed with considerable difficulty. Since both layers of gold need to

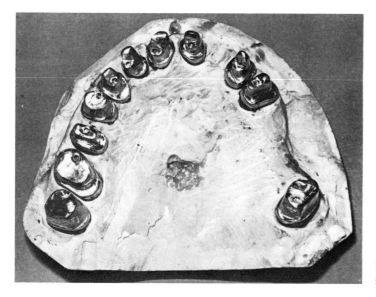

Fig. 680 Inner copings showing threaded sleeves.

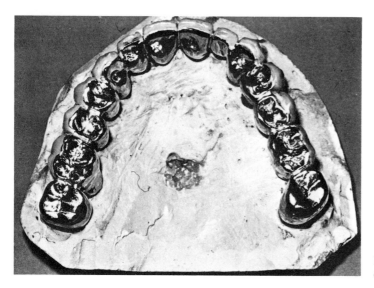

Fig. 681 Assembled prosthesis on the master cast.

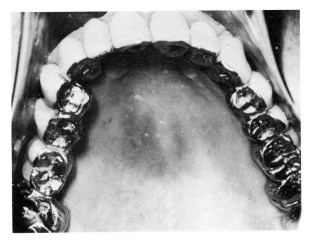

Fig. 682 Nine years later.

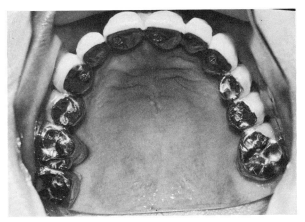

Fig. 683 Another example of the screw-retained telescopic prosthesis.

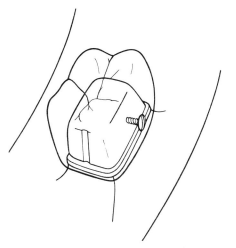

Fig. 684 A friction screw may be placed in the outer section of the prosthesis.

be kept as thin as possible, subsequent adjustment of the occlusal surfaces is difficult and in places impossible. Apart from the care in recording jaw relationships there is advantage in constructing a temporary acrylic resin bridge, for should lack of posterior occlusal support have led the patient to adopt a protruded mandibular posture, subsequent reversion to centric jaw relation might involve repreparing several teeth and reconstructing the restoration. The transitional prosthesis can be made on outlined preparations finished just short of the gingival margins.

These outlined preparations are useful in designing the restoration, for the cast can be surveyed to determine whether or not a common path of insertion can be provided. If this has been achieved, the inner copings can be made thin (usually 0·2 mm to 0·4 mm), and it remains to determine the size and position of the small recesses to be prepared for the threaded sleeves. Non-precious metal copings allowing casting thicknesses to be reduced to 0·15 mm may well simplify the technique.

If the surveyed cast (Fig. 685) shows no possible common path of insertion, several alternative treatments have to be considered:

1. To reprepare the teeth to provide a common path of insertion.

2. To build out the inner copings to provide a common path of insertion. This procedure increases the bulk of the final restoration and only small divergences can be corrected in this manner if overcontouring is to be prevented (Fig. 686). Small mesio-distal divergencies are simpler to correct than labio-palatal divergencies, particularly in anterior parts of the mouth.

Where wide divergences exist it may be possible to split the outer section by means of an intracoronal attachment. In this way two separate paths of insertion can be provided for the outer section (Figs. 687–689). If the prosthesis is designed as a splint, the junction must be rigid. This can only be achieved by employing an attachment of generous length and cross-section. A bracing arm should be employed as well.

The most convenient preparation is the full crown preparation with a shoulder width of about 1·5 mm. This shoulder need not be carried around the palatal or lingual surface of the teeth and, if it is prepared in these regions, it can be thin. It is important that the full width of the shoulder be carried through the proximal surfaces of posterior teeth. Apart from producing a better looking restoration, it provides space for the threaded sleeves if these are to be employed. The planning of the shoulder depends not

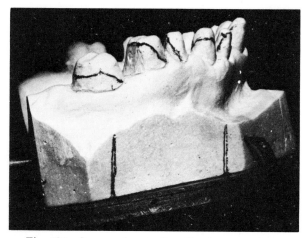

Fig. 685   Surveyed cast of outlined preparations.

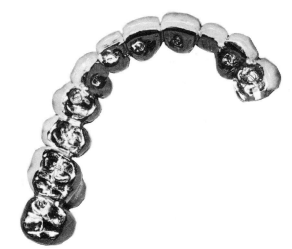

Fig. 688   Outer section to show female Crismani attachment and step for bracing arm.

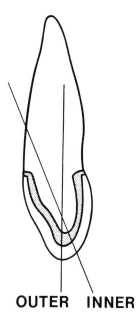

OUTER   INNER

Fig. 686 Attempting to correct labio-palatal divergences with the inner copings may lead to overcontouring.

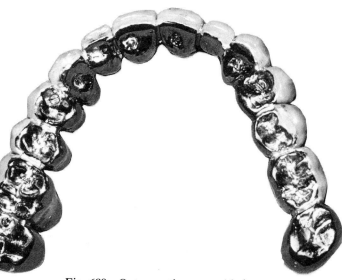

Fig. 689   Outer section assembled.

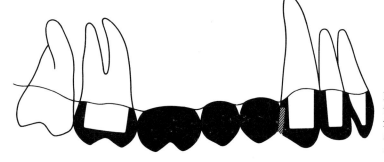

Fig. 687   Diagram to show how splitting the outer section of the prosthesis allows for considerable variation in abutment alignment without recourse to bulky inner copings.

only on the tooth contour, but upon the relation of the shoulder to the gingival margin. On the basis of experiments on dogs, Marcum (1967) has suggested the ideal finishing line to be at the level of the free gingival margin. It is naturally important that the periodontal tissues are sound before tooth preparation is begun, and that the surrounding soft tissues are not damaged during the course of the tooth preparation or while the impression is made.

A short 150° bevel on the shoulder may be useful in seating the inner copings, but this bevel has to be constructed with caution in the anterior labial aspects of the mouth if the appearance is not to suffer. The outer coping will seat down on part of the surface of the gold covering the bevel so that a short bevel will be virtually covered (Figs. 690, 691). If the bevel is less than 120° and more than 2 mm wide an exposed rim of gold is likely to show around the neck of the tooth (Figs. 692, 693).

Since the screw position should have been decided on the diagnostic cast, a small distal or preferably mesial box can be cut in the tooth preparation. A mesial angulation to the screw may simplify insertion and removal (Fig. 694).

Impression procedures depend largely upon the operator's personal preference; the result, not the technique, is important.

Recording jaw relations

While complex recording methods abound, a simple technique is to modify the system described by Dawson (1974); in principle the posterior teeth are prepared and every other anterior tooth. An impression is made and centric jaw relation recorded by means of a hard wax rim* that contacts the occlusal surfaces of the posterior teeth but does not touch the mucosa or anterior teeth. The master cast is now mounted on the articulator with this record. The impression of the unprepared teeth allows the anterior guidance angle to be set, or custom moulded in acrylic resin placed on the anteror guide table. The labial contours and incisal edge positions are also available to the technicians. Following preparation of all the teeth and a new impression, the cast of the impression is now mounted with the original wax record on the articulator.

Telescopic prostheses introduce a problem as it is usually necessary to produce a cast with all the preparations outlined for planning purposes. The answer lies in carefully constructed temporary acrylic resin crowns that reproduce the original

* Moyco Extra Hard Beauty Wax.

anatomy of the tooth. An alginate impression is made before tooth preparation and put aside taking the usual precautions to keep it damp. Following tooth preparation, a resin temporary crown material is placed in this impression, preferably with the aid of a syringe to avoid airblows, and the impression seated in the mouth. The temporary crown constructed should reproduce the anatomy of the original crown and can be used for production of the anterior guidance together with acting as a labial contour and incisal edge guide.

Facebow and eccentric records are naturally an important part of the jaw relation records.

As with any extensive restoration it is essential to establish the correct vertical relation before the centric relation record is made. Preliminary restorations as an aid to centric relation recording have been mentioned. Where insufficient posterior abutments remain for the occlusally supported wafer, a conventional occlusal rim may be employed.

Despite every care in recording jaw relations, it is advisable that they be checked once the metal castings have been constructed. The inner copings should be inserted and checked for extension and adaptation and then the outer structure slid into place over the copings. A check record is then made in fast-setting artificial stone. This record is made at centric jaw relation with the vertical dimension increased approximately 2 mm in a similar manner to the procedure employed for complete denture construction (Fig. 695). The lower cast is then remounted by means of this record on the articulator, the record removed, and the occlusion examined. It is normally found that little more than polishing certain sections of the prosthesis is necessary. More substantial errors, however, might involve remaking sections of the prosthesis, repositioning the screws and, in extreme cases, one of the abutments might need to be reprepared. While it is hoped that the corrections required will be small, it is far better they be carried out at this stage than after the entire prosthesis, together with its facings, has been completed. If the check record procedure is carried out with care, subsequent occlusal adjustments are virtually eliminated.

Cementation procedures

Cementation procedures are similar to those of other telescopic prostheses. There is a risk that slight malalignment of one of the copings during cementation might prevent the insertion of the outer structure. The inner copings should be positioned. Three or four can then be removed, dried, and

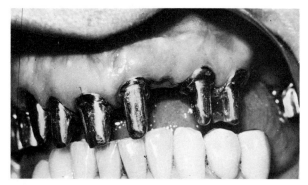

Fig. 690   Inner copings with short 60° bevels.

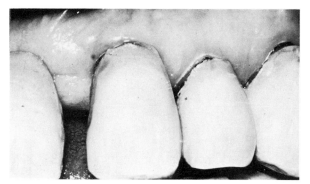

Fig. 693   The exposed rims of gold.

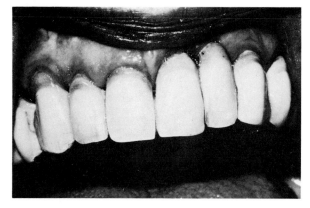

Fig. 691   Outer section covering the underlying copings.

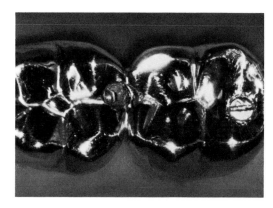

Fig. 694   A mesial angulation to the screw hole will simplify insertion and removal.

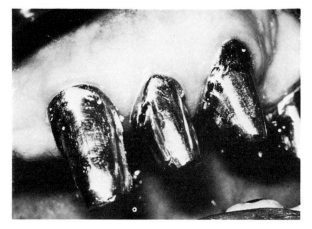

Fig. 692   Inner copings with long shallow bevels.

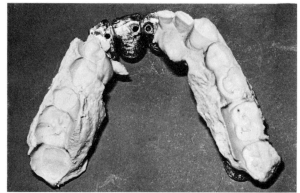

Fig. 695   The check record joined to the outer structure.

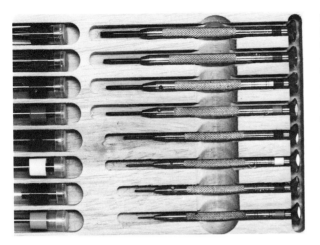

Fig. 696 A set of jeweller's screwdrivers useful for tightening screws on the cast and in the mouth. The screw heads may be removed from the handles where space is limited.

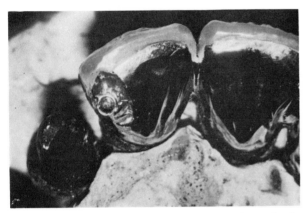

Fig. 697 Threaded sleeve in one section of the prosthesis.

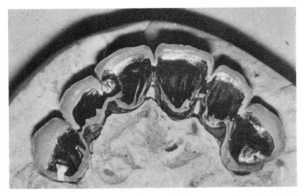

Fig. 698 The two sections of the prosthesis joined together.

cemented in place and the outer structure then slid into place before the cement sets. It is usually found convenient to cement up to four inner copings at a time and allow a period for the cement to be set before the outer structure is removed and the procedure repeated.

Manufacturers provide sets of special screwdrivers precisely adapted to the screws employed, thereby preventing damage to the screw heads (Fig. 696). Screws should not be inserted within half an hour of the cementation, to allow the cement to harden. When first inserted, the screws should be positioned in a sequence alternating from side to side, bearing in mind the possible danger of pulling the inner coping away from the abutment tooth. It is suggested that the screws be tightened gently and retightened over a period of the next few days. These screws may appear to loosen during this time, and this may be caused in part by slight realignment of the underlying roots. After a period of adjustment, usually two weeks or so, the screws are found to remain tight. During the tightening phase it is recommended that the screw heads be left unground, for if they are adjusted to blend with the cusp facets, subsequent tightening will alter this alignment.

Manufacturers of these attachments usually recommend that for posterior restorations the screw assembly should be positioned so that, when tightened, the slot in the screw head is at right-angles to the lateral path travelled by the opposing cusps in working side contacts and preferably out of contact. Few patients can feel the slot in the screw head because the head is counter-sunk.

Should it be required, the removal of the prosthesis usually presents few difficulties. The screws should be undone and placed in order on soft wax. There may be problems in removing the outer section if the copings have been designed to provide almost parallel-sided surfaces. It can then be surprisingly difficult to remove the restoration, for if one side is pulled down, the prosthesis jams. After the screws have been removed, an alginate or rubber base impression can be taken so that the prosthesis can be slid out of place in the impression along its designed pathway.

Screws may also be used for joining two non-aligned sections of a fixed prosthesis in a similar manner to that of intracoronal attachments (Figs. 697, 698). The overlapping pieces of metal should incorporate an anti-rotation device.

The small screws are delicate, easily lost, swallowed, or damaged. The slots in the screw heads are prone to mishandling with incorrect instruments.

Reliable and consistent long term results can only be achieved with detailed planning, regular inspection, and expert maintenance. It only takes one jammed, burnished, or damaged screw to defeat the entire purpose of the restoration.

Screw retainers for non-vital teeth

Provided that an effective post-retained diaphragm is constructed, the screw unit employed can be centrally placed and some of the size restrictions reduced. Amalgam cores, however, are best treated as vital teeth with respect to the screw units selected.

One system that has gained popularity consists of a precious metal block with a threaded screw-hole attached to a diaphragm. A removable section slides over the block and is screwed in position.

The Hruska unit is a good example of this type of attachment (Fig. 699) with two different sizes of block units available for anterior teeth, together with a block unit suitable for posterior teeth. Inserting the screw is simplified because the anterior block provides the screw with a palatally inclined path of insertion, while the posterior block provides a mesially inclined path of insertion (Figs. 700–703). Specially produced mandrels are available to ensure that the screw blocks are parallel to one another.

The Schubiger screw system is commendably versatile, basically consisting of a threaded stud on a base that can be soldered to a post diaphragm (Figs. 704–708). The unit to be attached by the screw is soldered to a special sleeve that slides over the screw thread and is then held in place by a matched nut screwed down over it. Since the sleeves have to slide over their respective threaded studs, it is important for these studs to be aligned. This procedure can be quite simply carried out on a surveyor using the paralleling mandrel supplied by the manufacturer. There are two sizes of Schubiger base available and for each of these bases a short or long sleeve may be obtained. The shorter sleeve nut unit is designed for securing a bar attachment to a root diaphragm. The bar is soldered to the sleeve which is then screwed down in the mouth. The Schubiger threaded stud has the same thread as the base of the Gerber stud units, so that if a root of a bar joint prosthesis is lost, the bar can be unscrewed and Gerber stud units screwed onto the remaining roots.

A longer sleeve/nut is available for screwing down a bridge onto several screw units (Fig. 709). This unit allows the construction of a rigid restoration removable by the dental surgeon for periodic inspection or replacement of facings. This system is

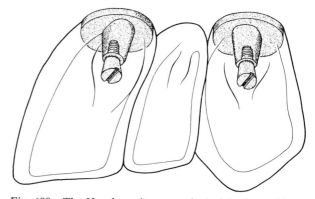

Fig. 699   The Hruska units are typical of the screw block system for joining a bridge to non-vital roots. The anterior blocks provide the screw with a palatally inclined path of insertion.

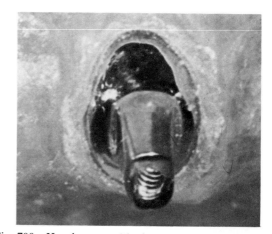

Fig. 700   Hruska screw block on an upper premolar root. This block provides the screw with a mesially inclined path of insertion.

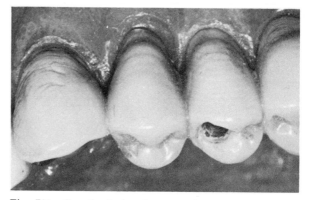

Fig. 701   Prosthesis in place, to show opening for the screw. The prosthesis is also retained by screws in the canine and in the second molar.

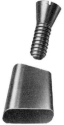
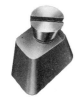

Fig. 702 Hruska screw block with palatal path of insertion for retaining screw.

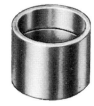
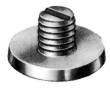

Fig. 704 The Schubiger screw system showing the sleeve to which the bar can be soldered.

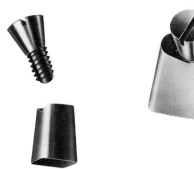

Fig. 703 Hruska screw block with mesial path of insertion for retaining screw.

particularly useful where the abutment teeth of a bridge require post preparations.

The Schubiger screw is comparatively large and centrally placed. The outer crowns are, therefore, securely held in place. Conventional telescopic prostheses can be retained by these units, or bars can be connected to the outer sections of the crowns (Fig. 710).

There is one important point concerning grinding the screw head flush with the facet of the crown through which it passes. Turning the screw alters its relationship to the crown facet as it cannot be exactly at right angles to its surrounding occlusal surface (Figs. 711, 712). The larger the screw the more important this aspect becomes. Grinding should therefore be carried out in the mouth and not on the master cast as the screw may not turn to precisely the same position and it is easier to screw the head tight before it has been ground.

Modification of a screw-retained bridge

Following tooth loss, it may be necessary to convert a screw-retained bridge to a bar prosthesis, or to a stud-retained denture. The standard size base of the

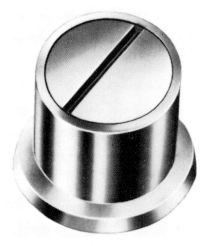

Fig. 705 The Schubiger system assembled.

Schubiger attachment allows considerable versatility in this respect, although the all-important biological considerations must not be overlooked. Unscrewing and removing the bridge leaves exposed the underlying screw base, but the problem remains of reproducing this section of the mouth so that a master cast can be made. This master cast is essential for the construction of the new prosthesis.

The correct friction cores (male sections) of the rigid Gerber attachments should be inserted on the exposed threaded projection in the patient's mouth with the retaining springs loosened. These female sections of the attachments are then placed over it with the retaining springs loosed. These female sections are to be used in a localising impression and auto-polymerising caps can be built over the female unit to enhance its stability in the impression. The localising impression should be made in plaster, wherever possible. The female sections of the Gerber attachment will be removed with the impression.

Before the impression is cast a special male section of the Gerber should be positioned. This section consists of a friction core and a threaded base. Unlike the normal Schubiger base, this unit has tagging incorporated so that when the impression is cast, the base becomes attached to the artificial

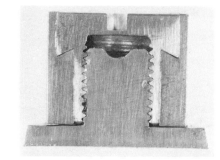

Fig. 708 Cross-sectional photograph of the shorter Schubiger sleeve/nut unit. The bar is soldered to the surrounding sleeve.

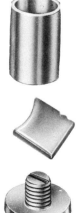

Fig. 709 The taller Schubiger screw/collar system. The sleeve is buried within the artificial abutment tooth, and the nut passes down through a hole in the occlusal surface to join it to the thread of the diaphragm.

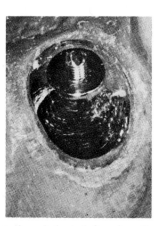

Fig. 706 The threaded stud forming the base of the Schubiger screw system.

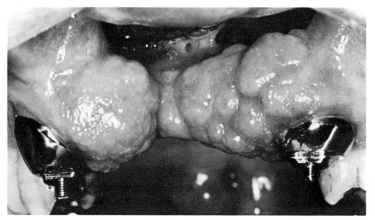

Fig. 707 Two Schubiger screws in the mouth. Versatility in treatment planning is possible with their use.

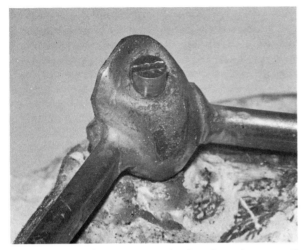

Fig. 710 Schubiger screw projecting through crown. It should not be trimmed on the master cast.

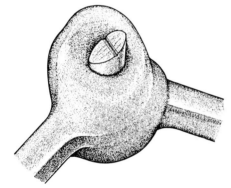

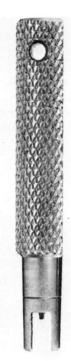

Fig. 712 Screwdriver specially designed for tightening or unscrewing the male sections of Gerber attachments.

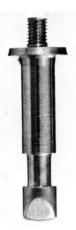

Fig. 713 Special Schubiger base with tagging for incorporation within a master cast.

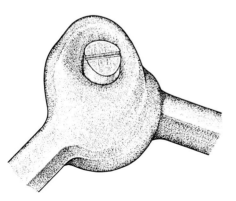

Fig. 711 Turning the screw alters its relationship to the cusp facet. For this reason the screw head should not be trimmed until final tightening in the mouth.

stone (Fig. 713). The master impression will thus incorporate two projecting Gerber attachments correctly localised.

When the friction cores are eventually placed in the mouth, a resin cement should be employed to prevent their subsequent loosening. A vent-hole allows the excess cement to escape.

The Schubiger and Gerber attachment systems are relatively strong and versatile. Where space permits there is much to recommend their use.

REFERENCES AND FURTHER READING

ABRAMS, L. and FEDER, M. (1962) Periodontal considerations for removable prosthesis. *Alpha Omega Fraternity (Sept.)*

AMSTERDAM, M. and ABRAMS, L. (1968) Periodontal prosthesis. In *Periodontal Therapy*, 4th ed., by Goldman, H. M. and Cohen, D. W. C. V. Mosby, St Louis, Mo.

BOTTGER, H. and GRUNDLER, H. (1970) *Die Praxis des Teleskop-systems*. Neuer Merkur, München

BREISACH, L. (1967) Esthetic attachments for removable partial dentures. *J. Prosth. Dent.*, *17*, 261

COHN, L. A. (1956) The physiological basis for tooth fixation in precision-attached partial dentures *J. prosth. Dent.*, *6*, 220

DAWSON, P. E. (1974) *Evaluation, Diagnosis, and Treatment of Occlusal Problems*. C. V. Mosby, St Louis, Mo.

GAERNY, A. (1969) *Der abnehmbare Interdentalraum-Verschluss (I.R.V.)*. Quintessenz, Berlin

HOFFMANN, M. and LUDWIG, P. (1973) Die teleskopierende Totalprothees im stark reduzierten Lückengebiss. *Dtsch. Zahnarztl Z.*, 28:2

ISAACSON, G. O. (1969) Telescope crown retainers for removable partial dentures. *J. prosth. Dent.*, *22*, 436

JORGENSEN, K. D. (1960) Factors affecting the film thickness of zinc phosphate cements. *Acta odont. scand.*, *18*, 479

JORGENSEN, K. D. and PETERSON, G. F. (1963) The grain size of zinc phosphate cement. *Acta. odont. scand.*, *21*, 255

KORBER, K. H. (1973) *Konuskronen-Teleskope*. 3 Aufl. Hüthig, Heidelberg

LANGE, F. (1955) Experiments on cementation of crowns. *Tandlaegebladet 50*, 181

McLEAN, J. W. (1969) Aluminous porcelain crowns. *Quart. Dent. Reb.*, *3*, 126

MARCUM, J. S. (1967) The effect of crown marginal depth upon gingival tissue. *J. prosth. Dent.*, *17*, 479

PALOMO, F. and PEDEN, J. (1976) Periodontal considerations of restorative procedures. *J. prosth Dent.*, *36:4*, 387

PEESO, F. A. (1916) *Crown and Bridgework for Students and Practitioners*. Lea & Febiger, Philadelphia

PREISKEL, H. W. (1967) Considerations of the check record in complete denture construction. *J. prosth. Dent.*, *18*, 98

PREISKEL, H. W. (1969) Telescopic prostheses. *Israel J. Dent. Med.*, *18*, 12

PREISKEL, H. W. (1971) Screw-retained telescopic prostheses. *Brit. Dent. J.*, *130*, 107

RATEITSCHAK, K. H. (1963) The therapeutic effect of local treatment on periodontal disease assessed upon evaluation of different diagnostic criteria. *J. Periodont.*, *35*, 540

SCHWEITZER, J. M. (1960) Gold copings for problematic teeth. *J. prosth. Dent.*, *10*, 163

SCHWEITZER, J. M. (1964) *Oral Rehabilitation Problem Cases: Treatment and Evaluation, Vol. 1*, pp. 234–240. C. V. Mosby, St Louis, Mo.

SCHWEITZER, J. M., SCHWEITZER, R. D. and SCHWEITZER, J. (1971) The telescoped complete denture. A resarch report at clinical level. *J. prosth. Dent.*, *26*, 357

SIMMONS, J. J. (1963) Swing-lock stabilization and retention. *Tex. Dent. J. 81*, 10

SINGER, F. and SCHON, F. (1966) *Partial Dentures*. Kimpton, London

STEIGER, A. A. and BOITEL, R. H. (1959) *Precision Work for Partial Dentures*, pp. 143–177. Stebo, Zürich

WAERHAUG, J. (1969) Justification for splinting in periodontal therapy. *J. prosth. Dent.*, *22*, 201

WEINBERG, L. A. (1969) New design for anterior unit built porcelain prostheses. *J. prosth. Dent.*, *21*, 1

WUEBBENHORST, A. M. (1970) Screw-type attachments for fixed partial dentures. *J. prosth. Dent.*, *24*, 275

YALISOVE, I. L. (1966) Crown and sleeve coping retainers for removable partial prostheses. *J. prosth. Dent.*, *6*, 1069

YALISOVE, I. L. (1972) The crown and sleeve coping retainer. *Alpha Omega*, Sept. p. 21

CHAPTER 13

Sectional Dentures

P. R. L'Estrange and **E. Pullen-Warner**

The sectional denture was designed to overcome many of the limitations of clasp-retained prostheses (Fig. 714). Sectional restorations are intended to supplement existing removable partial denture designs rather than to replace them (Figs. 715, 716). Although technical costs may be somewhat higher, sectional dentures have the following advantages over clasp-retained designs:

1. Better appearance.
2. Improved retention.
3. Ease of insertion and removal.
4. Complete restoration of the edentulous span and adjacent tissues.
5. Minimal mouth preparation.

The shape of anterior and posterior teeth often precludes the complete restoration of a space by a one-piece prosthesis and the appearance and retention will suffer. A common example occurs where the labial tissue in the region of the edentulous span

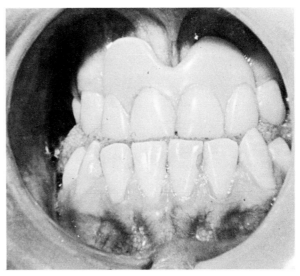

Fig. 715   Previous denture.

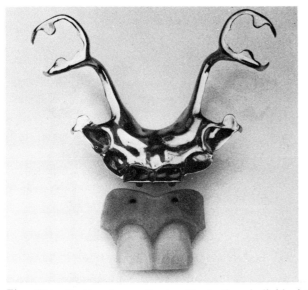

Fig. 714   Sectional prosthesis, illustrating individual parts.

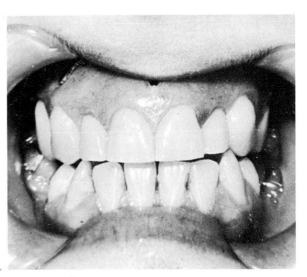

Fig. 716   Sectional restoration.

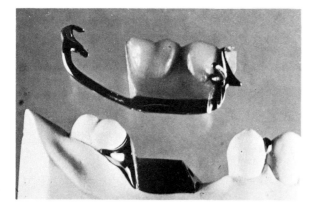

Fig. 717   Posterior sectional prosthesis – individual parts.

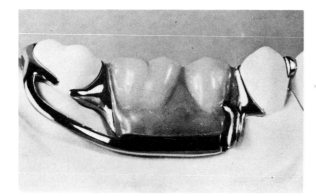

Fig. 718   Posterior sectional prosthesis – united prosthesis.

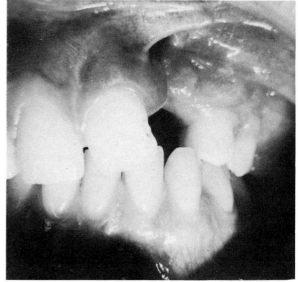

Fig. 719   Repaired anterior cleft.

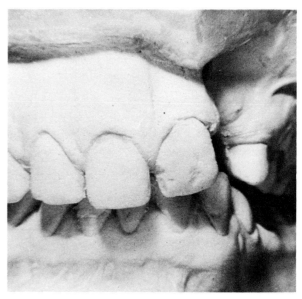

Fig. 720   Anterior cleft – artificial stone master cast.

is severely undercut, or where the space available for the restoration is small. Most of these problems can be overcome by using sectional prostheses. In some circumstances this type of restoration has advantages over the fixed prosthesis.

There are usually two parts to a sectional denture, each part having an individual path of insertion. The terms first and second parts are used relating to their sequence of insertion by the patient (Figs. 717, 718).

INDICATIONS FOR SECTIONAL DENTURES

Epileptics who require a removable prosthesis with maximum retention.

Cleft palate patients with a combination of soft tissue deficiency and abnormal tooth positions (Figs. 719–721).

Young patients who have suffered loss of permanent anterior teeth and where, because of age, crown preparations are contra-indicated. After orthodontic treatment a sectional prosthesis can provide a useful splint.

Instrument players. Wind instrument players may require positive anterior retention of a prosthesis to permit consistent use of an embouchure (Fig. 722).

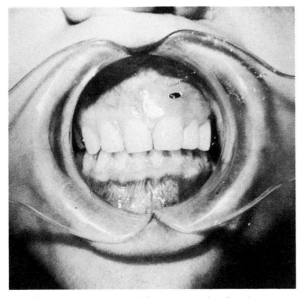

Fig. 721   Anterior cleft – restoration in place.

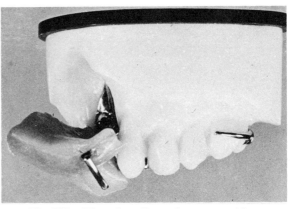

Fig. 723   Hinged appliance in open position.

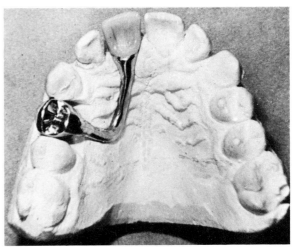

Fig. 724   Spring-bridge incorporating precision attachment.

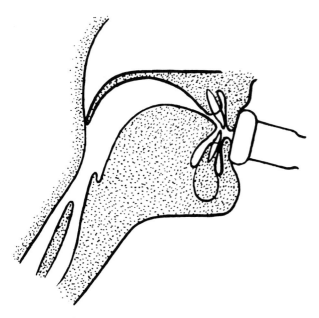

Fig. 722   Embouchure production.

Malangulation of the remaining teeth where adequate preliminary orthodontic therapy cannot be performed.

Appearance. The sectional denture can defy detection by close scrutiny.

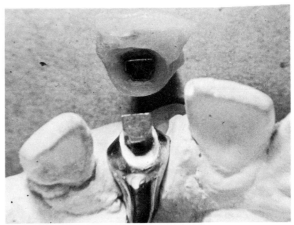

Fig. 725   Precision attachment and removal labial component.

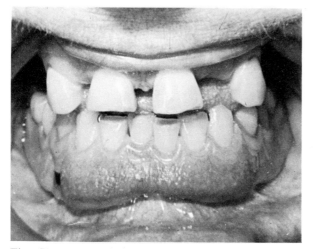

Fig. 726 Vertically hinged labial section similar to 'swing-lock' principle.

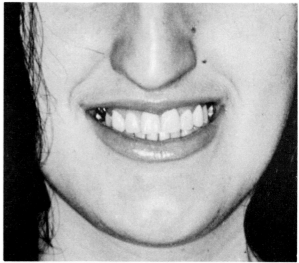

Fig. 728   Maxillo-mandibular skeletal base abnormality – restoration in place.

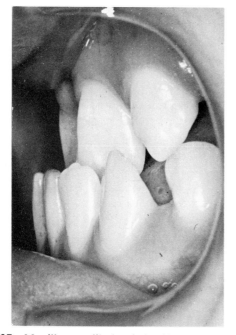

Fig. 727   Maxillo-mandibular skeletal base abnormality – anterior dental relationship.

Maxillo-facial prostheses. As an aid to post-operative reconstruction following maxillo-facial surgery (Fig. 723).

Bridgework. The sectional denture can be used in conjunction with fixed and removable restorations employing attachments (Figs. 724, 725).

Splinting. The sectional denture has an effective splinting action and can restore labial or buccal tissues as well (Fig. 726).

Maxillo-mandibular skeletal base abnormalities. Patients with Angle's Class III jaw relationships can often be given the appearance of those with a Class I dental relationship by means of a sectional prosthesis (Figs. 727, 728).

PRINCIPLES OF SECTIONAL DENTURE CONSTRUCTION

A simple wood joinery exercise shows the principles involved. In Fig. 729, '1' illustrates the area requiring restoration bounded by the surfaces 'a' and 'b'. A triangular-sectioned piece of wood 'á' is constructed to be placed against 'a' so that its exposed surface is parallel to that of 'b' (Fig. 729, '2' and '3'). Another piece of wood is prepared ('b'), the dimensions of which are complementary to the remaining space (Fig. 729, '4'). When these two pieces are assembled in the cavity, the space will be completely restored (Fig. 729, '5'). If a nail is driven through 'b' at an angle which will cause it to enter 'a', a union will be achieved that will effectively resist vertical displacement (Fig. 729, '6').

Consider now an anterior edentulous area as shown in Fig. 730. The shaded area adjacent to the edentulous span cannot be filled using the path of insertion indicated. If the cast is given a posterior tilt, a position will be reached where the areas previously undercut can now be fully engaged. In

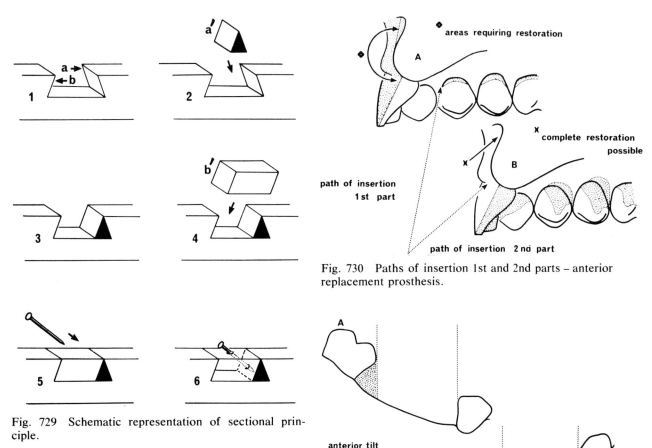

Fig. 729 Schematic representation of sectional principle.

Fig. 730 Paths of insertion 1st and 2nd parts – anterior replacement prosthesis.

Fig. 731 Paths of insertion 1st and 2nd parts – posterior replacement prosthesis.

anterior sectional denture construction the cast tilt illustrated in Fig. 730, 'A', represents the path of insertion of the first part and that shown in Fig. 730, 'B', the path of insertion of the second part. The first part will engage the palatal or lingual surfaces of the adjacent teeth and the second part will engage the proximal and labio-proximal tooth surfaces. In addition, the path of insertion for the second part permits complete restoration of labial soft tissue deficiencies.

When the posterior edentulous area illustrated in Fig. 731 'A' is to be restored, it will be seen that the shaded area adjacent to the molar tooth cannot be filled using the path of insertion indicated. If the cast is given a posterior tilt, a position will be reached where the entire mesial surface of the molar tooth can be engaged. The shaded area on the distal of the premolar cannot be engaged with the new path of insertion. In sectional denture construction the cast tilt illustrated in Fig. 731, 'B', represents the path of insertion of the first part, while that shown in Fig. 731, 'A' represents the path of insertion of the

second part. The first part will engage the entire mesial surface of the molar and the second part the entire distal surface of the premolar.

METHODS OF UNION

Two methods of union are commonly employed in anterior sectional denture construction:

1. Mechanical locking – PW Bolt (Fig. 732).

2. Frictional resistance – PW Split Post (Fig. 733).

The PW bolt*

This operates by introducing mechanical interference to the path of withdrawal of the second part. The design of the first and second parts is such that they give mutual support and are not entirely dependent on the bolt to resist displacing forces. The bolt is designed to function in many positions and attitudes, but adjustment to barrel and handle length is required to suit individual situations. The bolt barrel is secured within the flange by the use of self-curing acrylic resin.

Construction of the PW bolt

The bolt is constructed from wire and tubing. The principle of its action is similar to that of a rifle bolt – lift and slide (Fig. 734). Limitations of these movements are obtained by connecting facets cut into the bolt shank and forming a key-way (Fig. 732). The key-way is engaged by a retaining pin incorporated into the bolt barrel (Fig. 732). The guiding facets are completely enclosed within the bolt barrel, and ensure a trouble-free action. The bolt shank has a diameter of 1·3 mm. A sharp bend can be obtained in the wire to enable the handle to be formed without resorting to cutting and soldering, a process required if larger diameters are employed. The bolt must be kept small because of the limited space available.

The 1·3 mm diameter bolt gives adequate strength compatible with ease of location within the pontic area. Smaller diameter shank sizes can be employed, but are prone to failure after prolonged periods. As bolts may be used in a variety of positions in the dental arch, the slide facets are cut so that when the bolt lever is moved from the locked position, the bolt shank can slide to disengage the bolt boss from the second part. Easy bolt manipulation is quickly learned by the patient. Over 15 years we have found bolt failure to be extremely rare.

The PW split post

This device is a post split longitudinally. It consists of two half-round sections of 'Wiptam' wire, the flat surfaces of which are approximated to give the appearance of a round post (Fig. 733). The post is surrounded by a stainless steel tube incorporated within the second part. The post can be activated to provide frictional resistance with the tube. This simple and inexpensive method of attachment is readily incorporated into a removable prosthesis.

The split post provides an alternative means of fixation to the bolt. It has particular application in anterior tooth replacement where there is insufficient labio-palatal space to accommodate a bolt. It is an essential feature that the alignment of the split post coincides with the path of insertion and withdrawal of the second part. The bolt, however,

THE P-W DENTURE BOLT

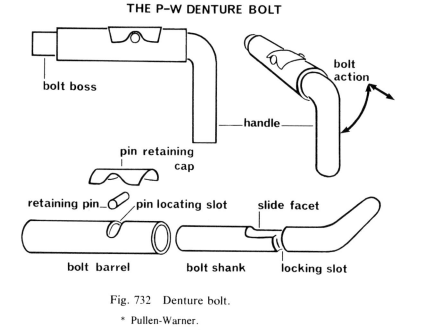

Fig. 732   Denture bolt.

* Pullen-Warner.

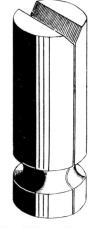

Fig. 733   Split post.

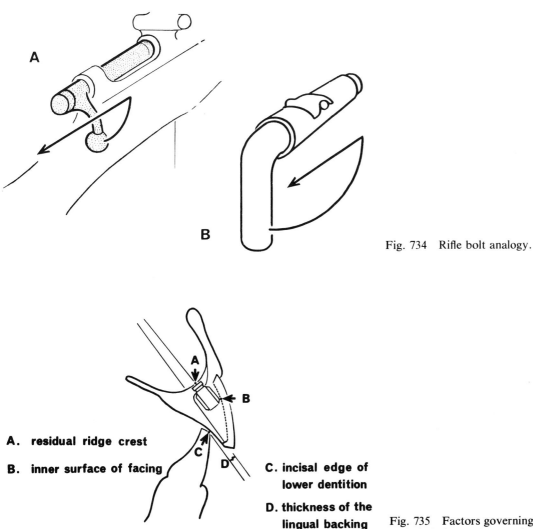

Fig. 734 Rifle bolt analogy.

A. residual ridge crest

B. inner surface of facing

C. incisal edge of
   lower dentition

D. thickness of the
   lingual backing

Fig. 735 Factors governing post-position and length-anterior replacement prosthesis.

is positioned so that the barrel direction opposes the path of insertion. The length of the post should be as great as possible to produce:

1. Maximum frictional resistance.
2. Ease of insertion (aids alignment).
3. Greater resistance to displacing forces.
4. Ease of adjustment when required.

Figure 735 illustrates the factors governing the maximum length of the post that can be employed.

1. The relationship of the inner surfaces of the pontic veneer to the residual ridge crest.

2. The angulation of the post to the residual ridge crest.

3. The relationship of the opposing dentition to the residual ridge crest.

4. The thickness of the palatal backing.

The more restricted the space available, the further to the labial will be the siting of the post to allow for the metal backing of the first part. Where possible, this space should be increased by reduction of the opposing dentition. It is recommended that the diameter of the split post should be 1·5 mm and the minimal overall length should be not less than 4 mm.

It is important to remember that all anterior sectional prostheses engage the same lingual and labial tooth surfaces irrespective of the method of union.

APPLICATION OF PRINCIPLES

1. Anterior replacement

Three sectional designs may be applied to anterior tooth replacement. The first type (Fig. 736) consists of two separate parts. It has a lingual section of all-metal construction engaging the lingual surfaces of the remaining anterior teeth. The path of insertion permits a spur to pass over the crest of the ridge and terminate in the sulcus incorporating a bolt hole to accept the bolt boss.

The spur is usually connected rigidly to the lingual casting but, where the labial tissue is severely undercut, the connection of the spur will be hinged (Fig. 738). The bolt hole is formed by casting around a length of stainless steel wire positioned in the wax pattern. The spur should be offset towards the midline to permit easy access to the bolt handle when it is in the closed position, and to give maximum barrel length (Fig. 737).

A 1·5 mm 'Wiptam' wire post is also placed in the wax pattern to be incorporated into the subsequent casting (Fig. 736). This wire post will eventually engage a stainless steel tube placed within the pontic crown included in the second part. The angle of this post is determined by the steepest undercut presented by either the mesio-labial surfaces of the teeth adjacent to the edentulous span, or the labial tissue of that span relative to the path of insertion of the first part. The post acts as a guide for the insertion of the second part, which consists of the pontic crown, labial flange, and bolt.

The second type (Fig. 738) incorporates a hinge that joins the lingual and labial sections together. Due to the manner in which the labial section swings into position, this type of denture is suitable for patients whose labial tissue is severely undercut, or whose loss of tissue is considerable. In this situation, a vertical bolt position can be used providing a better looking junction between the appliance and the adjacent natural tissues. A hinge axis should be sited as near to the incisal edge as possible. The hinge has a central bearing. This bearing is known as a cantilever hinge bearing and may be waxed or preformed. The limiting factor of this type of sectional denture is the labio-lingual dimension of the pontic crown.

The third type of sectional denture (Fig. 739) was devised to overcome the following limitations of bolt union in the restoration of small anterior edentulous spans:

1. Insufficient space in a labio-palatal direction, preventing extension of the labial spur over the most

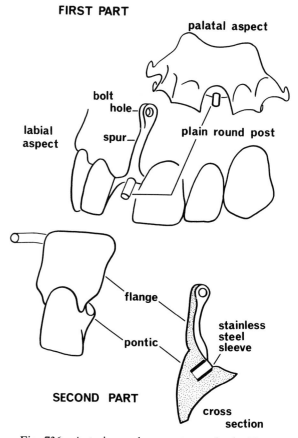

Fig. 736 Anterior replacement prosthesis, Type 1.

prominent contour of the edentulous area. The available space will be influenced by the degree of resorption of the edentulous alveolar ridge that has taken place and the desired position of the neck of the replacement tooth. The labial flange should give proper support to the upper lip, but must not be excessively thick. However, it must be thick enough to accommodate, and to disguise, the underlying spur.

2. Excessive elevation of the upper lip during smiling, leading to unsightly exposure of the bolt handle.

3. When replacing upper central incisors, location of the labial fraenum may prevent the use of a spur and the patient may not wish to undergo a fraenoplasty.

The obvious site for an alternative means of union is within the pontic crown. A small retentive device using the principle of frictional resistance is constructed from inexpensive materials, and known as the split post (Fig. 733).

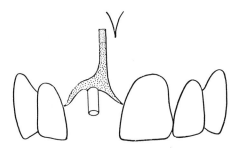

Fig. 737 Spur offset to mid-line.

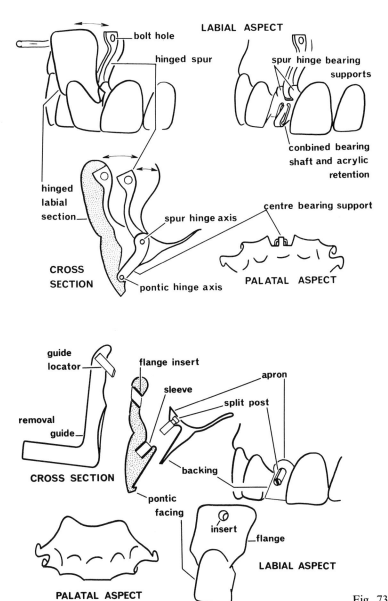

LABIAL ASPECT

bolt hole

hinged spur

spur hinge bearing
supports

conbined bearing
shaft and acrylic
retention

hinged
labial
section

spur hinge axis

centre bearing support

CROSS
SECTION

pontic hinge axis

PALATAL ASPECT

Fig. 738 Anterior replacement prosthesis,
Type 2.

guide
locator

flange insert

apron

sleeve

split post

removal
guide

backing

CROSS SECTION

pontic
facing

insert

flange

PALATAL ASPECT

LABIAL ASPECT

Fig. 739 Anterior replacement prosthesis, Type 3.

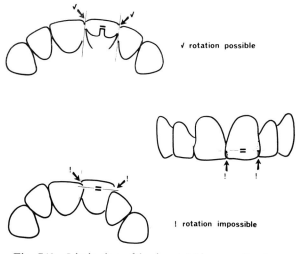

Fig. 740 Limitation of horizontal hinge application.

The *first part* is of all-metal construction and is designed to embrace the mesio-proximal surface of the posterior abutment from the lingual to the buccal aspect (Fig. 741). An arm traverses the edentulous span on its lingual aspect. This arm engages the mesio-lingual of the premolar, terminating with an occlusal rest on the mesio-occlusal surface of this tooth. An interdental spur is also provided between the lower right first premolar and the canine (Fig. 742).

The anterior surface of the part embracing the mesial aspect of the molar is made parallel to the distal infra-bulge surface of the premolar to create a distal guiding plane for the insertion of the second

Design factors

The success of these appliances depends on the complete restoration of the edentulous span and of the adjacent soft tissues. The following factors influence the final design of an anterior sectional denture:

1. The degree of alveolar resorption that has taken place.

2. The labio-lingual dimension of the replacement pontic crown and its inciso-cervical length.

The apparent depth of the sulcus and location of any fraenae may influence bolt position, or indicate use of a split post.

Where appearance requires an artificial tooth to overlap the adjacent natural tooth, a design consisting of two separate parts must be used. A sectional denture of Type 1 or Type 3 would be indicated. The Type 2 sectional denture would not be indicated, for when the labial section rotates the incisal edges will move palatally. This movement can only occur if the abutment teeth do not interfere with this rotation (Fig. 740).

2. Posterior replacement: first type (separate sections)

1. Unilateral

Unilateral posterior sectional dentures can be successfully employed. Where possible, more than two abutment teeth should be used to withstand the additional occlusal and lateral masticatory loads.

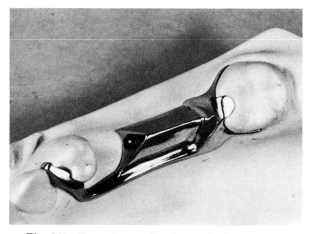

Fig. 741 Posterior sectional prosthesis – 1st part.

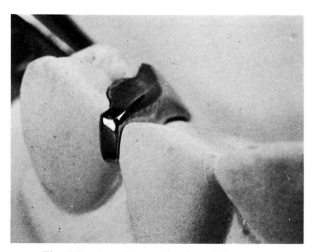

Fig. 742 Anterior termination of first part.

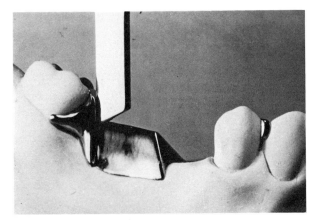

Fig. 743 First part – distal guiding plane alignment.

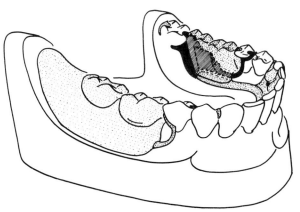

Fig. 746 Combination of a tooth-supported section and a distal extension base.

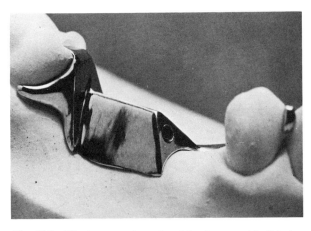

Fig. 744 First part – triangular ridge form and bolt hole.

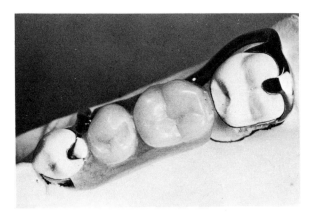

Fig. 745 Posterior sectional prosthesis – 2nd part – occlusal view.

part (Fig. 743). Extending forward from this surface, a triangular-sectioned ridge form is placed over the residual ridge crest to give increased lateral stability to the second part. It has a hole formed in its anterior face to accept the bolt boss (Fig. 744).

The *second part* is designed to embrace the distal aspects of both abutment teeth from their buccal to lingual surfaces, and also carries occlusal rests to be positioned on the disto-occlusal of each abutment. This framework will also carry the pontic teeth and flange together with the bolt (Fig. 745).

2. Bilateral

Bilateral partial dentures incorporating the sectional principle can be employed and the nature of the design will be specific for each case. Figure 746 illustrates a sectional design for the lower jaw with a tooth-supported section on the patient's left, and a distal extension base on the right. The first part is of orthodox design and the second part incorporates the lingual connector and distal extension.

Second-type (hinged sections)

These prostheses incorporate a hinge joining the sections together. They use buccal and lingual paths of insertion instead of the mesio-distal approaches employed with separate sections. Conditions may exist where mesio-distal paths of insertion are not possible due to the relationship of clinical crown height and length of the edentulous span. Furthermore, excessive resorption may have occurred on the buccal aspect, prohibiting a complete restoration.

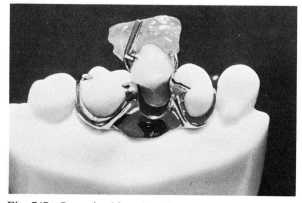

Fig. 747 Posterior hinged appliance replacing one tooth – open position.

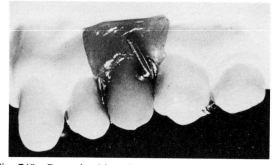

Fig. 748 Posterior hinged appliance replacing one tooth – closed position.

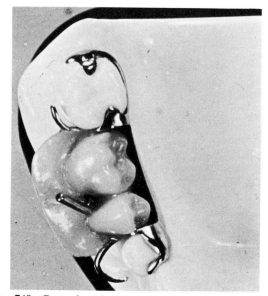

Fig. 749 Posterior hinged unilateral appliance replacing two teeth – open position.

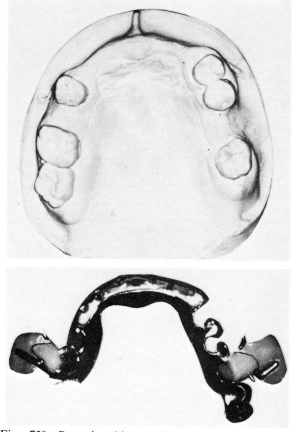

Fig. 750 Posterior hinged bilateral appliance – open position.

The hinge axis employed with this type of sectional denture lies mesio-distally and its supports are located close to the occlusal surfaces of the abutments. The hinged section carries the pontic teeth, the buccal flange, lateral stabilising arms, and the bolt (Figs. 747, 748). Both unilateral and bilateral hinged restorations can be constructed (Figs. 749, 750). Multiple edentulous spans can present difficulties requiring combinations of the various types discussed. The number of parts must be kept to a minimum, bearing in mind patient manipulation and future maintenance.

Variations in design

These variations may be attributed to the many combinations that can occur between the shape of the teeth and soft tissues adjacent to the edentulous span. Rotation or malalignment of one of the abutment teeth frequently complicates the design of the restoration.

The basic principles of sectional design must, however, be obeyed:

1. Complete restoration of the edentulous span.

2. Provision of a positive method of union so that the two parts form a rigid unit when assembled.

Anterior replacement

1. Bolt positions

Where possible, the bolt barrel should be positioned in the area of greatest resorption, or near to the border of the flange adjacent to the sulcus. Provided that the bolt lever is invisible during normal lip movements, the *horizontal position* is normally employed (Fig. 751a). Where fraenal attachments involve the normal site of the bolt, the *oblique position* can be used to advantage (Fig. 751b). The third, or *vertical position* (Fig. 751c) can be employed where there has been considerable tissue loss between the residual ridge crest and the sulcus. When this latter position is used, a spur is unnecessary and the bolt boss enters directly into the bolt hole in the first part (Fig. 752).

2. Hinged spurs

A hinge may be introduced between the main casting and the spur (Fig. 738). Before inserting the first part, the spur is rotated to prevent its impingement on the labial tissues. When the framework is in place, the hinged spur is moved into the undercut area, so that its terminal containing the bolt hole is placed in the correct position to receive the bolt boss. The spur terminal is shaped so that the fitting of the flange around it tends to hold the spur in its correct relationship to the bolt (Fig. 738). Failure to carry out this shaping can cause difficulty in closing the bolt, due to spur movement against the resilient labial tissue.

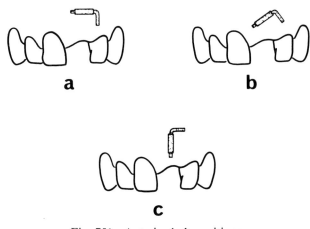

Fig. 751 Anterior bolt positions.

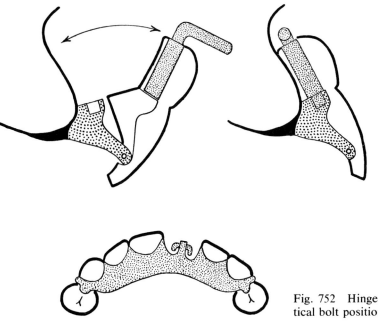

Fig. 752 Hinged anterior sectional prosthesis with vertical bolt position.

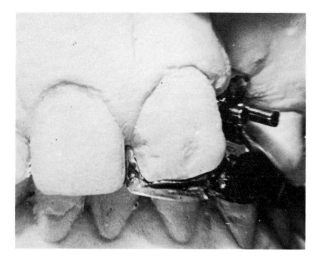

Fig. 753 The use of horizontal split posts in the restoration of an anterior defect.

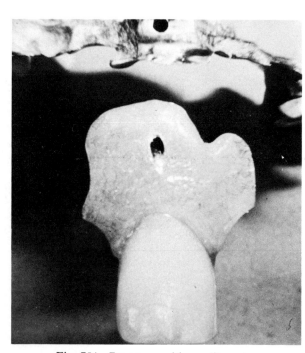

Fig. 754 Reverse position split post.

3. Split post positions

This method of union is most useful where minimal loss of the labial tissue has occurred. Split posts are normally positioned within the pontic crown (Fig. 735) but they have also been successfully employed

where a horizontal, or near horizontal, approach of the second part is required. This situation can occur with cleft palate patients and the split post may be positioned in the space created by the defect (Fig. 753). The use of this variation with post position enables complete restoration of the missing tissues.

Thin restorations can be retained by using the split post in a reverse position. Instead of the post being mounted on the main framework, it is placed to project from the inner aspect of the labial veneer and to enter a hole of corresponding diameter in the casting (Fig. 754). When this method is used, additional retention must be provided for the post to ensure its adequate fixation in the labial veneer (Fig. 755).

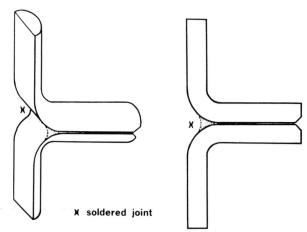

x soldered joint

Fig. 755 Additional retention for reverse position split post.

4. Variations incorporating the cantilever hinge bearing

This method of joining the second part to the main framework may be employed in the restoration of two central incisors (Fig. 756). When using two cantilever hinge bearings in the same base, care should be taken to ensure that *all* surfaces of the parent framework that might contact the hinged section are shaped to permit unobstructed rotation (Fig. 757). It is important to ensure the following:

(a) 'a' and 'b' must be parallel.

(b) The axes of 'c' and 'd' must coincide in order to form a common hinge axis.

(c) The tooth surfaces 'e' and 'f' must not be covered by the hinge section if they are incisal to the hinge axis.

Alternatively, the cantilever hinge bearing may be combined with an end bearing as illustrated in Fig. 758. In some instances, the whole anterior arch can be hinged using two centre bearings (Fig. 759a). The incisal edge of the hinged section close to the hinge axis must not impinge on the occlusal surface of the

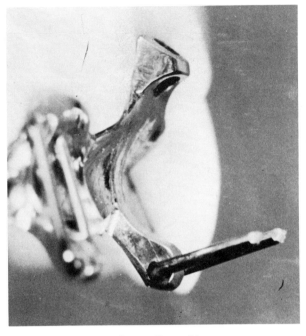

Fig. 756   Twin cantilever hinge supports.

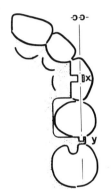
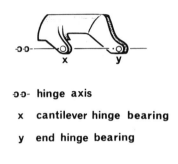

-ɔɘ- hinge axis

x   cantilever hinge bearing

y   end hinge bearing

Fig. 758   Combination of hinge supports.

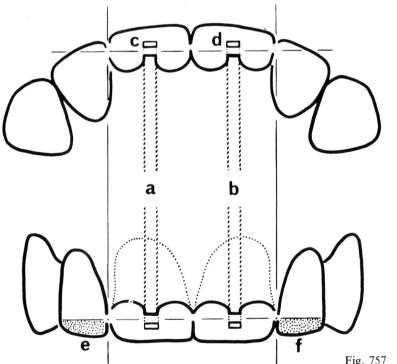

Fig. 757   Requirements for unobstructed rotation.

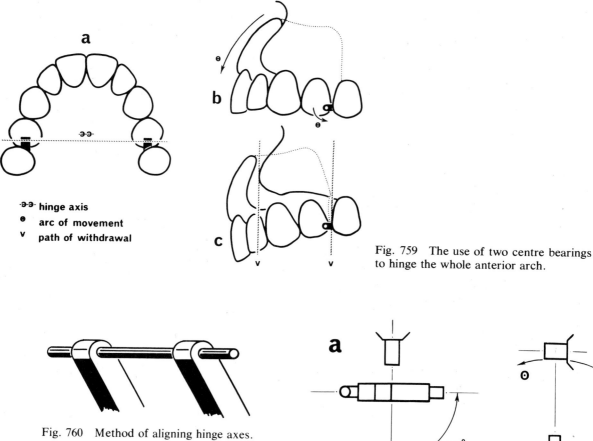

-ə-ə- hinge axis

ə arc of movement

v path of withdrawal

Fig. 759   The use of two centre bearings to hinge the whole anterior arch.

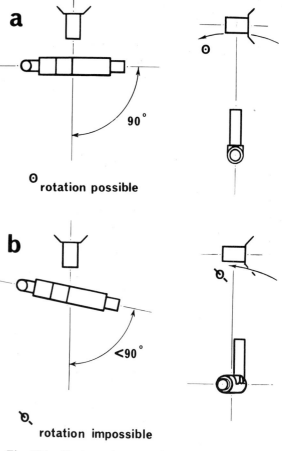

Fig. 760   Method of aligning hinge axes.

a

90°

ə **rotation possible**

b

<90°

rotation impossible

Fig. 761   Horizontal post and bolt relationship.

adjacent natural tooth before the flange is completely free from the undercut zone on the labial of the tissue, or the mesial surface of the abutment tooth (Figs. 759b and c).

Care must be taken with these designs to ensure that both hinge axes are aligned. This alignment is achieved by waxing into the pattern a straight piece of stainless steel wire of diameter 0·8 mm which is later removed from the casting (Fig. 760).

5. Variation in plain round post angulation

The plain round post may be used in a horizontal or near horizontal position (Fig. 761) in bolt-retained prostheses. It is important to note that axial rotation of the flange around the bolt boss is possible (Fig. 761a). This undesirable rotation may be prevented if the long axis of the bolt makes an angle of less than 90 degrees with the long axis of the post (Fig. 761b).

Posterior replacement

1. Bolt positions

In addition to the three variations in bolt positions already described, modifications of bolt position within the pontic or flange area are often required to permit the construction of a satisfactory appliance. The position of the bolt hole is determined by:

(a) the site of the edentulous span;

(b) the degree of resorption and its effect on hard and soft tissue contours;

(c) the necessity for access to the bolt handle by the patient, and

(d) appearance requirements, which dictate that the bolt handle should not be visible during maximal elevation of the lip in function.

2. Hinged first parts

Inclined abutment teeth can influence the design to the degree that it may become necessary to hinge the first part of the appliance. This will ensure complete restoration of the edentulous span and at the same time provide the necessary tooth support (Fig. 762). These appliances usually consist of individual sections, but can occasionally incorporate a further hinge to unite the second part to the first.

3. Sectional prostheses incorporating a vertical hinge

This type of denture provides an efficient means of splinting mobile teeth and may incorporate a periodontal veneer to improve the appearance. Another advantage of this restoration is its ability to provide effective retention from sites normally inaccessible to a clasp-retainer. This retention is provided without marring the appearance. A further application of this design is to the replacement of deficient labial tissue following maxillo-facial surgery. Several methods of union have been devised, a popular one being the 'Swing-Lock' prosthesis (Fig. 726).

Removal and adjustment aids for frictionally retained sectional dentures

Flange remover

The removal of bolt-retained sectional dentures presents no problems. Once the bolt is disengaged, the two parts readily separate. However, in the case of frictionally retained sectional dentures difficulty can be experienced in removing the labial flange. The patient should be instructed to hold the framework of the first part in place while removing the labial section. Upward pressure of the thumbs against the metal posteriors of the replacement teeth will achieve this aim. At the same time the index fingers can exert a downward and forward pressure on the labial flange. A flange remover may be constructed, consisting of clear acrylic resin and formed to the labial contours of the flange. The flange remover has an integral handle and engages the labial flange of the prosthesis (Fig. 763). This type of flange remover has also been used with attachment-retained prostheses.

From the inner aspect of the flange remover projects a 1·5 mm diameter stainless steel pin positioned to penetrate a small orifice high up in the flange of the labial section, above the high lip line (Fig. 764). The pin is placed so that, when viewed in sagittal section, it is at an angle of 90 degrees to

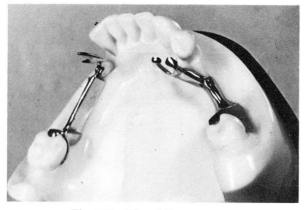

Fig. 762 Hinged first parts.

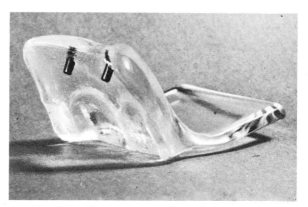

Fig. 763 Flange remover for split post design.

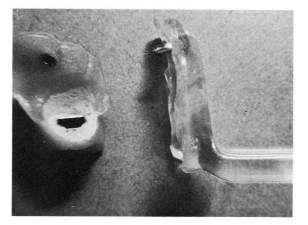

Fig. 764 Spring bridge – removable component and flange remover.

the long axis of the split post. When viewed from the labial aspect, the orifice in the labial flange should be in line with the long axis of the split post (Fig. 765). To minimise the effect of torque on a labial flange carrying two or more replacement teeth, two pins should be used. Both pins should be parallel to one another (Fig. 763).

Possible variations in fraenum shape and position may influence the placement of pins, but wherever possible an attempt should be made to site them so that an equal distribution of force is applied to the labial flange. To ensure accurate location and fit, together with minimal wear, the pins engage small lengths of 1·5 mm internal diameter stainless steel tubing inserted into the labial flange.

Adjustment control

A scalpel blade can be used to increase the retention provided by split posts, but this procedure needs to be carried out with care to avoid over-adjustment. A simple adjustment aid can be constructed to simplify this procedure (Fig. 766).

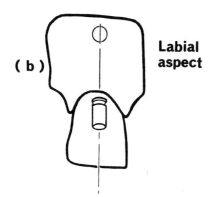

Fig. 765 Sagittal section and frontal view of flange remover (template) and labial component.

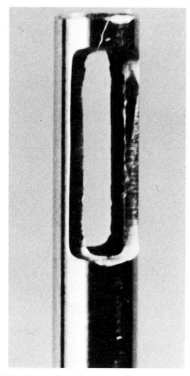

Fig. 766 Control tube for split post adjustment.

The framework is placed on the surveyor with the split post vertical. This is most conveniently carried out with the framework seated on its original master cast, but impression compound can be used if this cast is not available.

The adjustment control tube is now placed in the surveyor chuck and is then seated over the split post and secured (Fig. 767). A scalpel blade can now be inserted through the slot and adjustment carried out with complete safety. Clinical experience has shown the need for adjustments at yearly intervals. Should frictional resistance still be insufficient this will indicate that the stainless steel sleeve incorporated in the labial section is worn and in need of renewal.

Labial flanges

Self-curing acrylic resins simplify labial flange construction. These flanges should be shaped to provide complete restoration of the missing natural tissues. These contours will result in greater extension than is normally employed and they will have thin edges mesially and distally (Fig. 768). If the correct colouring has been selected, the flanges will defy detection at normal conversational distances.

CONCLUSIONS

Sectional dentures have considerable and worthwhile advantages over conventional one-piece partial dentures. They seldom require significant mouth preparation, while the appearance and retention is usually extremely good. The technical procedures involved use materials readily available in any dental laboratory and do not require specialised equipment. These prostheses should be considered when restoring any partially dentate mouth.

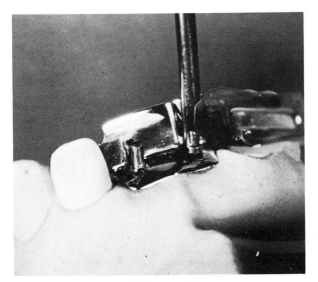

Fig. 767   Split post adjustments.

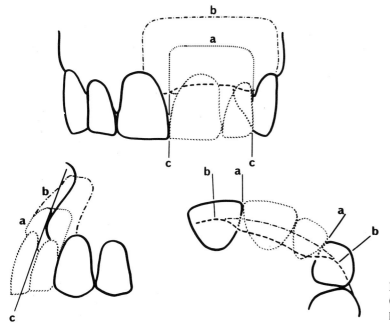

Fig. 768   Flange outlines for conventional (a) and sectional (b) prostheses. (c) is the path of insertion.

MATERIALS USED IN SECTIONAL DENTURE CONSTRUCTION

'Krupp' products: 'Wipla' stainless-steel tubing and wire. 'Wiptam' (cobalt/chromium) wire, and hinges (preformed). (Friedrich Krupp, GmbH, Widia-Fabrik, Wipla Dental-Werkstätten, Essen, W. Germany.)

Cobalt chromium alloys: Any alloy that does not require a casting mould temperature in excess of 1000 °C.

Teeth: 'Myerson' facings. (Lang Dental Manufacturing Co., Chicago, Illinois, U.S.A.)

Acrylic base: 'Jet' self-curing acrylic resin.

Materials: 'Myerson' Dentine powders.
            'Caulk' Opaquers. (The L. D. Caulk Company, Milford, Del., Toronto, Ontario, Canada.)

REFERENCES AND FURTHER READING

L'ESTRANGE, P. R. and PULLEN-WARNER, E. (1969) *Dent. Practit.*, *19*, 379

L'ESTRANGE, P. R. and PULLEN-WARNER, E. (1969) *Dent. Practit.*, *20*, 135

L'ESTRANGE, P. R. and PULLEN-WARNER, E. (1972) Sectional dentures. The use of the horizontal split post in the treatment of cleft palate patients. *Dent. Practit.*, *22*, 271

PULLEN-WARNER, E. (1964) *Dent. News (Lond.)*, *2*, 1

PULLEN-WARNER, E. (1965) *Dent. News (Lond.)*, *2*, 12

PULLEN-WARNER, E. and L'ESTRANGE, P. R. (1978) *Sectional Dentures: A Clinical and Laboratory Manual.* John Wright, Bristol

Appendix

This book concerns the principles of attachment application, employing individual units as examples. The reader should thus be enabled to assess the relative merits of manufactured units and apply them to the restoration of his patient's mouth. Attachment designs change from time to time but the principles are unlikely to vary. The following list may not be complete and is provided solely for the convenience of readers.

Attachment Manufacturers

Ancorvis,
Galleria del Oro 3,
Bologna, Italy.

Ceka N. V.
Maria Henriettalei 6–8 bus 5,
B2000, Antwerpen, Belgium.

Cendres et Métaux SA,
Rue de Boujean 122,
Biel-Bienne 2501, Switzerland.

Columbia Dentoform Corporation,
49 East 21st Street,
New York,
N.Y. 10010, U.S.A.

Degussa,
Geschäftsbereich Dental,
6 Frankfurt (Main), Germany.

J. F. Jelenko & Co. Inc.,
170 Petersville Road,
New Rochelle, New York 10801, U.S.A.

Cav. G. Lipparini,
Piazza Calderini 2/2,
Bologna, Italy.

Métaux Précieux SA,
Avenue du Vignoble 2,
CH-200 Neuchâtel, Switzerland.

Precision Attachments Ltd.,
1114 Hillside Road,
West Vancouver 237, B.C. Canada.

APM Sterngold,
320 Washington Street,
Mt. Vernon, New York, 10553, U.S.A.

The J. M. Ney Co.,
Maplewood Avenue,
Bloomfield, Connecticut, 06002, U.S.A.

Ultratek Attachments and Technology Inc.,
1041 Shary Circle,
Concord, California 94518, U.S.A.

Usine Genevoise De Dégroississage d'Or,
Place Volontaires 4,
CH-1211, Geneva 11, Switzerland.

Whaledent International,
237 Fifth Avenue,
New York, NY 10001, U.S.A.

Attachment Selectors

Bell International Inc.,
1320 Marston Road,
Burlingame, CA. 90401, U.S.A.

Index

290